W9-APO-420

Edited by

ARTHUR G. STEINBERG, Ph.D.

Francis Hobart Herrick Professor of Biology,
Department of Biology, and
Professor of Human Genetics,
Case Western Reserve University, 2119 *abington Rd.*
Cleveland, Ohio 44106

ALEXANDER G. BEARN, M.D.

Professor and Chairman,
Department of Medicine,
Stanton Griffis Distinguished Medical Professor,
Cornell University Medical College;
Physician-in-Chief, The New York Hospital, 525 E 68th St
New York, New York 10021

ARNO G. MOTULSKY, M.D.

Professor of Medicine and Genetics,
Director, Center for Inherited Diseases,
University of Washington, *School of medicine*
Seattle, Washington 98195

BARTON CHILDS, M.D.

Professor of Pediatrics,
The Johns Hopkins University, *Johns Hopkins Hospital*
Baltimore, Maryland 21205

Progress in

MEDICAL
GENETICS

NEW SERIES

Volume II

1977

W. B. SAUNDERS COMPANY

Philadelphia, London, Toronto

W. B. Saunders Company: West Washington Square
                          Philadelphia, PA   19105

                          1 St. Anne's Road
                          Eastbourne, East Sussex BN21 3UN, England

                          1 Goldthorne Avenue
                          Toronto, Ontario M8Z 5T9, Canada

Progress in Medical Genetics — New Series, Volume II   ISBN   0-7216-8588-9

Last digit is the print number: 9   8   7   6   5   4   3   2   1

FOREWORD

Volume II of the new series of *Progress in Medical Genetics* continues to review fields of rapid change in human and medical genetics. In keeping with previous volumes, there is a mixture of articles of clinical significance, disease mechanisms, and human variation. The first article, by D. J. H. Brock, describes methods for the antenatal diagnosis of neural tube defects. The measurement of α-fetoprotein in amniotic fluid to diagnose open neural tube defects in fetuses carried by women who have had a previous child with this distressing syndrome is reviewed, along with the advantages and disadvantages of its measurement in the serum of women who have not had an affected child. Rapid progress is being made, and it is Dr. Brock's view that we may look forward to a time when every pregnancy may be profitably tested.

Most previous volumes of *Progress in Medical Genetics* have contained one or more articles of immunological significance. For this volume, Andrew McMichael and Hugh McDevitt have contributed a comprehensive discussion of the association between the HL-A system and disease. The major histocompatibility complexes of both mouse and man are reviewed, giving the evidence for linkage relationships between the H_2 system and immune response genes in the mouse and the probability that such genes exist in man as well. This is followed by a summary of published articles revealing frequencies of the various HL-A types in many diseases. The authors favor the idea that these associations actually have to do with immune response genes whose relationship to the HL-A type is maintained by linkage disequilibrium.

E. S. Gershon, S. D. Targum, L. R. Kessler, C. M. Mazure, and W. E. Bunney, Jr., have provided an exhaustive review of the genetic predisposition to manic depressive disease. Few of us outside the field of psychiatry are aware of the difficulty investigators have experienced in gaining acceptance among psychiatrists for the idea that the genotype is important in the genesis of psychotic behavior. Despite such difficulties, a good deal of progress has been made in showing the relation of the genes to this behavioral abnormality and in separating out the various types by genetic means.

The next article, by H. H. Kazazian, Jr., S. Cho, and J. A. Phillips, III, describes advances in the description of disease at the level of changes in messenger RNAs, using the thalassemia syndromes as examples. The capacity to isolate and characterize messenger RNA provides a further degree of resolution of the effects of mutations.

Gebhard Flatz and Hans Werner Rotthauwe have given us a splendid review of the problem of lactase malabsorption. They choose this term, as opposed to lactase deficiency or lactose intolerance, because the latter conjure up thoughts of disease, and, as the paper shows convincingly, the malabsorbers are in the majority in the world. Thus to see lactose malabsorption as a disease would be to say that the usual state is the abnormal one. The paper includes a review of molecular mechanisms, clinical details, formal genetics, and the geographic distribution of this trait, and we are provided speculations on the causes of the various frequencies and distributions of the genes involved.

The final paper is a review of chromosome heteromorphisms by Patricia Jacobs. This useful article covers descriptions of types, frequencies, geographical distributions, and uses of these variations as genetic markers. She also points out that they probably are of only minimal, if any, clinical significance.

The Editors wish to acknowledge their gratitude to the authors of these excellent papers for the labor and care they have expended on them. Readers will find them a rewarding experience.

A.G.S.
A.G.B.
A.G.M.
B.C.

CONTENTS OF *PROGRESS IN MEDICAL GENETICS*, VOLUME I

CONTENTS

Biochemical and Cytological Methods in the Diagnosis of Neural Tube Defects

D. J. H. BROCK

Department of Human Genetics, University of Edinburgh, Western General Hospital, Edinburgh, Scotland

INTRODUCTION

For most of the past decade prenatal diagnosis has been concerned mainly with cytogenetic disorders, and in particular with the early detection of Down's syndrome in mothers who are at risk because of advanced age. A quantitatively less important, but nonetheless scientifically significant, corollary to these studies has been the attempt to diagnose metabolic disorders early in pregnancy. Recently, however, it has become possible to diagnose the neural tube defects through measurements of alphafetoprotein and other parameters in the amniotic fluid, and in some parts of the world this has become of equal importance with the determination of fetal karyotype. Furthermore, since determinations of alphafetoprotein concentration in maternal blood allow the early recognition of a certain proportion of cases of both spina bifida and anencephaly, it has now become possible, at least in theory, to apply prenatal diagnosis to all pregnant women and thus to make an attack on the incidence of one of the more serious groups of congenital malformations. Since hitherto prenatal diagnosis has been an enterprise oriented toward reassuring patients who have a known and defined risk of bearing an abnormal child, this new development has serious medical, scientific, and ethical implications. This review will be concerned with assessing the current state of knowledge of prenatal diagnosis of the neural tube defects and with considering the consequences of the new procedures.

THE NEURAL TUBE DEFECTS

Description

Defects of closure of the neural tube account for the great majority of central nervous system malformations. The most common anomalies are anencephaly with or without spina bifida and the various forms of spina bifida cystica. Spina bifida occulta, although apparently common, is rarely associated with neurological or musculoskeletal disturbances. Less common forms of neural tube defect are hydrocephaly, exencephaly (a congenital exposure of the brain), encephalocele (hernia of the brain), and iniencephaly (congenital absence of the neck). All are superbly described by Warkany (1971). The etiological relationship between anencephaly and spina bifida cystica is well established, but their relationship to the less common neural tube defects is not yet clear.

Anencephaly is a lethal condition in which the brain is amorphous and the vault of the skull is absent. About three-quarters of anencephalics are stillborn, and virtually all die within hours or days of birth. Many have an associated spina bifida, but from the point of view of this review, the combined condition will be classified as anencephaly. There is a great preponderance of females in anencephalic fetuses, the ratio ranging from 3:1 up to 7:1 (Nakano, 1973).

Cases of spina bifida cystica are usually subdivided into meningoceles and myeloceles. In meningoceles, the meninges herniate out of the spinal canal, whereas the cord remains in its normal position. In myeloceles the neural plate has locally failed to close over completely to form a tube, and the cord tissue with some degenerative changes lies on the surface. Meningoceles have been estimated to account for between 5 and 10 per cent of the total cases of spina bifida cystica (Laurence, 1974).

From the point of view of prenatal diagnosis, it is convenient to divide the neural tube defects into open and closed lesions. A closed lesion is defined as a malformation in which there is a full-thickness skin cover. An open lesion is defined as one in which meninges or neural elements lie exposed on the surface whether these be covered by a membrane or not. Most cases of anencephaly and myelocele spina bifida represent open lesions, whereas the majority of meningocele spina bifidas and encephaloceles are closed lesions. However, the correlation between the open and closed terminology required by prenatal diagnosticians and the various subdivisions of the neural tube defects is not an exact one and remains to be clarified by further careful pathological studies.

Occurrence

The geographical distribution of the neural tube defects varies widely. Incidence rates are complicated by seasonal fluctuations, by long-term trends, and by doubtful statistics from areas where compulsory registration of congenital malformations is not demanded. In most surveys, the incidence of anencephaly has been found to be roughly equivalent to that of spina bifida cystica, and the figures given in Table 1 are to some extent based on this assumption.

Highest frequencies are found in the North and West of the British Isles, particularly in Scotland, Wales, and Northern Ireland. Elwood (1970) has shown that the incidence of anencephaly in Northern Ireland during the years 1950 to 1966 ranged from a low of 3.18 per 1000 in 1953 to 5.23 per 1000 in 1961, with an overall rate of

Table 1.   Approximate Incidence Rates for Neural Tube Defects*

Area	Period Studied	Incidence Rate per 1000
Northern Ireland (Belfast)	1950–1966	7.9
South Wales	1956–1961	7.7
Scotland	1961–1972	5.6
England (London)	1938–1953	3.1
Germany (Munich)	1929–1941	1.7
France	1945–1955	1.1
Sweden (Lund)	1923–1945	1.1
Canada (Quebec)	1956–1965	2.9
U.S.A. (Providence)	1885–1965	3.1
U.S.A. (Boston)	1930–1965	2.0
U.S.A. (Chicago)	1950–1959	1.4
India (Bombay)	1946–1955	1.5
Japan (Nagasaki and Hiroshima)	1948–1954	1.3
Brazil (São Paulo)	1961–1964	1.2
West Indies (Jamaica)	1956–1967	0.8
Uganda (Kampala)	1953–1955	0.7

*Data compiled from Nakano, 1973.

3.95 per 1000. This suggests a combined incidence for neural tube defects of about 8 per 1000. Carter et al. (1968) reported a combined rate for spina bifida and anencephaly of 7.67 per 1000 for South Wales over the period 1956 to 1961. Fedrick (1976) has shown an incidence rate for anencephaly of 2.8 per 1000 in Scotland during the 12-year period 1961 to 1972, suggesting a combined rate for neural tube defects of about 6 per 1000. Conversely, low frequencies have been shown in most black populations, whether in West Africa, the United States, the West Indies, or Britain (Leck, 1972). Low rates are also found among Asians (with the exception of Sikh Indians) and in South America. Intermediate rates have been reported from most parts of Europe outside the British Isles (Nakano, 1973). In the United States the highest rates appear to occur in the Northeast, with an incidence of 1.6 per 1000 for anencephaly being reported from Rhode Island (MacMahon and Yen, 1971). That incidence rates can depend on both ethnic group and locality has been shown by the data of Naggan and MacMahon (1967) in their study in Boston, where it was found that rates for children of Irish ancestry were three times greater than for the whole group but considerably lower than those reported in Ireland itself. Neural tube defects in descendants of migrants tend to move from the pattern observed in their home country toward that of the host country (Morton et al., 1967; Naggan, 1971), but there appears to be a much greater contrast between black and white populations (Leck, 1969).

Recurrence Risks

In estimating recurrence risks from empirical studies, it has been shown that anencephaly, iniencephaly, encephalocele, myelocele, and meningocele may be treated as having a common etiology (Carter, 1976), although this approach has been criticized by Holmes et al. (1976). Recurrence risks after a single affected sib range from 4.5 to 5.6 per cent (Carter, 1974), and there is little difference whether the index patient had spina bifida or anencephaly. The recurrence risk is lower when the birth frequency of neural tube defects in the population is lower, and it is probable that the relative risks based on British data are overestimates for most other populations. The recurrence risk after two affected sibs is of the order of 10 per cent. If either of the parents is a surviving patient with spina bifida cystica, the risk to their children is about 4.5 per cent (Carter, 1976). Other empirical risks are shown in Table 2 and include calculations for more complicated family histories (Smith, 1973). It should be noted that because there is a U-shaped relationship between both birth order and maternal age and the incidence of neural tube defects, the older mother has a slightly increased risk of bearing an affected infant, although the magnitude of this effect is not yet clear.

ALPHAFETOPROTEIN

Using paper electrophoresis, Bergstrand and Czar (1956) discovered a new protein in the serum of early human fetuses. It had alpha$_1$ mobility and was not detectable in adult or neonatal serum and so was given the name alphafetoprotein (AFP) or, more correctly, alpha$_1$-fetoprotein. Since other fetoproteins have been described, the World Health Organization and International Agency for Research on Cancer defined AFP as the first alpha-globulin to appear in

Table 2. Empirical Risk of Neural Tube Defect (NTD) in Various Family Situations*

Family History	Risk (%)	Reference
One child with NTD	5	Carter et al., 1968
Two children with NTD	10	Carter and Roberts, 1967
Three children with NTD	21	Smith, 1973
Parent with NTD	4.5	Carter, 1976
One child with multiple vertebral anomalies	5	Wynne-Davies, 1975
One child with spinal dysraphism	4	Carter et al., 1976

*Based on U.K. incidence rates. Risks will be lower in areas where NTD incidence is lower.

mammalian serum during development and the dominating serum protein in early embryonic life. It reappears in adult serum during certain pathological states, primarily hepatomas and teratomas, and so correctly belongs to the category of oncofetal antigens. Currently, there is some dispute as to whether the low levels of AFP detectable in the sera of normal, healthy adults are real or artifactual (Nørgaard-Pedersen and Axelsen, 1976). The fact that no one has yet detected antibodies to AFP in human serum suggests that low levels of the protein may be continuously synthesized throughout life.

In early embryogenesis, AFP is produced first by the yolk sac and later by the liver (Gitlin and Boesman, 1967; Gitlin and Perricelli, 1970). Traces are also made in the fetal gastrointestinal tract (Gitlin et al., 1972) and possibly, although by no means certainly, in the placenta (Furth and Adinolfi, 1969). The cellular site of synthesis appears to be the hepatocytes or precursors of hepatocytes (Adinolfi et al., 1975).

AFP is present in human fetal sera from as early as 6 weeks of gestation (Gitlin and Perricelli, 1970). Concentrations rise quite rapidly, reaching a peak at the end of the first trimester, at which time levels of up to 3 to 4 mg per ml have been found (Gitlin and Boesman, 1966; Furth and Adinolfi, 1969; Brock, 1974), thus making it second only to albumin in terms of quantitative importance. Thereafter, although net AFP synthesis remains constant until about the thirtieth week of in utero life, the rapidly expanding fetal blood volume causes a steady decrease in concentration (Gitlin and Boesman, 1967). At birth the AFP concentration in cord serum from normal mature infants is between 10 and 150 μg per ml (Gitlin and Boesman, 1966; Furth and Adinolfi, 1969). The serum AFP concentration in newborn babies falls rapidly in the first few weeks and is usually not greatly different from the adult level by 6 months of age (Masseyeff et al., 1974). Apparent concentrations of AFP in normal adult serum lie between 2 and 20 ng per ml, about 10^{-5} times the concentration found in the 13-week fetus. Concentrations comparable to those found in fetal serum have been reported in fetal cerebrospinal fluid (Brock and Sutcliffe, 1972; Adinolfi et al., 1975). AFP can be detected in normal human amniotic fluid throughout gestation (Gitlin and Boesman, 1966; Brock and Sutcliffe, 1972) at about one hundredth of the level found in fetal serum at the corresponding gestation (Brock, 1976a). It is also detectable in fetal urine throughout gestation at levels high enough to suggest that this is a major origin of the amniotic fluid AFP.

AFP has been successfully purified a number of times (Nishi, 1970; Ruoslahti and Seppälä, 1971, Masseyeff, 1972; Nørgaard-Pedersen, 1972), the usual starting material being fetal, neonatal, or hepatoma serum. It is a typical globulin of molecular weight be-

tween 61,000 and 75,000 (Nishi, 1970; Adinolfi et al., 1971; Masopust et al., 1971; Ruoslahti and Seppälä, 1971; Ruoslahti et al., 1971;
Hirai et al., 1973), consisting of a single polypeptide chain and containing about 3 per cent carbohydrate. In physical properties it is
remarkably similar to albumin, and it is extraordinarily difficult to
remove residual traces of albumin from purified AFP. Heterogeneity
of AFP can be demonstrated by isoelectric focusing (Alpert et al.,
1972) or by differential affinity for concanavallin A (Smith and
Kelleher, 1973). This is thought to represent secondary modifications
of the primary polypeptide chain through removal of neuraminic acid
residues, and its significance is yet to be assessed. No genetic
variants of AFP have yet been described, and the protein appears to
be identical whatever the source of purification (Nishi, 1970; Ruoslahti et al., 1971; Hirai et al., 1973).

The different methods of measuring AFP have been well reviewed (Nørgaard-Pedersen, 1976; Adinolfi et al., 1975). All methods
depend on a specific antiserum which is usually raised by injecting
experimental animals with fetal, neonatal, or hepatoma sera. Such
antisera may contain traces of antibodies against other, as yet un-
described, fetal proteins. For quantitation of the mg per ml concentrations in fetal and hepatoma serum and the μg per ml concentrations in amniotic fluids, gel immunoprecipitation methods are
suitable, the most commonly used being radial immunodiffusion and
rocket immunoelectrophoresis (Fig. 1). For the ng per ml concentrations in adult serum, more sensitive techniques are necessary. The
most widely employed methods are radioimmunoassay, immunoau-
toradiography, and enzyme-linked immunoassay, but there are pro-
ponents for both complement fixation and hemagglutination. The
choice of assay depends on the technical facilities available and the
daily number of samples to be examined. Since automated radioimmunoassay is specific, precise, and cheap, it has been most widely
employed in the various trials of maternal serum AFP in relation to
prenatal detection of neural tube defects.

In addition to its value in prenatal diagnosis, AFP has been of
clinical importance in a number of other pathological states. These
include a number of malignant conditions: primary liver carcinomas
(Tatarinov, 1964; Abelev, 1971), secondary liver carcinoma (Masseyeff, 1972), teratocarcinomas of the testes and ovaries (Abelev et
al., 1967), and gastric and pancreatic carcinomas, some of which had
associated liver metastases (McIntire et al., 1975). Nonmalignant
conditions in which raised AFP concentrations have been described
include acute and chronic hepatitis (Abelev, 1971), Indian childhood
cirrhosis (Nayak et al., 1972), nonspecific cirrhoses and fatty liver
degeneration (Ruoslahti et al., 1974), hereditary tyrosinemia
(Bélanger, 1973), and ataxia-telangiectasia (Waldmann and McIntyre,

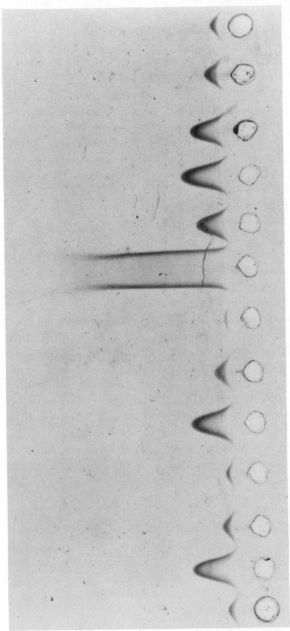

Figure 1. "Rocket" immunoelectrophoretic determination of amniotic fluid AFP. The open-topped rocket is from a pregnancy in which the fetus had a neural tube defect.

1972). A report that measurement of serum AFP will allow detection of cystic fibrosis of the pancreas, as well as symptomless carriers of a single dose of the cystic fibrosis gene (Chandra et al., 1975), has not been confirmed (Brock et al., 1975a).

The function of AFP remains elusive. Early suggestions that it binds estrogens have been confirmed for mouse and rat (Nunez et al., 1971; Uriel et al., 1972) but not apparently for man (Savu et al., 1974; Swartz et al., 1974), presumably because in man sex hormones are carried by the beta-globulin fraction of serum. The suggestion that AFP is a fetal homologue of albumin has obvious attractions, because the two proteins are so remarkably similar in solubility, molecular weight, electrophoretic mobility, isoelectric point, dye binding properties (Endo et al., 1974), and amino acid sequence (Ruoslahti and Terry, 1976). Fetospecific alphaglobulins, closely related to albumin, have been found in all mammals so far examined (Gitlin and Boesman, 1967), but this tells little of the actual physiological function of this class of fetal proteins.

Current thinking is that AFP is involved in immunoregulation during fetal development. Lymphocyte response to phytohemagglutinin, concanavallin A, and rabbit anti-human thymocyte serum is inhibited by AFP, as is the one-way mixed lymphocyte culture test (Murgita and Tomasi, 1975; Yachnin, 1976). Immunofluorescence studies point to the presence of AFP receptors on the surface of a subpopulation of T-cell lymphocytes in mice (Dattwyler et al., 1975). Since the fetus is genetically distinct from its mother (in immunological terms, a foreign object), it has been suggested that AFP may function by assisting the fetus in withstanding immune rejection. This is supported by the finding that injection of anti-AFP antisera into pregnant rats, mice, and rabbits produces both miscarriages and congenital abnormalities (Smith, 1972; Slade, 1973; Mizejewski and Grimley, 1976). However, the mechanism of these induced abortions remains unknown, and there is still no direct evidence that AFP is involved with protection of the fetus from immunological attack by its mother in humans.

PRENATAL DIAGNOSIS OF NEURAL TUBE DEFECTS THROUGH AMNIOTIC FLUID STUDIES

Amniotic Fluid Alphafetoprotein

Discovery of the Value of Alphafetoprotein. In 1964, Stewart and Taylor reported raised bilirubin concentrations in full-term amniotic fluids from anencephalic stillbirths. Confirmation of this observation (Cassady and Cailliteau, 1967; Lee and Wei, 1970) suggested that there was substantial leakage or transudation of blood and blood components from the fetal circulation into the fluid in these massive open lesions. Bilirubin, however, is a low molecular weight compound with a rapid turnover and can furthermore originate from either fetal or maternal circulation. What was needed as an unambiguous marker of a neural tube lesion was a high molecular weight compound of known fetal origin. AFP was the obvious choice.

Using frozen-stored material, Brock and Sutcliffe (1972) assembled a large series of amniotic fluids from pregnancies in which the outcome had been an infant with a neural tube defect. The series comprised 31 cases of anencephaly, 2 cases of spina bifida, and 3 cases of hydrocephaly, all between 26 and 42 weeks of pregnancy. Although the cases of spina bifida and hydrocephaly had AFP concentrations within the normal range, a large majority of the anencephalic fluids had grossly elevated AFP concentrations. Furthermore, one case of myelocele spina bifida, in which the fluid had been taken at 13 weeks of pregnancy, had an AFP level more than 5 times the upper limit of the normal range. This suggested that both the major forms of neural tube defect would be diagnosable from AFP measurements early enough in pregnancy to make a safe termination possible. Within a few months Brock and Scrimgeour (1972) were able to confirm this by measurements made on an amniotic fluid from an 18-week anencephalic pregnancy. By one of those curious quirks of the timing of scientific discoveries, the initial publication was somewhat overshadowed by the furious debate which was then raging over the recently advanced hypothesis of Renwick (1972), that spina bifida and anencephaly were caused by a teratogenic substance derived from blighted potatoes.

Confirmation of the Value of Amniotic Fluid AFP. The response to the initial reports was rapid. Seppälä and Ruoslahti (1973c), who had much experience with AFP determinations, but in a low neural tube defect area, claimed that the high AFP concentrations indicated fetal distress rather than a central nervous system lesion per se. However, within a few months Lorber et al. (1973) and Seller et al. (1973) prospectively diagnosed cases of anencephaly on the basis of amniotic fluid AFP concentrations supported by ultra-sonar scan, terminated the pregnancies, and confirmed their diagnoses. Nevin et al. (1973) then showed greatly increased AFP concentrations in two further early cases of spina bifida, the amniotic fluids having been obtained for other purposes and stored in the frozen state. It was left to Allan et al. (1973) to perform the first prospective diagnosis of spina bifida on the basis of amniotic fluid AFP concentration, without the benefit of other confirmatory measurements. The scene was thus set for a general introduction of this new parameter into prenatal diagnostic studies. The first report of its use outside the British Isles appeared a year later (Milunsky and Alpert, 1974).

   Sensitivity of Amniotic Fluid AFP. AFP concentrations in amniotic fluids from pregnancies in which the fetus has a neural tube defect are usually very high indeed (Fig. 2). Anencephalic values tend to be higher than those in spina bifida, in accordance with the theory that the protein leaks from the lesion into the surrounding

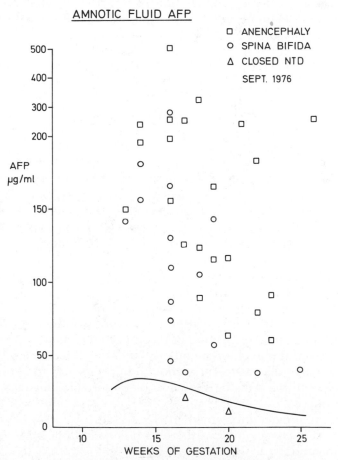

Figure 2.   Amniotic fluid AFP concentrations in diagnostic amniocentesis samples in which the fetus had a neural tube defect. The solid line represents the upper limit of the normal range. (The author's experience to September 1976.)

fluid. A compilation of published data in 1975 showed that 33 out of 33 cases of anencephaly had values outside the normal range, whereas for spina bifida the figures were 36 out of 40 (Brock, 1976b). If "rocket" electrophoresis is the assay method used, neural tube defects often reveal themselves as open peaks, making precise quantitation largely redundant (Fig. 1). However, less clear-cut but nonetheless abnormal values may sometimes be observed with small, open spina bifidas.

Amniotic fluid AFP will not, however, allow the detection of all types of neural tube defect. This was first pointed out by Laurence et al. (1973), who reported a large, slack occipital encephalocele with a normal amniotic fluid AFP value at 16 weeks. Nevin et al. (1974) reported a case of iniencephaly and Stewart et al. (1975) a case of closed lumbar meningocele, both with normal AFP values before the twentieth week of pregnancy. There is now a general belief that a closed neural tube defect will not be detectable through assay of AFP in amniotic fluid, and this is borne out by the data in Table 3, in which only 1 out of 9 cases of closed spina bifida was more than two standard deviations above the mean. It is not yet clear what proportion of the total number of cases of neural tube defects is represented by the closed lesions. It is generally reckoned at between 5 and 10 per cent (Laurence, 1974), although studies on maternal serum AFP suggest that it may be substantially larger. It is also not yet clear how serious these failures will be. Many will be represented by the comparatively harmless meningocele spina bifidas; but as Laurence (1974) has pointed out, encephaloceles and small, skin-covered myelocele spina bifidas are serious disorders, and may cause great distress to mothers who were expecting to be protected against the birth of a child with a neural tube defect.

Specificity of Amniotic Fluid AFP. Measurements of amniotic fluid AFP have been criticized on the grounds of their relative non-specificity, it being suggested that the association of other fetal conditions with raised values compromises the usefulness of this diagnostic tool. A close inspection of the reported facts does not support this criticism. It must be remembered that the objective of AFP analysis is to make diagnoses early enough in pregnancy to permit termination should the fetus be shown to be abnormal. Thus observations that amniotic fluid AFP is raised in Fallot's tetralogy in the third trimester of pregnancy (Seppälä, 1975) has little bearing on the specificity of AFP assay until such time as this condition can be shown to be associated with an elevated value at or around the sixteenth week of pregnancy. Likewise, the observations that AFP may be grossly elevated after intrauterine fetal death (Table 3) can hardly be

Table 3. Fetal Conditions, Other Than Anencephaly and Spina Bifida, in Which Elevated Amniotic Fluid AFP Concentrations Have Been Reported

Condition	Gestation (Trimester)	AFP*	Reference
1. Intrauterine death (missed abortion)	3rd	R	Seppälä and Ruoslahti, 1973a
	2nd ⎱	R ⎱	Wisniewski et al., 1974
	1st ⎰	R ⎰	
2. Rh isoimmunization	3rd	R	Seppälä and Ruoslahti, 1973d
	2nd	R&N	Brock et al., 1975c
3. Hydrocephalus	3rd	N	Brock and Sutcliffe, 1972
	3rd	R	Seppälä and Unnerus, 1974
4. Turner's syndrome	1st	R	Seller et al., 1974a
	2nd	R	Milunsky and Alpert, 1974
	2nd	R	Hunter et al., 1976
	2nd	N	Seller, 1976
5. Exomphalos	1st and 2nd	N	Brock and Sutcliffe, 1973
	3rd	R	Bruijn and Huisges, 1975
	2nd	R	Nevin and Armstrong, 1975
	2nd	R	Kunz and Schmid, 1976
6. Congenital nephrosis	3rd	R	Seppälä and Ruoslahti, 1973a
	2nd	R	Kjessler et al., 1975
	2nd	R	Seppälä et al., 1976
7. Duodenal atresia	3rd	R	Leschot and Treffers, 1975
	2nd	R	Weinberg et al., 1975
8. Esophageal atresia	3rd	R	Seppälä, 1973
9. Sacrococcygeal teratoma	2nd	R	Schmid and Muhlethaler, 1975
10. Meckel's syndrome	2nd	R	Seller, 1975a
11. Annular pancreas	3rd	R	Ainbender and Hirschhorn, 1976
12. Fallot's tetralogy	3rd	R	Seppälä, 1975
13. Pilonidal sinus	2nd	R	Jandial et al., 1976
14. Congenital skin defects	3rd	R	Leschot and Treffers, 1975
	2nd	R	Fitzsimmons et al., 1976

*R, raised; N, normal.

taken as reducing the value of this diagnostic technique. Good obstetrical practice should include listening for the fetal heart both before and after amniocentesis; if this precaution is overlooked or if there are difficulties in obtaining a good fetal echogram, the high AFP values associated with fetal demise should be of value in the proper management of the pregnancy. In considering the specificity of the AFP test, it is necessary to ask whether a high AFP value invariably means a neural tube defect or whether it might also indicate a mild abnormality or even a normal fetus.

Unfortunately the data on other fetal abnormalities are still sparse (Table 3). Much of the information is unhelpful in that it was made late in pregnancy, and there are doubts as to whether these conditions will be associated with high values at a time when amniocentesis is performed for prenatal diagnosis. Hydrocephaly is such an example. In other situations, such as Turner's syndrome, some of the relevant observations were made in amniotic fluid aspirated from the intact sacs of spontaneous abortions (Seller et al., 1974a), in which high values are often encountered even in the absence of fetal abnormality (Allan et al., 1973; Brock et al., 1975c). Probably the most reliable data come from the observations on congenital nephrosis first made by Kjessler et al. (1975). This is of particular significance, because congenital nephrosis is inherited as a Mendelian recessive and mothers who have already had affected children have a 1 in 4 risk of recurrence. This is thus the first inborn error of metabolism to become diagnosable through nonenzymatic protein measurements made in the amniotic fluid supernatant.

In several of the other conditions shown in Table 3, the tentative conclusion must be that some but not all cases will be associated with elevated values. Thus in exomphalos (omphalocele) both normal and increased values have been observed. In the duodenal and esophageal atresias elevated values will probably depend on the extent of the impairment of fetal swallowing (Brock, 1976d). In Meckel's syndrome, also inherited as an autosomal recessive, increased amniotic AFP is to be expected if the associated neural tube defect is an open one, although it is reported that in most cases the lesion is closed (Warkany, 1971). The recent report on a fetus with a small pilonidal sinus, in whom both serum and amniotic fluid AFP were greatly raised, is a disturbing one, because this condition is unlikely to be sufficiently serious to warrant termination of pregnancy (Jandial et al., 1976).

Far and away the most common sources of apparent false positive amniotic fluid AFP values are those deriving from fluids contaminated with fetal blood. AFP levels in fetal serum parallel those in amniotic fluid quite closely over time, but with concentrations between 100- and 200-fold higher (Fig. 3). This means that the admixture of a comparatively small amount of fetal blood with the amniotic fluid can increase the AFP value to a point at which it mimics the values found in neural tube defects. Once this problem is recognized, there is little difficulty in avoiding it. Current practice in many laboratories is to set aside an aliquot of whole amniotic fluid from

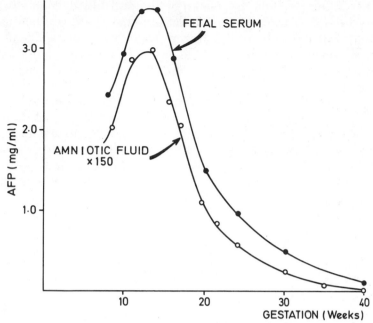

Figure 3. Comparative AFP concentrations in amniotic fluid and fetal serum.

any sample in which there is visible blood contamination. Should the AFP value be elevated, the cell button is then examined for the presence of fetal red cells either by Kleihauer test or electrophoresis, which will show the characteristic band of hemoglobin F, or by the use of commercially available antisera, which are directed specifically against hemoglobin F. Contaminated samples with moderately raised AFP values which contain a major proportion of fetal blood should be rejected and a fresh amniocentesis called for. Attempts to calculate the relative contribution of the AFP deriving from the fetal serum to the total which has been measured must sometimes fail, because fetal AFP concentrations vary quite widely early in gestation. It seems most likely that mixing of fetal blood and amniotic fluid occurs in the amniocentesis syringe owing to penetration of fetal blood vessels in the placenta. When this is the case, it can be anticipated that a second amniocentesis within a week or 10 days should produce a clear uncontaminated sample. It has been suggested that in severe cases of anencephaly there is natural bleeding from the lesion into the amniotic fluid so that amniotic fluids from such pregnancies may show the presence of fetal blood (Milunsky and Kimball, 1976). However, the AFP values in anencephaly are usually so high that fetal blood contamination is irrelevant.

One other problem associated with fetal blood contamination should be emphasized. Many laboratories have large collections of amniotic fluids stored in the frozen state which have been subsequently used in constructing the normal range of amniotic fluid AFP values throughout gestation. The difficulty in using such material is that these fluids will have been centrifuged and stored as cell-free supernatants. If any of them have been contaminated by fetal blood, and if the sample has been correctly handled so that there has been little lysis of the fetal red cells, there will be no way of detecting the presence of fetal serum in the amniotic fluid. Such samples will therefore give much higher values of amniotic fluid AFP than would be obtained in "clean" fluids. Construction of a normal range from such samples could therefore give a misleadingly wide spread of apparent values.

When allowance has been made for fetal blood–contaminated samples, it is still difficult to estimate the true proportion of genuine false positives. As has been pointed out by Wald and Cuckle (1976), much depends on the accepted upper limit of the normal range. Data from my laboratory show that if the cut-off point is 3 standard deviations above the mean for the gestational period, the false positive rate is about 0.5 per cent. If the cut-off is raised to 5 standard deviations above the mean, the false positive rate drops to 0.1 per cent, with only a small increase in "missed" spina bifidas. These figures are of considerable importance in view of the fact that it is now widely recommended that all amniotic fluid samples be subjected to AFP analysis, whatever the reason for amniocentesis. Since the most common indications for amniocentesis remain advanced maternal age or a previous history of chromosome abnormality, neural tube defects will be encountered infrequently in these samples. It is therefore of the greatest importance that the false positive rate in AFP assay be kept as low as possible lest more normal pregnancies than those in which the fetus has a neural tube defect be identified as abnormal.

The significance of low amniotic fluid AFP values is still unclear. Data from fluids aspirated from the intact sacs of spontaneous abortions suggest that very low or undetectable values may be found in cases of blighted embryo or empty sac (Allan et al., 1973). Although it is unlikely that such pregnancies will proceed beyond the end of the first trimester, Ainbender and Hirschhorn (1976) have reported a case in which an amniocentesis was performed because of uncertainty whether there was a pregnancy present in an enlarged uterus. Amniotic fluid AFP was below the detectable limit, and after direct visualization of the uterus, which revealed a placenta and no fetus, the pregnancy was terminated. The absence of other reports of empty sacs among amniocentesis samples in large compilations of data suggests that this phenomenon will be rarely encountered. A more common but spurious low AFP situation comes from misdirected amniocenteses (cystocentesis), in which fluid is aspirated from the maternal urine rather than from the amniotic fluid. Although the difference between maternal urine and amniotic fluid should be fairly obvious, this problem has caused at least one misdiagnosis of an open spina bifida (Field and Kerr, 1975). Various methods have been suggested for checking amniotic fluids; sharp odor, low pH, and a comparative absence of cells should be characteristic of maternal urine (Brock, 1975a), as will be low concentrations of albumin and glucose (Labstix reagent strip) and high concentrations of urea or potassium (Pirani et al., 1976; Guibaud et al., 1976). However, the amniotic fluid AFP value has by now become sufficiently characteristic that a concentration below 1 μg per ml at 15 or 16 weeks' gestation should alert the laboratory technician to the possibility of a misdirected amniocentesis.

Beta-Trace Protein

Soon after the discovery of the value of amniotic fluid AFP in diagnosing neural tube defects, Macri et al. (1973) introduced another protein with apparently similar usefulness. They showed that an antigen with properties similar to beta-trace protein of human CSF could be observed in the amniotic fluid of Lewis rats with experimentally induced spina bifida in the fetus. Using antiserum against human beta-trace protein, they claimed to have identified a precipitin reaction in the amniotic fluid from an anencephalic fetus at 32 weeks of pregnancy (Macri et al., 1974b). Later, using the same antiserum, they were able to detect beta-trace protein in the amniotic fluids of 15 cases of open neural tube defect but not in 110 control samples (Macri et al., 1974a). The new test, for which it was claimed there was a much higher specificity than for amniotic fluid AFP (Weiss et al., 1974), was promoted vigorously in the United States (Milunsky, 1975; Milunsky et al., 1975). The feeling was that since beta-trace protein occurs at highest concentrations in CSF, its elevation in amniotic fluid might be more indicative of lesions involving the spinal column than of other fetal abnormalities.

In Europe, experience was rather different. Olsson et al. (1974) showed that beta-trace protein was measurable in normal amniotic fluids at concentrations ranging from 3.6 to 13.3 μg per ml and also in normal human serum at levels of 2.6 to 6.0 μg per ml. They pointed out that since the antiserum used by Macri and his group had been absorbed with amniotic fluid and human serum, it could not be capable of measuring beta-trace protein. Subsequently Brock and Olsson 1976), using a highly specific antiserum to beta-trace protein, compared concentrations in 19 pregnancies in which the outcome was an infant with a neural tube defect and concentrations in 19 matched controls. There was no significant difference in the mean beta-trace protein values for the pathological samples when compared with the controls, and there were no striking differences in the values within individual matched pairs. When AFP was measured in the same samples, the differences between normal and pathological material were very striking indeed (Fig. 4). The conclusion seems inescapable that Macri and his colleagues have not been measuring beta-trace protein, and this has now been confirmed (Macri, 1975). Exactly what they are measuring is awaited with considerable interest. However, doubts may be expressed about the possibility of finding a useful

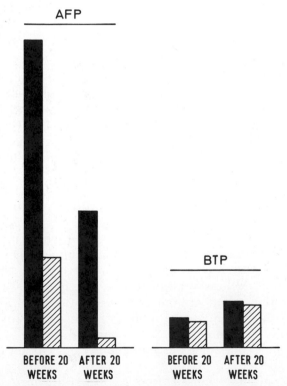

Figure 4. Mean AFP and beta-trace protein (BTP) concentrations in matched neural tube defect (solid bars) and control (hatched bars) amniotic fluids.

Table 4. Individual Proteins in Maternal Serum and Amniotic Fluid as Percentage of Total Protein; Results Represent Average of 11 Determinations on Different Fluids and Sera[*]

Protein	Molecular Weight	Maternal Serum	Amniotic Fluid
Transferrin	90,000	18.1	16.9
Post-albumins	50,000	8.3	8.3
Albumin	68,000	42.1	63.0
Ceruloplasmin	140,000	1.0	0.4
IgA	150,000	3.0	0.6
IgG	150,000	20.2	7.3
IgM	950,000	1.3	0
Alpha$_2$-macroglobulin	800,000	6.4	0
Beta-lipoprotein	2,400,000	1.9	0

[*]Adapted from Usategui-Gomez, 1974.

marker of neural tube defects early in pregnancy with an antiserum which has been raised against adult human CSF.

High Molecular Weight Proteins

It has been demonstrated immunologically that the bulk of amniotic fluid protein early in pregnancy derives from the maternal circulation (Sutcliffe and Brock, 1973). There is, however, an upper limit on the molecular weight of maternally derived proteins in early amniotic fluid, probably lying somewhere between 200,000 and 300,000 daltons (Table 4). Thus high molecular weight proteins are not normally found in amniotic fluid when conventional immunodiffusion or immunoelectrophoretic techniques are used in measurement, or unless the fluid is contamined with blood.

Brock (1975b) argued that if such proteins were indeed excluded from normal amniotic fluids, their presence could indicate a breakdown in one of the permeability barriers of the materno-fetal unit. The most obvious such breakdown is in the neural tube defects, in which much evidence had already suggested substantial leakage from the fetal circulation into the fluid. Measurement of the high molecular weight protein, alpha$_2$-macroglobulin (molecular weight, 850,000 daltons) confirmed that this was indeed the case. In 33 pregnancies in which the outcome was an infant with an open neural tube defect, alpha$_2$-macroglobulin concentration ranged from 1.3 to 50 μg per ml, but was undetectable in matched controls. Similar observations were made in the case of IgM (900,000 daltons) and beta-lipoprotein (2,500,000 daltons), although discrimination was best for alpha$_2$-mac-

roglobulin (Brock, 1976e). It is also the easiest of the three high molecular weight proteins to measure by rocket immunoelectrophoresis
using a commercial antiserum.

Another high molecular weight protein not found in normal amniotic fluids is fibrinogen. Purdie et al. (1975), noting that amniotic
fluid has fibrinolytic potential, measured the concentrations of fib-
rin/fibrinogen degradation products (FDP) in amniotic fluids from
normal pregnancies and those complicated by fetal neural tube defects. They observed that the concentrations of FDP in normal amniotic fluids were essentially independent of gestation and that those
in 5 cases of spina bifida and 6 cases of anencephaly in the second
trimester were substantially raised above normal. This observation
has been confirmed by Weiss et al. (1976), who did not, however,
find as clear a distinction between the neural tube defects and the
normal pregnancies. Purdie et al. (1975) discarded blood-contamin-
ated amniotic fluids in which the criterion for contamination was 1
part whole blood in 2^{18} parts of amniotic fluid. This wholly unrealis-
tic measure of contamination would exclude most amniotic fluids
taken by early amniocentesis. As in the case of alpha$_2$-macroglobulin,
IgM, and beta-lipoprotein, contamination of amniotic fluid by maternal blood distorts results sufficiently to render them void. This is a
serious drawback of this methodology, because a substantial proportion of amniocentesis fluids contains visible amounts of maternal
blood.

Fetal Macrophages

When amniotic fluid cells are plated out onto glass or plastic sur-
faces for the purpose of in vitro culture, they adhere comparatively
slowly and are usually left undisturbed for a period of days. Sutherland et al. (1973) noted that fluids from pregnancies in which the
fetus had a neural tube defect contained comparatively high proportions of cells that became firmly fixed in as little as 12 to 24 hours.
They showed that the cells had the properties of macrophages and
that they were fetal in origin. A simple counting procedure was
devised for their estimation, and this has been successful in identifying 8 cases of anencephaly and 6 cases of spina bifida before the
twentieth week of pregnancy (Nelson et al., 1974; Sutherland et al.,
1975; Brock, 1976a). However, a number of puzzling false positives
have been encountered (large numbers of macrophages in pregnancies which have subsequently turned out to be normal), and this lack
of specificity prevents quantitative macrophage estimation from

being used as a primary method for diagnosis of neural tube defects. Nonetheless it is of value as an adjunct to AFP assay and also in distinguishing between elevated AFP concentrations which are due to accidental contamination of amniotic fluid by fetal blood and those which are due to the presence of a fetus with neural tube defect (Sutherland, 1975).

The nature and origin of the glass-adherent cells found in amniotic fluids in which the fetus has a neural tube defect are by no means clear. Some are obviously macrophages, as judged by their ability to phagocytose sensitized sheep red cells and also from their characteristic ultrastructure under the electron microscope. Presumably these originate from the CSF or from the vascularized tissue surrounding the open neural tube lesion. If they originate from the CSF, one might expect to find other cells characteristic of neural tissue in the amniotic fluid in these conditions. Likewise, if the glass-adherent cells originate from vascularized tissue, one might expect to find high counts in other conditions in which an exposed fetal lesion occurs, such as exomphalos.

SCREENING FOR NEURAL TUBE DEFECTS

Maternal Serum AFP

Although the categories of mothers at increased risk of bearing children with neural tube defects are now well established (Table 2), complete ascertainment of these families, together with adequate counseling and monitoring of the pregnancies through amniotic fluid AFP, would have a comparatively small impact on the overall incidence of these abnormalities. More than 90 per cent of infants with anencephaly and spina bifida are born to mothers who have no previous history to suggest increased risk. Unless early amniocentesis were to become routine in all pregnancies (which, given its uncertain risk to the fetus and the load that such a policy would throw on obstetrical services, seems unlikely), screening through amniotic fluid AFP assay is impossible. Likewise, screening all pregnancies through a noninvasive technique such as ultrasonography is presently not feasible. Although it is claimed that both anencephaly and spina bifida are detectable by ultrasonar scan before the twentieth week of pregnancy (Campbell, 1974; Campbell et al., 1975), it is clear that the procedure is highly operator dependent and extremely time consuming if any kind of reliability is to be achieved. It is possible, indeed likely, that improvements in ultrasonar technology will alter this situation in the near future. In such a case a routine scan of all pregnant women at around the sixteenth week of gestation, which could locate the placenta, fix fetal age, exclude the possibility of twins, and detect several types of serious congenital abnormality, would become the method of choice for the prenatal diagnosis of neural tube defects. For the present, however, screening for spina bifida and anencephaly must depend on rapid chemical tests made in the maternal body fluids.

The possibility of maternal serum AFP measurements being used in screening for neural tube defects was predicted by Brock and Sutcliffe (1972). The protein, believed to be absent from normal adult serum, had been reported to reappear in the blood of pregnant women (Foy et al., 1970). However, Ruoslahti and Seppälä (1972), using a sensitive radioimmunoassay, demonstrated the presence of AFP in normal serum and showed that it rose sharply during pregnancy (Seppälä and Ruoslahti, 1972a; 1973b). They also reported greatly increased concentrations in the sera of mothers whose infants died in utero and in cases of threatened abortion (Seppälä and Ruoslahti, 1972b). Although these findings could be interpreted in terms of increased AFP transfer from the fetal circulation through the placenta to the maternal circulation, an alternative explanation was that the maternal serum levels correlated with increased amniotic fluid AFP. If this were the case, it could confidently be anticipated that the very high levels of amniotic fluid AFP observed early in gestation with anencephaly and spina bifida should also be reflected in increased maternal serum levels.

The first report of raised maternal serum AFP levels in pregnancies in which the fetuses had anencephaly was made by Hino et al. (1972), although only in the third trimester. A similar finding was made by Leek et al. (1973), again late in pregnancy. Of more relevance to prenatal diagnosis was the observation by Brock et al. (1973) of increased maternal serum AFP at 16 weeks and again at 21 weeks in a pregnancy which, after amniocentesis and confirmatory amniotic fluid AFP determination, was terminated to yield a fetus with anencephaly. Within a few months a number of papers were published directed toward assessment of this new diagnostic procedure (Harris et al., 1974; Seller et al., 1974b; Brock et al., 1974; Wald et al., 1974). All were guarded in their conclusions, but the consensus was that measurement of maternal serum AFP would allow the early detection of some but by no means all cases of neural tube defects. It was clear that serum measurements were to be seen as a preliminary screen, and that whenever high values were found follow-up should include ultrasonar scan, amniocentesis, and confirmatory amniotic fluid AFP determination. A workshop was convened in London to compare results and to discuss refinements of assay techniques (Editorial, 1974). It was decided to institute a collaborative study (the U.K. Collaborative Study on AFP in Relation to Neural Tube Defects), which, by pooling of results, might define the prospects and limitations of the AFP screening technique.

Sensitivity of Maternal Serum AFP

During the years in which data for the Collaborative Study were being collected, a number of publications on maternal serum AFP appeared (Cowchock and Jackson, 1974; Leek et al., 1974; Nevin, 1974; Malmqvist et al., 1975; Vince et al., 1975; Macri et al., 1975; Campbell et al., 1975; Cowchock and Jackson, 1976; Nørgaard-Pedersen and Schultz-Larsen 1976). Two, however, had a considerable influence on the setting up of prospective intervention trials. The first, which was a compilation of data from Edinburgh and Oxford, reported on maternal serum AFP concentrations between 8 and 22 weeks of gestation in 62 pregnancies which had resulted in an infant with a neural tube defect (Brock et al., 1975b). It pointed out that before the end of the first trimester, screening for neural tube defects through maternal serum AFP was essentially useless. This was a major drawback in contemplating the use of the technique, particularly in the United Kingdom, where most women first register at antenatal clinics at about the tenth week of pregnancy and thereafter do not return until well into the third trimester. The second point made by Brock et al. (1975b) was that if the ninety-eighth percentile of the normal range was used as the upper limit of normal, 80 per cent of cases of anencephaly but only 40 per cent of open spina bifida had elevated values. Since any form of contemplated screening would be directed primarily against reducing the incidence of spina bifida, this was a somewhat discouraging finding. Shortly thereafter a more optimistic paper appeared (Leighton et al., 1975) in which 51 pregnancies associated with fetal neural tube defects had been examined. Their claim that the detection rate for open spina bifida was 92 per cent was strongly criticized by Seller (1975b), who pointed out that within the relevant gestational period only 5 cases of open spina bifida had been tested. In contrast, Brock et al. (1975b) had evaluated 17 cases of open spina bifida within the same period. A compilation of published cases reported in the literature at this time showed that 15 out of 32 cases of spina bifida had given rise to elevated maternal serum AFP values between 15 and 20 weeks of pregnancy (Brock, 1976c).

Table 5.   Cases of Anencephaly in Which Maternal Serum AFP Was Above
the 96th, 97th, 98th, and 99th Percentiles of the Normal Range*

Gestation (Weeks)	Number of Cases	99th	98th	97th	96th
10–12	15	2 (13%)	2 (13%)	2 (13%)	2 (13%)
13–15	34	15 (44%)	17 (50%)	18 (53%)	20 (59%)
16–18	46	36 (78%)	39 (85%)	41 (89%)	41 (89%)
19–21	17	17 (100%)	17 (100%)	17 (100%)	17 (100%)

*Preliminary data from the U.K. Collaborative Study.

Preliminary data from the U.K. Collaborative Study are shown in
Tables 5 and 6. Sera from 112 pregnancies in which the fetus had
anencephaly and 77 in which it had open spina bifida have been
analyzed in terms of various percentiles of the normal range for the
laboratory concerned. In both tables it is apparent that detection efficiencies improve strikingly as pregnancy progresses (Fig. 5), and
that the power of screening diminishes sharply if carried out before
the end of the fifteenth week. It is also noteworthy that moving the
upper limit of normal from the ninety-sixth to the ninety-ninth percentile does not greatly decrease the ability to pick out either anencephaly (89 per cent down to 78 per cent at 16 to 18 weeks) or open
spina bifida (78 per cent down to 63 per cent at 16 to 18 weeks).

Specificity of Maternal Serum AFP

In setting the upper limit of the normal range at the ninety-
eighth percentile, 2 per cent of all pregnancies will be initially registered as having abnormal values. These are not true false positives in
the sense that the upper limit of normal can be adjusted according to
the detection efficiency required (Tables 5 and 6). They are perhaps
better named as "pseudo-positives." Among the 2 per cent within this

Table 6.   Cases of Open Spina Bifida in Which Maternal Serum AFP Was
Above the 96th, 97th, 98th, and 99th Percentiles of the Normal Range*

Gestation (Weeks)	Number of Cases	99th	98th	97th	96th
10–12	17	1 (6%)	1 (6%)	1 (6%)	2 (12%)
13–15	23	5 (22%)	6 (26%)	7 (31%)	10 (44%)
16–18	27	17 (63%)	19 (70%)	21 (78%)	21 (78%)
19–21	10	5 (50%)	5 (50%)	6 (60%)	6 (60%)

*Preliminary data from the U.K. Collaborative Study.

DETECTION EFFICIENCY IN PERCENT

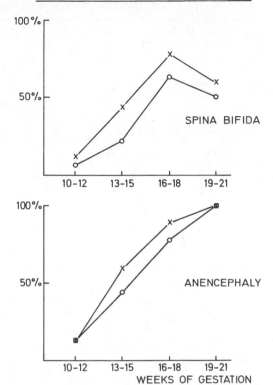

Figure 5. Maternal serum AFP detection efficiency for spina bifida and anencephaly, using the ninety-sixth percentile (×) and the ninety-ninth percentile (○) as the upper limit of normal.

abnormal category will be some pregnancies which do not simply represent the upper end of the normal distribution or a neural tube defect, but rather some other physiological or pathological state. The most common of these is, of course, an incorrectly stated gestation as the normal median value for serum AFP increases by about 10 per cent, for each week between 12 and 21 weeks of gestation.

Recognizing other possible causes of elevated serum AFP is of some importance (Table 7). The most frequently encountered is likely to be multiple pregnancy (Garoff and Seppälä, 1973; Ishiguro, 1973; Vince et al., 1975). Wald et al. (1975), on the basis of ten pregnancies, pointed out that the geometric mean level for twin pregnancies was 2.1 times that for singletons. In triplet pregnancies the level was even higher. Multiple pregnancies should be easily recognized on ultrasonar scan before any amniocentesis is contemplated, so that this group of high values is of advantage in the management of the pregnancy. Likewise, an intrauterine death should be recognized before amniocentesis by the absence of a fetal heartbeat.

Table 7. Elevated Maternal Serum AFP Levels Not Associated with
Neural Tube Defects (See Text)

Condition	Gestation
Multiple pregnancy	2nd and 3rd trimesters
Threatened abortion	1st, 2nd, and 3rd trimesters
Intrauterine death	1st, 2nd, and 3rd trimesters
Severe Rh isoimmunization	3rd trimester
Toxemia	3rd trimester
Fetal distress (anoxia)	3rd trimester
Congenital nephrosis	2nd and 3rd trimesters
Exomphalos	2nd and 3rd trimesters
Blood sample taken immediately after amniocentesis	2nd trimester

Several of the other conditions in Table 7, such as fetal distress, toxemia, and severe Rh isoimmunization, have contributed to raised values only in the third trimester of pregnancy and seem unlikely to complicate early screening programs. Potentially the most serious is threatened abortion (Garoff and Seppälä, 1975, Vince et al., 1975). The problem here is that if a woman with a high serum AFP has an amniocentesis and subsequently aborts, the tendency will be to assume that the high serum value was indicating a threatened abortion and that the amniocentesis should never have been carried out. However, by a careful analysis of retrospective data, Wald et al. (1977) have shown that clinical symptoms of threatened abortion appear at almost the same time as, and never more than a few days later than, the elevation of serum AFP. Since there is always a gap between the reporting of a serum AFP result and completion of the arrangements for amniocentesis, it should be clear to the obstetrician when he is dealing with a case in which high serum AFP was indicating threatened abortion.

In a large series comprising 3048 completed pregnancies on which serum AFP was determined in the fourteenth to twentieth week of gestation, Kjessler et al. (1976) observed 124 raised values, i.e., exceeding 3 log standard deviations above the mean for the pregnancy week. A majority of these raised values resulted in normal singleton births. Of the remaining 46 cases, 19 resulted in spontaneous abortion, 17 in multiple births, 6 in premature single births, 2 in intrauterine death, 1 in an ectopic pregnancy, and 1 in an induced abortion. This experience is rather different from the author's prospective intervention study, in which a very small number of spontaneous abortions have been observed.

Implications of Screening

It is apparent that screening for neural tube defects using maternal serum AFP has a number of serious disadvantages. The most obvious of these is the incomplete nature of the test. As long as screening misses a substantial proportion of pregnancies in which the fetus is affected, it will be on difficult ground. Whatever decisions are made about publicizing the new test, there is no doubt that the knowledge that screening is being carried out will gradually permeate the public consciousness and generate an expectation among mothers that they are being protected against one of the more devastating infant abnormalities, which the screening test is unable to justify. This in turn could create a backlash which will further diminish its effectiveness. It will have to be recognized from the outset that serum AFP detection of neural tube defects is less than 100 per cent efficient and that this is due to biological variations in pregnant women and not to technical imperfections in the assay. There are obvious hopes that the efficiency of the test will rise with more practice, and indeed it is curious that the various prospective intervention trials being conducted in the United Kingdom seem to be recording much higher detection efficiencies for spina bifida than had been anticipated. Possibly this is because the blood test is being performed later in pregnancy when the pick-up rate is much higher (Tables 5 and 6).

A second major disadvantage of screening is that the upper limit of the normal range has to be set in such a way that between 1 and 5 per cent of all pregnancies will be initially classified as abnormal. Some of these will have high values owing to wrong dates, some to other conditions as shown in Table 7, and some to the presence of a fetal neural tube defect. However, the majority may be uncomplicated pregnancies lying at the upper end of normal biological variation. Communicating the fact of a high value to such a patient will be a matter of extreme delicacy. Obstetricians will seldom know in advance what a patient's reaction will be to the suggestion of amniocentesis and possible termination of pregnancy. The patient must be approached in such a way that if she is firmly opposed to abortion she can continue her pregnancy without excessive worry. One way of handling such a situation is to treat all high serum AFP values as indicating incorrectly specified gestations until proved otherwise, and to ask mothers to cooperate through a second blood sample and an ultrasonar scan in fixing fetal age more precisely. This will allow the obstetrician a chance to exclude cases of high serum values which are due to wrong dating and, if the ultrasonar scan is efficient, those due to multiple pregnancy. It should also allow him to approach the question of amniocentesis with his patient in a noncommittal way.

If an amniocentesis is performed because of an elevated serum AFP, the calculations in Table 8 allow an estimate of the proportion of times amniotic fluid AFP will confirm a neural tube defect. Much depends on a high detection rate in serum AFP being maintained. Thus if the Boston incidence of neural tube defects of 2 per 1000 is used (Table 1), screening at the ninety-eighth percentile will yield one abnormal fetus in 12 amniocenteses at 80 per cent detection efficiency and one abnormal fetus in 17 amniocenteses at 60 per cent efficiency (Table 8). If the ninety-eighth percentile is used, the proportion of confirmations will be even higher. It must be remembered that

Table 8. Theoretical Implications of Maternal Serum AFP Screening for Neural Tube Defects (NTD)

1. If the 98th percentile of the normal range is taken as the upper limit, then 20 in every 1000 pregnancies will be subject to amniocentesis. If the local incidence of neural tube defects is 3 per 1000 and the detection efficiency of screening is 67 per cent, then 2 out of the 3 neural tube defects will be detected. Therefore 20 amniocenteses yield 2 neural tube defects, yielding an amniocentesis per NTD "rate" of 10.0.

2. If the 99th percentile is used, there will be 10 amniocenteses per 1000 pregnancies. If the local incidence is 5 per 1000 and the detection efficiency is 80 per cent, then 4 out of 5 neural tube defects will be detected. This gives an amniocentesis per NTD "rate" of 10/4 or 2.5.

Local Incidence Rate per 1000	Detection Efficiency (%)	Cases Detected per 1000	Amniocenteses per NTD
98th percentile as upper limit of normal (20 amniocenteses per 1000 pregnancies):			
6	80	4.8	4.2
4	80	3.2	6.3
2	80	1.6	12.5
6	60	3.6	5.5
4	60	2.4	8.3
2	60	1.2	16.7
99th percentile as upper limit of normal (10 amniocenteses per 1000 pregnancies):			
6	80	4.8	2.1
4	80	3.2	3.1
2	80	1.6	6.3
6	60	3.6	2.8
4	60	2.4	4.2
2	60	1.2	8.3

one abnormal fetus in 20 amniocenteses is the present figure in the United Kingdom for women who have previously had a child with a neural tube defect.

Carrying out serum AFP testing at the right stage in gestation is of great importance. This raises different problems according to the pattern of antenatal health care. In the United Kingdom, where almost all women deliver in hospital, the time of first registering at the antenatal clinic depends very much on the pressure on obstetric services. When it is high, women tend to book early; when it is low, they tend to be later. But in most areas only a small proportion of women would actually register between the sixteenth and eighteenth weeks of pregnancy and thus make themselves available for a blood test at the most appropriate time. For others a second visit to the hospital will have to be arranged, thus making antenatal care even more hospital oriented than it is at the moment. The logistics of allowing blood collection to be performed by family doctors is complex and to be avoided if it can be. In a prospective intervention trial in which various types of blood collection have been compared, the performance of family doctors has been disappointing (Brock et al., unpublished data). In the United Kingdom, where there is a general move to give family doctors a larger share in the care of their pregnant patients, the prospects of a nationwide policy of screening for neural tube defects is a move in the opposite direction.

One question of great importance which is extraordinarily difficult to answer is whether the cases of spina bifida detected as a result of screening are those that would have survived the neonatal months to become a burden on their families. It is possible that high serum AFP is found only in conjunction with lesions so serious that the infant would be unlikely to be born alive or to survive the first days of life. Unfortunately it is becoming increasingly difficult to answer this question, because many centers have adopted intervention screening and are terminating a proportion of the pregnancies, a factor which will seriously distort obtaining complete information on the survival and degree of handicap of infants associated with high maternal serum AFP levels in utero. The only data that have bearing on this particular problem are those collected by Wald (1976). He has examined the degree of handicap in 9 infants with spina bifida who survived for 6 months or longer and on whom a serum AFP determination had been made. Three of the infants with moderate or severe handicap had AFP values above the ninety-eighth percentile, and could therefore be scored as detectable. Four infants with moderate or severe handicap had levels below the ninety-eighth percentile, and would therefore have escaped detection. The remaining two in-

fants with minimal or no handicap had normal values. Although no
real conclusions can be drawn from such a limited set of data, the direction in which it points is mildly reassuring, particularly when it is
remembered that this screening was performed at a time when the
best gestational week had not been identified. More complete data,
however, are urgently needed and will have to be collected from
areas where intervention screening is not being carried out.

The disadvantages of serum AFP screening for neural tube
defects are considerable and raise the question of whether it is a
worthwhile procedure. For some time it has been reckoned that such
screening could be easily justified on economic grounds, because of
the very low cost of the AFP radioimmunoassay. However, recently
Hagard et al. (1976) conducted a sophisticated cost-benefit analysis
of screening for spina bifida, taking a particular area of Western
Scotland and the United Kingdom health care services as their
model. Assuming a detection efficiency of 80 per cent for open spina
bifida, they argued for a benefit-cost index (the total benefit of the
screening program divided by its total costs) of 1.86 in a population
incidence area of approximately 3 per 1000. Large numbers of assumptions have to be made in analyses of this type (which depend
on health care patterns in the country concerned), and one of the
most contentious is applying a financial discount rate of 10 per cent.
This assumes that a dollar spent today would be 10 per cent more
valuable in a year's time because of investment; it takes no account
of inflation. If a 5 per cent discount rate were used, the benefit-cost
index would rise to 3.06. However, if the sensitivity of the detection
method dropped to 40 per cent (the findings of the largest single laboratory determination of efficiency so far made [Brock et al., 1975b]),
the benefit-cost index would drop to 1.0 in a 3 per 1000 incidence
area. In other words the costs of the screening program, both direct
and indirect, would be as great as the economic benefits from detecting and aborting early spina bifidas. In lower incidence areas the
index would drop even lower. Where health services are essentially
private, as in the United States, a rather different benefit-cost index
might emerge.

It is obvious from these figures that screening for neural tube
defects cannot be justified on the ground of economic benefit alone,
except in very high incidence areas. However, few medical programs
are assessed solely on these terms. Certainly no other antenatal diagnostic endeavor could get anywhere near the figures for neural tube
defects, and yet there is no doubt that such endeavors will go on. What
has to be considered instead is the burden of the disorder to family,
community, and physician. This is an emotional area in which the facts

arc impossible to quantify. However, the author has n
devastating consequences of a child with spina bifida
lies are so considerable that an efficient program of sc
neural tube defects by serum AFP is justifiable in most con
which have the resources to provide it.

References

Abelev, G. I. 1971. Alpha-fetoprotein in ontogenesis and its association with malignant tumors. Adv. Cancer Res., *14*:295–358.

Abelev, G. I., I. V. Assecritova, N. A. Kravesky, S. D. Perova, and N. I. Perevodchi-kowa. 1967. Embryonal serum alpha-globulin in cancer patients: Diagnostic value. Int. J. Cancer 2:551–558.

Adinolfi, A., M. Adinolfi, and S. Cohen. 1971. Isolation and characterisation of human foetal α-globulin (α_1F) from foetal and hepatoma sera. Biochim. Biophys. Acta *251*:197–207.

Adinolfi, A., M. Adinolfi, and M. H. Lessof. 1975. Alpha-fetoprotein during development and in disease. J. Med. Genet. *12*:138–151.

Ainbender, E., and K. Hirschhorn. 1976. Routine alphafetoprotein studies in amniotic fluid. Lancet *1*:597–598.

Allan, L. D., M. A. Ferguson-Smith, I. Donald, E. M. Sweet, and A. A. M. Gibson. 1973. Amniotic fluid alpha-fetoprotein in the antenatal diagnosis of spina bifida. Lancet 2:522–525.

Alpert, E., J. W. Drysdale, K. J. Isselbacher, and H. Schur. 1972. Human α-fetoprotein: Isolation, characterization and demonstration of microheterogeneity. J. Biol. Chem. *247*:3792–3798.

Bélanger, L. 1973. Tyrosinémie héréditaire et alpha-1-foetoprotéine. II. Recherche tissulaire comparée de l'alpha-foetoprotéine dans deux cas de tyrosinémie héréditaire. Considérations sur l'ontogenèse de la foetoprotéine humaine. Path. Biol. *21*:457–463.

Bergstrand, C. G., and B. Czar. 1956. Demonstration of a new protein fraction in serum from the human fetus. Scand. J. Clin. Lab. Invest. 8:174–179.

Brock, D. J. H. 1974. The molecular nature of alphafetoprotein in anencephaly and spina bifida. Clin. Chim. Acta 57:315–320.

Brock, D. J. H. 1975a. Antenatal misdiagnosis of neural tube defects. Lancet 2:495.

Brock, D. J. H. 1975b. Alpha$_2$-macroglobulin in the antenatal diagnosis of anencephaly and spina bifida. Clin. Genet. 8:297–301.

Brock, D. J. H. 1976a. The prenatal diagnosis of neural tube defects. Obstet. Gynec. Surv. *31*:32–40.

Brock, D. J. H. 1976b. Prenatal diagnosis—chemical methods. Brit. Med. Bull. *32*:16–20.

Brock, D. J. H. 1976c. Screening for neural tube defects. Lancet *1*:46–47.

Brock, D. J. H. 1976d. Mechanisms by which amniotic fluid alphafetoprotein may be raised in fetal abnormality. Lancet 2:345–346.

Brock, D. J. H. 1976e. Protein measurements in the antenatal diagnosis of spina bifida. Hum. Hered. 26:401–408.

Brock, D. J. H., A. E. Bolton, and J. M. Monaghan. 1973. Prenatal diagnosis of anencephaly through maternal serum alphafetoprotein measurement. Lancet 2:923–924.

Brock, D. J. H., A. E. Bolton, and J. B. Scrimgeour. 1974. Prenatal diagnosis of spina bifida and anencephaly through maternal plasma—alphafetoprotein measurement. Lancet *1*:767–769.

Brock, D. J. H., J. C. Manson, J. A. Raeburn, A. E. Bolton, and N. M. McCrae. 1975a. Serum alpha-fetoprotein in cystic fibrosis. Brit. Med. J. 2:392.

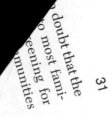

6. Comparison of alphafetoprotein and betatrace
of anencephaly and spina bifida. Clin. Genet.

972. Early prenatal diagnosis of anencephaly.

Bolton, N. J. Wald, R. Peto, and S. Barker.
screening for neural defects by maternal
195–196.
M. Nelson. 1975c. Amniotic fluid alphafe-
diagnosis of central nervous system dis-

phafetoprotein in the antenatal diagnosis
?:197–199.
natal diagnosis of anencephaly. Trans.

..phalocele and raised alphafetoprotein

...al Detection of Fetal Abnormality by Ultrasonic Diag-
...ects. Moltulsky, A., and W. Lenz (Eds.), pp. 240–247. Amster-
...crpta Medica.

Ca...ppell, S., J. Pryse-Davies, T. M. Coltart, M. J. Seller, and J. D. Singer. 1975. Ul-
trasound in the diagnosis of spina bifida. Lancet 1:1065–1068.

Carter, C. O. 1974. Clues to the aetiology of neural tube malformations. Dev. Med.
Child. Neurol. 16: suppl. 32, 3–15.

Carter, C. O. 1976. Genetics of common single malformations. Brit. Med. Bull. 32:21–
26.

Carter, C. O., P. A. David, and K. M. Laurence. 1968. A family study of major central
nervous system malformations in South Wales. J. Med. Genet. 5:81–91.

Carter, C. O., K. A. Evans, and K. Till. 1976. Spinal dysraphism: Genetic relation to
neural tube malformations. J. Med. Genet. 13:343–350.

Carter, C. O., and J. A. F. Roberts. 1967. The risk of recurrence after two children with
central nervous system malformations. Lancet 1:306–307.

Cassady, G., and J. Cailliteau. 1967. The amniotic fluid in anencephaly. Am. J. Obstet.
Gynec. 97:395–399.

Chandra, R. K., K. Madhavankutty, and R. C. Way. 1975. Serum α-fetoprotein levels in
patients with cystic fibrosis and their parents and siblings. Brit. Med. J., 1:714–
715.

Cowchock, F. S., and L. G. Jackson. 1974. Maternal serum alpha-fetoprotein and anencephaly. Lancet 2:48.

Cowchock, F. S., and L. G. Jackson. 1976. Diagnostic use of maternal serum alphafetoprotein levels. Obstet. Gynec. 47:63–68.

Dattwyler, R. J., R. A. Murgita, and T. B. Tomasi. 1975. Binding of α-fetoprotein to
murine T cells. Nature 256:656–657.

Editorial. 1974. Towards the prevention of spina bifida. Lancet 1:907.

Elwood, J. H. 1970. Anencephalus in Belfast. Brit. J. Prev. Soc. Med. 24:78–88.

Endo, Y., K. Kanai, S. Iino, and T. Oda. 1974. Dye-binding properties of AFP. In
L'Alpha-foeto-protéine, (Ed.). Masseyeff, R. Paris, Inserm.

Fedrick, J. 1976. Anencephalus in Scotland 1961–1972. Brit. J. Prev. Soc. Med.
30:132–137.

Field, B., and C. Kerr. 1975. Antenatal diagnosis of neural tube defects. Lancet 2:324.

Fitzsimmons, J. S., G. M. Filshine, A. S. Hill, and R. Kime. 1976. Antenatal diagnosis
of trisomy 13 with unexpected increase in alphafetoprotein. J. Med. Genet.
13:400–412.

Foy, H., A. Kondi, and C. A. Linsell. 1970. Fetoprotein in pregnant African women.
Lancet 2:663–664.

Furth, R. Van, and M. Adinolfi. 1969. In vitro synthesis of the foetal α_1-globulin in
man. Nature 222:1296–1299.

Garoff, L., and M. Seppälä. 1973. Alpha-fetoprotein and human placental lactogen

31

levels in maternal serum in multiple pregnancies. J. Obstet. Gynaec. Brit. Comm. 80:695–700.

Garoff, L., and M. Seppälä. 1975. Prediction of fetal outcome in threatened abortion by serum placental lactogen and alpha-fetoprotein. Am. J. Obstet. Gynec. 121:257–261.

Gitlin, D., and M. Boesman. 1966. Serum α-fetoprotein, albumin, and γG-globulin in the human conceptus. J. Clin. Invest. 45:1826–1838.

Gitlin, D., and M. Boesman. 1967. Sites of serum α-fetoprotein synthesis in the human and in the rat. J. Clin. Invest. 46:1010–1016.

Gitlin, D., and A. Perricelli. 1970. Synthesis of serum albumin, prealbumin, α-fetoprotein, $α_1$-antitrypsin and transferrin by the human yolk sac. Nature 228:995–997.

Gitlin, D., A. Perricelli, and G. M. Gitlin. 1972. Synthesis of α-fetoprotein by liver, yolk sac, and gastrointestinal tract in the human conceptus. Cancer Res. 32:979–982.

Guibaud, S., M. Bonnet, A. Durie, J. M. Thoulon, and M. Dumont. 1976. Amniotic fluid or maternal urine. Lancet 1:746.

Hagard, S., F. Carter, and R. G. Milne. 1976. Screening for spina bifida. A cost-benefit analysis. Brit. J. Prev. Soc. Med. 30:40–53.

Harris, R., R. F. Jennison, A. J. Barson, K. M. Laurence, E. Ruoslahti, and M. Seppälä. 1974. Comparison of amniotic fluid and maternal serum alpha-fetoprotein levels in the early antenatal diagnosis of spina bifida and anencephaly. Lancet 1:429–433.

Hino, M., Y. Koki, and S. Nishi. 1972. Alpha-fetoprotein in pregnant women. Igaku no Ayumi 82:512–513.

Hirai, H., S. Nishi, H. Watabe, and Y. Tsukada. 1973. Some chemical, experimental, and clinical investigations of alpha-fetoprotein. Gann Monogr. Cancer Res. 14:19–33.

Holmes, L. B., S. G. Driscoll, and L. Atkins. 1976. Etiologic heterogeneity of neural tube defects. New Eng. J. Med. 294:365–369.

Hunter, A., J. L. Hammerton, T. Baskett, and E. Lyons. 1976. Raised amniotic fluid alphafetoprotein in Turner syndrome. Lancet 1:598–599.

Ishiguro, T. 1973. Alpha-fetoprotein in twin pregnancy. Lancet 2:1214.

Jandial, V., H. Thom, and J. Gibson. 1976. Raised alphafetoprotein levels associated with minor congenital defect. Brit. Med. J. 3:22–23.

Kjessler, B., S. G. O. Johansson, G. Lidbjork, and M. Sherman. 1976. Alphafetoprotein Levels in Maternal Serum in Early Pregnancy. In Protides of the Biological Fluids, Vol. XXIV, Abstracts, p. 82.

Kjessler, B., S. G. O. Johansson, M. Sherman, K. H. Gustavson, and G. Hultqvist. 1975. Alpha-fetoprotein in antenatal diagnosis of congenital nephrosis. Lancet 1:432–433.

Kunz, J., and J. Schmid. 1976. Amniotic alphafetoprotein and omphalocele. Lancet 1:47.

Laurence, K. M. 1974. Fetal malformations and abnormalities. Lancet 2:939–941.

Laurence, K. M., A. C. Turnbull, R. Harris, R. F. Jennison, E. Ruoslahti, and M. Seppälä. 1973. Antenatal diagnosis of spina bifida. Lancet 2:860.

Leck, I. 1969. Ethnic differences in the incidence of malformation following migration. Brit. J. Prev. Soc. Med. 23:166–173.

Leck, I. 1972. The aetiology of human malformations and insights from epidemiology. Teratology 5:303–307.

Lee, T. Y., and P. Y. Wei. 1970. Spectrophotometric analysis of amniotic fluid in anencephalic pregnancies. Am. J. Obstet. Gynec. 107:917–920.

Leek, A. E., P. C. Leighton, M. J. Kitau, and T. Chard. 1974. Prospective diagnosis of spina bifida. Lancet 2:1511.

Leek, A. E., C. F. Ruoss, M. J. Kitau, and T. Chard. 1973. Raised alpha-fetoprotein in maternal serum with anencephalic pregnancy. Lancet 2:385.

Leighton, P. C., Y. B. Gordon, M. J. Kitau, A. E. Leek, and T. Chard. 1975. Levels of alpha-fetoprotein in maternal blood as a screening test for neural tube defects. Lancet 2:1012–1015.

Leschot, N. J., and P. E. Treffers. 1975. Elevated amniotic fluid alphafetoprotein without neural tube defects. Lancet 2:1141.

Lorber, J., C. R. Stewart, and A. Milford Ward. 1973. Alpha-fetoprotein in antenatal diagnosis of anencephaly and spina bifida. Lancet 1:1187.

MacMahon, B., and S. Yen. 1971. Unrecognized epidemic of anencephaly and spina bifida. Lancet 1:31–33.

Macri, J. N. 1975. Personal communication.

Macri, J. N., M. S. Joshi, and M. I. Evans. 1973. An antenatal diagnosis of spina bifida in the Lewis rat. Nature–New Biol. 246:89–90.

Macri, J. N., R. R. Weiss, and M. S. Joshi. 1974a. Beta-trace protein and neural tube defects. Lancet 1:1109–1110.

Macri, J. N., R. R. Weiss, M. S. Joshi, and M. I. Evans. 1974b. Antenatal diagnosis of neural tube defect using cerebrospinal fluid proteins. Lancet 1:14–15.

Macri, J. N., R. R. Weiss, N. A. Starkorsky, K. W. Elligers, and D. B. Berger. 1975. Maternal serum alpha-fetoprotein and prospective screening. Lancet 2:719–720.

Malmqvist, E., J. Lindsten, B. Nørgaard-Pedersen, B. Hellstrøm, and B. Sundberg. 1975. Elevated levels of alpha-fetoprotein in maternal serum and amniotic fluid in two cases of spina bifida. Clin. Genet. 7:176–180.

Masopust, J., H. Tomasova, and L. Kotal. 1971. Some physicochemical characteristics of human α_1-fetoprotein. Protides Biol. Fluids 18:37–42.

Masseyeff, R. 1972. Revue genérale. Human alphafetoprotein. Path. Biol. 20:703–725.

Masseyeff, R., C. Bonet, J. Drouet, P. Sudaka, and C. Lalanne. 1974. Radioimmunoassay of alphafetoprotein. I. Technique and serum levels in the normal adult. Digestion 10:17–28.

McIntire, K. R., T. A. Waldmann, C. G. Moertel, and V. L. W. Go. 1975. Serum α-fetoprotein in patients with neoplasms of the gastrointestinal tract. Cancer Res. 35:991–996.

Milunsky, A. 1975. The Prevention of Genetic Disease and Mental Retardation, pp. 221–263. Philadelphia, W. B. Saunders Co.

Milunsky, A., and E. Alpert. 1974. The value of alphafetoprotein in the prenatal diagnosis of neural tube defects. J. Pediat. 84:889–893.

Milunsky, A., and M. E. Kimball. 1976. Alphafetoprotein assay in all amniocentesis samples. Lancet 2:209.

Milunsky, A., J. N. Macri, R. R. Weiss, E. Alpert, D. McIsaac, and M. I. Joshi. 1975. Prenatal detection of neural tube defects; comparison between alphafetoprotein and beta-trace protein assays. Am. J. Obstet. Gynec. 122:313–315.

Mizejewski, G. J., and P. M. Grimley. 1976. Abortogenic activity of antiserum to alpha-foetoprotein. Nature 259:222–224.

Morton, N. E., C. S. Chung, and M. P. Mi. 1967. Genetics of Interracial Crosses in Hawaii. Monographs on Human Genetics. 3. Basel, Karger.

Murgita, R. A., and T. B. Tomasi. 1975. Suppression of the immune response by α-fetoprotein. J. Exp. Med. 141:440–452.

Naggan, L. 1971. Anencephaly and spina bifida in Israel. Pediatrics 47:577–583.

Naggan, L., and B. MacMahon. 1967. Ethnic differences in the prevalence of anencephaly and spina bifida in Boston. New Eng. J. Med. 277:1119–1123.

Nakano, K. K. 1973. Anencephaly: A review. Dev. Med. Child. Neurol. 15:383–400.

Nayak, N. C., V. Chawla, A. N. Malaviya, and R. K. Chandra. 1972. α-Fetoprotein in Indian childhood cirrhosis. Lancet 1:68–72.

Nelson, M. M., M. T. Ruttiman, and D. J. H. Brock. 1974. Predictive value of amniotic fluid macrophages in gross C.N.S. defects. Lancet 1:504.

Nevin, N. C. 1974. Amniotic fluid and maternal serum alpha-fetoprotein determinations in neural tube defects. Dev. Med. Child Neurol. 16:122–125.

Nevin, N. C., and M. J. Armstrong. 1975. Raised alphafetoprotein levels in amniotic fluid and maternal serum in a triplet pregnancy in which one fetus had an omphalocoele. Brit. J. Obstet. Gynaec. 82:826–828.

Nevin, N. C., S. Nesbitt, and W. Thompson. 1973. Myelocele and alphafetoprotein in amniotic fluid. Lancet 1:1383.

Nevin, N. C., W. Thompson, and S. Nesbitt. 1974. Amniotic fluid alphafetoprotein in the antenatal diagnosis of neural tube defects. J. Obstet. Gynaec. Brit. Comm. 81:757–760.

Nishi, S. 1970. Isolation and characterization of a human fetal α-globulin from the sera of fetuses and a hepatoma patient. Cancer Res. 30:2507–2513.

Nørgaard-Pedersen, B. 1972. Purification and sensitive immunoelectrophoretical detection and quantitation of human α_1-foetoprotein. Clin. Chim. Acta 38:163–170.

Nørgaard-Pedersen, B. 1976. Human alpha-fetoprotein. Scand. J. Immunol. Suppl. 4:45.

Nørgaard-Pedersen, B., and N. H. Axelsen. 1976. Alpha-fetoprotein–like activity in sera from patients with malignant and nonmalignant disease and from healthy individuals. Clin. Chim. Acta 71:343–347.

Nørgaard-Pedersen, B., and P. Schultz-Larsen. 1976. Reference interval for maternal serum alpha-fetoprotein. Clin. Genet. 9:374–377.

Nunez, E., F. Engelman, C. Bennassayag, and M. Jayle. 1971. Identification and preliminary purification of fetal protein-binding estrogens in serum of the newborn rat. C. R. Hebd. Seanc. Acad. Sci. (Paris) 273:831–837.

Olsson, J. E., M. S. Sherman, and B. Kjessler. 1974. Beta-trace protein in neural tube defects. Lancet 2:347–348.

Pirani, B. B. K., T. A. Doran, and R. J. Benzie. 1976. Amniotic fluid or maternal urine. Lancet 1:303.

Purdie, D. W., P. W. Howie, W. Edgar, C. D. Forbes, and C. R. M. Prentice. 1975. Raised amniotic fluid FDP in fetal neural tube anomalies. Lancet 1:1013–1014.

Renwick, J. H. 1972. Hypothesis. Anencephaly and spina bifida are usually preventable by avoidance of a specific but unidentified substance present in certain potatoes. Brit. J. Prev. Soc. Med. 26:67–88.

Ruoslahti, E., M. Salaspuro, H. Pihko, L. Anderson, and M. Seppälä. 1974. Serum alpha-fetoprotein: Diagnostic significance in liver disease. Brit. Med. J. 2:527–529.

Ruoslahti, E., and M. Seppälä, 1971. Studies of carcino-fetal proteins: Physical and chemical properties of human α-fetoprotein. Int. J. Cancer 7:218–225.

Ruoslahti, E., and M. Seppälä. 1972. α-Fetoprotein in normal human serum. Nature 235:161–162.

Ruoslahti, E., M. Seppälä, H. Pihko, and P. P. Vuopio. 1971. Studies of carcino-fetal protein. II. Biochemical comparison of α-fetoprotein from human fetuses and patients with hepatocellular cancer. Int. J. Cancer 8:283–288.

Ruoslahti, E., and W. D. Terry. 1976. α-Fetoprotein and serum albumin show sequence homology. Nature 260:804–805.

Savu, L., G. Vallette, E. Nunez, M. Azria, and M. F. Joyle. 1974. A Comparative Study on the Binding of Free Estrogens by Serum Proteins During Development in Several Mammalian Species. In L'Alpha-Fòeto-Protéine, Masseyeff, R. (Ed.), Paris, Inserm. pp. 75–83.

Schmid, W., and J. P. Muhlethaler. 1975. High amniotic fluid alpha-1-fetoprotein in a case of fetal sacrococcygeal teratoma. Hum. Genet. 26:353–354.

Seller, M. J. 1975a. Case Report: Prenatal diagnosis of a neural tube defect: Meckel syndrome. J. Med. Genet. 12:109–110.

Seller, M. J. 1975b. Screening for neural tube defects. Lancet 2:1141.

Seller, M. J. 1976. Raised amniotic fluid alpha-fetoprotein in Turner syndrome. Lancet 1:807.

Seller, M. J., S. Campbell, T. M. Coltart, and J. D. Singer. 1973. Early termination of anencephalic pregnancy after detection of raised alpha-feto-protein levels. Lancet 2:73.

Seller, M. J., M. R. Creasy, and E. D. Alberman. 1974a. Alpha-fetoprotein levels in amniotic fluids from spontaneous abortions. Brit. Med. J. 2:624–525.

Seller, M. J., J. D. Singer, T. M. Coltart, and S. Campbell. 1974b. Maternal serum-alpha-fetoprotein levels and prenatal diagnosis of neural-tube defects. Lancet 1:428–429.

Seppälä, M. 1973. Increased alphafetoprotein in amniotic fluid associated with a congenital esophageal atresia of the fetus. Obstet. Gynec. 42:613–614.

Seppälä, M. 1975. Fetal pathophysiology of human alphafetoprotein. Ann. N.Y. Acad. Sci. 259:59–73.

Seppälä, M., P. Aula, J. Rapola, O. Karjalainen, N. P. Huttunen, and E. Ruoslahti. 1976. Congenital nephrotic syndrome: Prenatal diagnosis and genetic counselling by estimation of amniotic fluid and maternal serum alphafetoprotein. Lancet 2:123–125.

Seppälä, M., and E. Ruoslahti. 1972a. α-Fetoprotein in normal and pregnancy sera. Lancet 1:375–376.

Seppälä, M., and E. Ruoslahti. 1972b. Alpha-fetoprotein in abortion. Brit. Med. J. 4:769–771.

Seppälä, M., and E. Ruoslahti. 1973a. Alpha-fetoprotein: Physiology and pathology during pregnancy and application to antenatal diagnosis. J. Perinat. Med. 1:104–113.

Seppälä, M., and E. Ruoslahti. 1973b. Alpha-fetoprotein in maternal serum: A new marker for detection of fetal distress and intrauterine death. Am. J. Obstet. Gynec. 115:48–52.

Seppälä, M., and E. Ruoslahti. 1973c. Alpha-fetoprotein in antenatal diagnosis. Lancet 1:155.

Seppälä, M., and E. Ruoslahti. 1973d. Alpha-fetoprotein in Rh-immunized pregnancies. Obstet. Gynec. 42:701–706.

Seppälä, M., and H. A. Unnerus. 1974. Elevated amniotic fluid alphafetoprotein in fetal hydrocephaly. Am. J. Obstet. Gynec. 119:270–272.

Slade, B. 1973. Antibodies to α-foetoprotein cause foetal mortality in rabbits. Nature 246:493.

Smith, C. 1973. Implications of Antenatal Diagnosis. In Antenatal Diagnosis of Genetic Disease, Emery, A. E. H. (Ed.). London, Churchill-Livingstone.

Smith, C. J., and P. C. Kelleher, 1973. α_1-Fetoprotein: Separation of two molecular variants by affinity chromatography with concanavallin A-agarose. Biochim. Biophys. Acta 317:231–235.

Smith, J. A. 1972. Alpha-fetoprotein: A possible factor necessary for normal development of the embryo. Lancet 1:851.

Stewart, A. G., and W. C. Taylor. 1964. Amniotic fluid analysis as an aid to the antepartum diagnosis of haemolytic disease. J. Obstet. Gynaec. Brit. Common. 71:604–608.

Stewart, C. R., A. M. Ward, and J. Lorber. 1975. Amniotic fluid alpha$_1$-fetoprotein in the diagnosis of neural tract malformations. Brit. J. Obstet. Gynaec. 82:257–261.

Sutcliffe, R. G., and D. J. H. Brock. 1973. Immunological studies on the nature and origin of the major proteins in amniotic fluid. J. Obstet. Gynaec. Brit. Comm. 80:721–727.

Sutcliffe, R. G., D. J. H. Brock, and J. B. Scrimgeour. 1972. Origin of amniotic fluid group-specific component. Nature 238:400.

Sutherland, G. R. 1975. Antenatal misdiagnosis of spina bifida. Lancet 2:280–281.

Sutherland, G. R., D. J. H. Brock, and J. B. Scrimgeour. 1973. Amniotic fluid macrophages and anencephaly. Lancet 2:1098.

Sutherland, G. R., D. J. H. Brock, and J. B. Scrimgeour. 1975. Amniotic fluid macrophages and the antenatal diagnosis of anencephaly and spina bifida. J. Med. Genet. 12:135–137.

Swartz, S. K., M. S. Soloff, and R. R. Suviano. 1974. A Comparison of the Estrogen Binding Activity of Rat and Human AFP. In L'Alpha-foeto-protéine, Masseyeff, R. (Ed.). Paris, Inserm.

Tatarinov, Y. S. 1964. Detection of embryo-specific alphaglobulin in the blood sera of patients with primary liver tumour. Vop. Med. Khim. 10:90–91.

Uriel, J., B. de Nechaud, and M. Dupiers. 1972. Estrogen-binding properties of rat, mouse and man fetospecific serum proteins. Demonstration by immuno-autoradiographic methods. Biochem. Biophys. Res. Commun. 46:1175–1180.

Usategui-Gomez, M. 1974. Immunoglobulins and Other Protein Constituents of Amniotic Fluid. In Amniotic Fluid, Physiology, Biochemistry and Clinical Chemistry, Natalson, S., A. Scommegna, and M. B. Epstein (Eds.). New York, Wiley.

Vince, J. D., T. J. McManus, M. Ferguson-Smith, and J. G. Ratcliffe. 1975. A semi-automated serum alphafetoprotein radioimmunoassay for prenatal spina bifida screening. Brit. J. Obstet. Gynaec. 82:718–727.

Wald, N. J. 1976. The Detection of Neural Tube Defects by Screening Maternal Blood. In Prenatal Diagnosis, Boue, A. (Ed.). Paris, Inserm.

Wald, N. J., S. Barker, H. Cuckle, D. J. H. Brock, and G. Stirratt. 1977. Maternal serum AFP and spontaneous abortion. Brit. Med. J., in press.

Wald, N. J., S. Barker, R. Peto, D. J. H. Brock, and J. Bonnar. 1975. Maternal serum α-fetoprotein levels in multiple pregnancy. Brit. Med. J. 1:651–652.

Wald, N. J., D. J. H. Brock, and J. Bonnar. 1974. Prenatal diagnosis of spina bifida by maternal serum alphafetoprotein measurement: A controlled study. Lancet 1:765–767.

Wald, N. J., and H. Cuckle. 1976. Routine testing for alphafetoprotein in amniotic fluid. Lancet 1:1292.

Waldmann, T. A., and K. R. McIntire. 1972. Serum alphafetoprotein levels in patients with ataxia-telangiectasia. Lancet 2:1112–1115.

Warkany, J. 1971. Congenital Malformations. Chicago, Year Book Medical Publishers.

Weinberg, A. G., A. Milunsky, and M. J. Harrod. 1975. Elevated amniotic fluid alphafetoprotein and duodenal atresia. Lancet 2:496.

Weiss, R. R., J. N. Macri, and C. Merskey, 1976. FDP in amniotic fluid as marker for neural tube defects. Lancet 1:304.

Weiss, R. R., J. N. Macri, N. Tejani, R. Tillitt, and L. I. Mann. 1974. Antenatal diagnosis and lung maturation in anencephaly. Obstet. Gynaec. 44:368–372.

Wisniewski, L., Z. Skrzydlewski, and J. Orciuch. 1974. Alphafetoprotein in amniotic fluid in early normal pregnancy and intra-uterine fetal death. Brit. Med. J. 3:742.

Wynne-Davies, R. 1975. Congenital vertebral anomalies: Aetiology and relationship to spina bifida cystica. J. Med. Genet. 12:280–288.

Yachnin, S. 1976. Demonstration of the inhibitory effect of human alphafetoprotein on in vitro transformation of human lymphocytes. Proc. Nat. Acad. Sci. U.S.A. 73:2857–2861.

2

The Association Between the HLA System and Disease*

Andrew McMichael
Hugh McDevitt

Division of Immunology, Department of Medicine, Stanford University School of Medicine, Stanford, California

*This work was supported in part by an NIH Grant AI 11313. Dr. McMichael is sponsored by a Medical Research Council Travelling Fellowship from the United Kingdom.

39

INTRODUCTION

The association between products of the human major histocompatibility complex (MHC), or HLA (*Human Leukocyte Antigen*) system, and diseases poses one of the most intriguing problems in human immunology. Approximately forty diseases have been shown to be associated with an increased frequency of particular alleles of this gene complex. This relationship between disease susceptibility and the HLA system may extend even further because, if the identifiable genes are merely marker genes, the demonstration of an association depends on the existence of linkage disequilibrium between the marker gene and the true susceptibility gene (McDevitt and Bodmer, 1974). The HLA system illustrates to an extraordinary degree the phenomena of genetic polymorphism and linkage disequilibrium. These characteristics may have no simple explanation, but the clear involvement of this system in the pathogenesis of so many varying maladies suggests that diseases themselves may have contributed to the present observed features of the system.

The functions of the MHC are not entirely understood. It was first demonstrated as a genetic system controlling expression of the major barrier to transplantation of tissues. That the MHC might have an identifiable physiologic function came first from studies by Lilly (1966, 1971), who showed that susceptibility to Gross virus leukemia in mice was genetically controlled and linked to the mouse MHC (H-2). Shortly thereafter came the surprising findings of McDevitt and Sela (1965) and later Benacerraf and coworkers (McDevitt and Benacerraf, 1969; Ellman et al., 1970) that the immune response to certain synthetic peptide antigens was under the control of single autosomal dominant genes that were not immunoglobulin structural genes and that mapped in the MHC (McDevitt et al., 1972). Subsequent work has shown that this genetic complex may control other aspects of the body's defense system, including cellular immune responses and the complement system (for a detailed discussion, see Katz and Benacerraf, 1976b).

In order to understand the mechanisms that might underlie the disease associations, it will be necessary to review in some detail the genetics of the MHC and functional studies in experimental animals, notably the mouse, as well as in man.

THE MHC IN THE MOUSE AND OTHER EXPERIMENTAL ANIMALS

The Regions

H-2K and D. The study of histocompatibility antigens developed in parallel with transplantation experiments. Several inbred

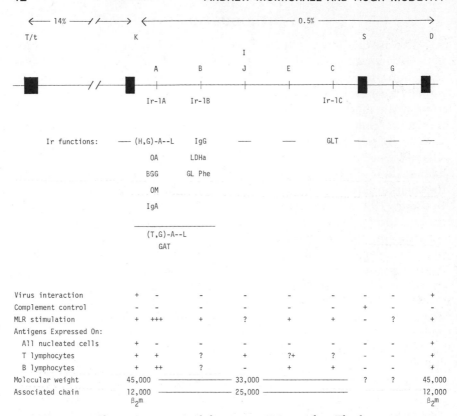

Figure 1. Chromosome map of the mouse *H-2* complex. The known properties of each component are indicated. Abbreviations: (T,G)-A--L: (Tyr,Glu)-Ala--Lys. (H,G)-A--L: (His-Glu)-Ala--Lys. OA: ovalbumin. BGG: bovine gamma globulin. OM: ovomucoid. IgG: mouse immunoglobulin G allotype. LDHa: lactic dehydrogenase. GL Phe: Glu-Lys-Phe. IgA: mouse immunoglobulin A allotype. GLT: glu-lys-tyr. GAT: glu-ala-tyr. β_2m: β_2 microglobulin.

mouse strains were developed in the early part of this century in order to transplant and propagate tumors. It was suggested by Haldane (1933) that failure of such transplants to grow in mouse strains other than the strain of origin was because of an immune reaction to alloantigens. This was later clearly demonstrated by Gorer (1937) and was shown to be true for transplantation of normal tissues also (Medawar, 1944). Following this discovery of a genetically controlled transplantation barrier, Snell (1948) set about a precise analysis by breeding congenic mouse strains that had single histocompatibility differences. These mice, together with the serological methods developed by Gorer's group (Gorer and O'Gorman, 1956), have made it possible, by cross-immunization, to raise antisera against different genetic regions of the mouse major histocompatibility (*H–2*) complex. In this way a very detailed dissection of this genetic region has been achieved (Fig. 1).

The mouse *H–2* complex is the major transplantation barrier; differences between donor and recipient for these antigens result in the most rapid rejection of a graft. Other histocompatibility systems exist, possibly as many as 500 (Snell, 1974); and it is likely that any cell surface protein, whether its primary function is structural, enzymatic, or a receptor, is potentially a transplantation antigen if it exists in polymorphic forms.

The nomenclature of *H–2* is derived from the early assumption that *H–2* was a single locus. Thus *H–2* types, actually haplotypes, are known by letters—e.g., BALB/c mice are *H–2^d*, C57 mice are *H–2^b*, C3H are *H–2^k*, and A strain mice are *H–2^a*. Subsequent study revealed that recombination between H–2 antigenic specificities occurred, indicating that *H–2* was actually more than one locus. In 1971, it was postulated by Klein and Shreffler (1971) that there were two loci controlling the H–2 antigens. An analysis of recombinant H–2 haplotypes supported this hypothesis. The two loci were designated *H–2K* and *H–2D*.

The *H–2K* and *D* loci are now known to be separated by a recombination distance of 0.5 percent. Their products are to some extent serologically cross-reactive, so that Klein and Shreffler (1971) postulated that they might have arisen by gene duplication. K and D products have a similar tissue distribution, being found on the surface of all nucleated cells so far examined. Their products are extremely polymorphic; 68 H–2 haplotypes are known in inbred mice. As these are derived from related breeding stock (Klein, 1975), the whole polymorphism in the species is probably extremely great. Studies of wild mouse populations indicate an enormous degree of polymorphism.

The *K* and *D* antigens have been shown to be glycoproteins of molecular weight 45,000 (reviewed by Nathenson and Cullen, 1974). They are found on the cell surface in close association with B$_2$ microglobulin, molecular weight 12,000, which has close sequence homology with an immunoglobulin heavy chain constant region domain*

---

*Immunoglobulins were shown by Gally and Edelman (1972) to be made up of repeating units on domains of approximately 110 amino acids, each containing an intrachain disulfide loop. Each domain shows some sequence homology and may thus have arisen by gene duplication from an ancestral single gene. Each variable region comprises one domain, the constant region of light chain is one domain, and the constant region of heavy chains includes three or four domains, depending on immunoglobulin class.

(Cunningham and Berggard, 1974). The H–2 molecule therefore appears to be expressed on the cell surface as a two chain monomer. Evidence from the human shows that β_2 microglobulin is not polymorphic, and that it is coded for by a gene on a different chromosome from the MHC (Jones et al., 1976). Some progress has been made in sequencing K and D antigens (Silver and Hood, 1976). There appears to be strong sequence homology between K and D, strongly supporting the idea of origin by gene duplication.

   Ia Antigens.   Although out of historical sequence, it is convenient to continue to describe serologically defined components of the *H–2* system. Interest in the region of *H–2* between *K* and *D* was provoked by the finding that genes controlling the immune response *(Ir* genes) to protein antigens mapped there at three distinct loci. It was then found that there were a series of cell surface antigens of restricted tissue distribution that also mapped between *K* and D (Hauptfeld et al., 1973; Sachs and Cone, 1973; David et al., 1973; Götze et al., 1973; Hämmerling et al., 1974). They mapped in the same region as the *Ir* loci *(Ir–1A, 1B, Ir–IC)* and were thus named *I* region-*a*ssociated, or *Ia* loci. Three loci were originally defined: *I–A*, *I–B*, and *I–C*, corresponding to *Ir–1A, Ir–1B,* and *Ir–1C*, the immune response gene loci (Fig. 1). They are expressed primarily on lymphocytes but are not present on all classes. The Ia–A and C antigens are most easily detected on B lymphocytes, which are the progenitors of antibody-forming cells. It is not certain whether they are present on T lymphocytes, which serve a regulatory function. Recently, new *I* regions have been found, *I–E* (Colombani et al., 1976) and *I–J* (Murphy et al., 1976; Tada et al., 1976). The latter is of great interest, because I–J determinants appear to be expressed only on a subpopulation of T lymphocytes, suppressor cells (Murphy et al., 1976; Tada et al., 1976). (For a detailed explanation of these lymphocyte subclasses, see pages 46 to 50.)

   An important experimental function of these antigens was found by Meo et al. (1973), Widmer et al. (1973), Lonai and McDevitt (1974b), and Fathman et al. (1974) to be to stimulate in the mixed lymphocyte reaction. When lymphocytes from two cell donors are mixed, both populations will undergo blastogenesis and synthesize DNA if they differ at the MHC (Bain et al., 1964; Bach and Hirschhorn, 1964). In mice the strongest stimulatory determinants were found to be antigens of the *I* region (Bach et al., 1972). The biological role of this phenomenon is not understood, but this reaction has had important applications in the study of the human equivalent of the *I* region (see pages 53 to 60).

   Chemical studies on the Ia antigens showed that they are glycoproteins of molecular weight 33,000 and 25,000 Daltons

(Schwartz and Cullen, 1976) and that the antigenic determinants are in the protein part of the molecule (Cullen et al., 1975). Recent work in the guinea pig, mouse (Schwartz et al., 1976), and human (Snary et al., 1977) has revealed that Ia antigens have a two-chain structure, 33,000 and 25,000. By analogy with studies on the human (Barnstable et al., 1977) it appears that only the 33,000 component, which carries the alloantigenic determinants, is genetically controlled by the MHC.

Early sequence data (Silver and Hood, 1976) and two-dimensional gel analysis (Jones, 1976) of Ia antigens in mice suggest that there is heterogeneity in Ia in the individual. This is not surprising if the *I* region is composed of 5 or more loci. However, because of the possibility that Ia antigens might, as the product of *Ir* genes, be the T cell antigen receptor, it is critical to know whether the Ia heterogeneity is large enough to account for the high degree of specificity shown by *Ir* genes (see pages 46 to 49). It is clear that the recombination distances in the mouse Ia region are large enough to contain several hundred genes.

The S Region.   An early finding in mouse *H–2* genetics was that there was a serum protein, a β-globulin called Ss, whose quantitative expression was linked to the *H–2* system. Later a sex linked protein, Slp, with allotypic* variants, was found. The *Ss–Slp* system mapped between *K* and *D* (Shreffler and David, 1972). The *I* region was later found to map between *K* and *Ss* (McDevitt et al., 1972).

Hinzova et al. (1972), Demant et al. (1973), and Capkova and Demant (1974) showed that the level of serum complement activity was linked to this *S* region of *H–2*, and Hansen et al. (1975) showed that Ss was probably a component of the complement system. It has now been shown that Ss is immunologically closely related to human C4 (Meo et al., 1975). Ss may thus be a structural gene for one of the three polypeptide chains of C4. An interesting speculation is that it might be the 33,000 molecular weight γ chain, and might therefore have been derived from *Ia* genes by duplication.

Population Genetics of the H–2 System.   It has already been indicated that the H–2 antigens are highly polymorphic cell surface proteins.

Analyses of wild mice have revealed some interesting findings. Mice live in demes of 7 to 12 mice controlled by a dominant male. Within a deme the *H–2* type is fairly homogeneous (Klein, 1975). A linked genetic system, the *T/t* system, has been found to play an important role in mouse population genetics. T/t mutants show several

---

*An allotype is a serologically defined genetically determined variant that is found within a species, in contrast to xenotypes which are variants between species.

fascinating features, descriptions of which are beyond the scope of this review (see Bennett, 1975, and Artzt and Bennett, 1975). Two phenomena of relevance are segregation distortion and crossover suppression between T/t (near the centromere) and H–2 (14 centimorgans further to the right) (Artzt and Bennett, 1975). As T/t mutants are very common in wild mouse populations, this may have a profound effect on forcing heterozygosity at *H–2* because the T/T and t/t genotypes are both lethal.

Functional Studies on the H–2 Complex

Immune Response (Ir) Genes. In 1965, McDevitt and Sela described an immune response gene that was an autosomal dominant which controlled the level of antibody response to a synthetic peptide antigen (T,G)–A--L. This peptide has sidechains of poly-D,L-*a*lanine on a poly-L-*ly*sine backbone, with amino termini of *ty*rosine and *g*lutamic acid. Subsequently, other *Ir* genes were found and were shown to be linked to *H–2* (McDevitt and Benacerraf, 1969; Benacerraf and McDevitt, 1972), and similar MHC linked *Ir* genes were found in guinea pigs (Ellman et al., 1970). Because *Ir* genes were not linked to immunoglobulin allotypes (heavy chain markers) they could not control immunoglobulin specificity. The *Ir* gene for (T,G)-A--L mapped between *H–2K* and *D* (McDevitt et al., 1972). Similar analyses for several other antigens under *Ir* gene control showed that they map in three distinct regions: *Ir–1A, Ir–1B,* and *Ir–1C* (Fig. 1). In order to understand the possible mechanisms by which *Ir* genes function, it is necessary to review briefly the sequence of events that follows challenge of an animal with a foreign protein antigen.

It has been shown that two basic lymphocyte types are involved in the antibody response (Claman et al., 1966; Miller and Mitchell, 1969; Mitchison, 1971a, b) (Fig. 2). One population, B (bone marrow derived) lymphocytes, recognizes "hapten" determinants on the immunogen, proliferates, matures to plasma cells, and secretes antibody. Each B cell is clonally restricted to the expression of a single immunoglobulin "species" (with a unique pair of variable regions) on its cell surface as an antigen receptor. Its progeny secrete the same antibody (Burnett, 1959). Triggering of a B cell to antibody production requires two signals (Bretscher and Cohn, 1970); one is provided by antigen binding to the receptor; the other is provided by T (thymus derived) lymphocytes. The latter signal, however, can be bypassed by the use of adjuvants (Strober, 1970) or injection of allogenic cells (Kreth and Williamson, 1971; Katz, 1972) and may be

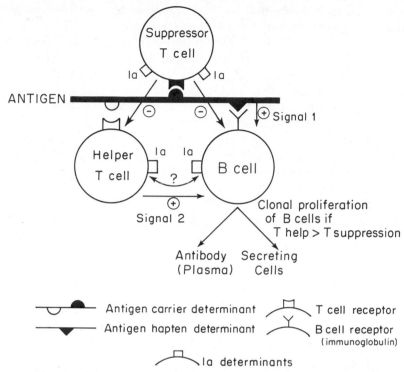

Figure 2. Schematic representation of the humoral immune response.

unnecessary when the antigen has multiple repeating units, as in some carbohydrate antigens (Basten and Howard, 1973). In an early antibody response, the antibody is of the IgM class and its production may be T cell independent in some cases. Later antibody is IgG, whose production is almost always T cell dependent and which gradually increases in affinity with time (Eisen and Siskind, 1964).

T cells are thymus processed lymphocytes. Helper T cells recognize a different set of (carrier) determinants on the antigen. The nature of the T cell receptor is controversial. Direct attempts to demonstrate surface immunoglobulin on T cells have given variable results (Vitetta et al., 1972; Marchialonis, 1974). Recently, however, Eichmann and Rajewsky (1975) and Wigzell and Binz (1976) have shown that helper T cells may express at least the variable part of immunoglobulin molecules on their surface. It is not clear whether T cells actually synthesize this immunoglobulin or acquire it from B cells. However, their findings suggest that immunoglobulin variable regions form at least part of the T cell receptor for antigen. The nature of the associated constant region is uncertain, but it must be assumed to be a heavy chain constant region because the coupling of V regions to C regions can occur only in the cis configuration (Hood, 1972).

Ir genes were shown (McDevitt and Benacerraf, 1969; Benacerraf and McDevitt, 1972) to be operative at the level of T cells, probably controlling antigen recognition, or interaction with B cells and macrophages, or both. Responsiveness is dominant, and *Ir* genes show considerable specificity. The *Ir* gene product could therefore be a T cell receptor (Benacerraf and McDevitt, 1972). However, the specificity presents considerable problems. *H–2* linked *Ir* genes can, for instance, distinguish between the ordered side chain sequences Glu-Glu-Tyr (G-G-T-) and Glu-Tyr-Tyr-Glu (G-T-T-G-) on the Ala-Lys (A--L) backbone of (T,G)-A--L (Seaver et al., 1976). At least 40 protein antigens have been shown to be under *Ir* gene control. It seems probable that all protein antigens will be found to be under *Ir* gene control, although for complex proteins the use of limiting antigen doses may be necessary to demonstrate this, possibly because they have multiple and varied carrier antigenic determinants (Vaz et al., 1971). Thus the *Ir* gene specificity repertoire may be as precise as that of immunoglobulin variable regions. It is not certain whether this degree of specificity is controlled by several hundred gene loci with multiple alleles at each, whether it represents interaction of two or more multi-allelic gene products, or whether there is somatic mutation of the *Ir* genes (as has been proposed for variable region genes) or somatic modification of products of *Ir* genes. Interaction of a relatively small number of *Ir* gene products with the T cell immunoglobulin variable regions would be one possible way of reconciling the data on the specificity of *Ir* genes, their possible receptor function, and the putative T cell immunoglobulin.

Recently it has been shown that the immune response to certain antigens is under the control of two *Ir* genes (Dorf et al., 1975; Melchers and Rajewsky, 1975; Munro and Taussig, 1975; Schwartz et al., 1976). These genes can be mapped in separate regions of the MHC, between *K* and *D*. Taussig and Munro in their experiments show that one is operative at the T cell level, the classic *Ir* gene for (T,G)-A–L, and the other is operative at the level of the B cell. These *Ir* genes therefore appear to control T cell–B cell interactions. Schwartz et al. (1976) have demonstrated that two *Ir* genes are required for T cell recognition of glu,lys,phe terpolymer, although this does require the presence of macrophages so that one or both genes could be expressed on that cell population. Benacerraf and Dorf (1976) have shown that interaction between *Ir* genes in the cis configuration is more efficient than in the trans situation. In addition, it appears that both genes must be expressed in interacting T and B cell populations (Katz and Benacerraf, 1976a, b). The situation is thus potentially complex; it is possible that as the *I* region of the *H–2* complex is dissected further (see below) and new regions are identified, more antigens under two *Ir* gene or multiple *Ir* gene control will be found.

The overall picture that is emerging, therefore, may be summarized as follows. *Ir* genes are dominantly expressed as a helper T cell function. In some instances two *Ir* genes are necessary for a particular immune response. The high degree of specificity demonstrable in *Ir* gene regulation of immune responsiveness strongly suggests that they may act either alone or in combination with immunoglobulin variable regions, as the T cell receptor.

Immune Suppression (Is) Genes. In recent months it has become apparent that immune suppression may also map in the *I* region of the *H–2* complex. The helper function of T cells in antibody responses has already been described. Gershon and Kondo (1971), Baker et al. (1974), and Herzenberg et al. (1975) initially demonstrated that specific suppression of immune responses was controlled by T cells. As suppressor T cells have been demonstrated in many varying types of experimental systems (Zembala and Asherson, 1973; Waldmann et al., 1974; Tada et al., 1976; McMichael and Sasazuki, 1977), it is now apparent that they are probably ubiquitous regulators of the immune response, acting in opposition to T helper (or amplifier) cells (Fig. 2).

Kapp et al. (1974) and Benacerraf and Dorf (1976) first showed that a specific immune suppression function mapped in the *I* region of *H–2*, i.e., an immune suppression (*Is*) gene. It has now been shown that suppressor T cells carry surface markers (Ia antigens) that map in the *I-J* region of the *H–2* (Murphy et al., 1976; Tada et al., 1976). The *I* region may thus control both antigen specific helper and suppressor T cell regulation of immune responses to a large number of antigens.

The relationship between *Ir* genes or *Is* genes and Ia antigens is unclear. *Ir* and *Is* genes are measured as a function in assays, in vivo or in vitro, which may involve several complex events. Ia antigens can be directly analyzed. It is possible therefore that Ia antigens are the *Ir* or *Is* gene products. It was suggested by Benacerraf and Mc-Devitt (1972) that the *Ir* gene product might be the T cell receptor, either alone or in conjunction with immunoglobulin variable regions. Although the heterogeneity of Ia antigens would be consistent with this hypothesis, the tissue distribution of I-A, B, and C antigens on B cells rather than T cells is not. It has been suggested, primarily by Katz and Benacerraf, that Ia antigens mediate B and T cells interac-

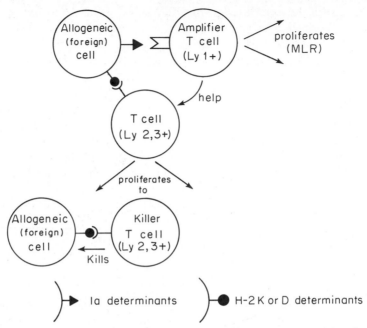

Figure 3. Schematic representation of the cellular immune response with generation of cytotoxic T cells. Ly-1,2,3 or non-MHC surface markers (Cantor and Boyse, 1975).

tion. Their series of experiments show that when T and B cells from different mouse strains are mixed, they will collaborate only if they are identical in the *I-A* and *I-B* region (Katz and Benacerraf, 1976a). A similar requirement has been shown for immune suppression (Tada et al., 1976). This is currently a field of much active research interest and controversy (Katz and Benacerraf, 1976b). As will be discussed in the following sections, the relationship between *Ia* and *Ir* is of some importance in predicting the mechanisms underlying HLA and disease associations.

    Cellular Immune Response.   A second type of immune response is the "cellular response" (Fig. 3). Antibody is not produced, and B cells appear not to be involved. In one type of response "killer" lymphocytes are generated, which can be shown to be a subset of T cells by non-MHC surface markers (Cantor and Boyse, 1975). In another type, lymphocytes mediating delayed hypersensitivity (DH) cells are generated (Miller et al., 1976). The effector cells are again a T cell subset. Generation of these effector T cells is probably dependent on amplifying or helper T cells. These immune responses also appear to be under control of the same kind of immune response genes as antibody responses (Schmitt-Verhulst and Shearer, 1975).

Killer T cells were first demonstrated to be active against transplanted histoincompatible tissue and could be demonstrated in an experimental system *in vitro*, the cell mediated lympholysis (CML) assay (Hayry and Defendi, 1970; Solliday and Bach, 1970; Lightbody et al., 1971). In these experiments two cell populations (one irradiated to prevent its proliferative response) are mixed, and after four days the sensitized responder cells can be shown to kill specifically ^{51}Cr labeled target cells of the sensitizing type. The initial recognition of foreignness in this mixed lymphocyte culture may reflect *I* region differences (Alter et al., 1973), but the targets in the killing assay are products of the *K* and *D* loci or closely linked genes (Eisjvoogel et al., 1973) (Fig. 3).

In an important series of experiments, Blanden et al. (1975) and Doherty and Zinkernagel (1975) have shown that virus infected mouse target cells can be killed by T cells of an infected animal. They further showed that T cells of infected mice of a different strain could kill the infected target cells, but only if the killer cells and target cells share *H–2K* or *D* regions (Fig. 4). Products of the *K* and *D* loci may therefore be directly involved in this kind of immune response, but the possibility that closely linked genes are involved remains.

In a parallel series of experiments, Shearer et al. (1975) have shown the *D* and *K* identity between sensitizing and target cells is also required for CML to occur when killer cells have been generated against chemically modified (by trinitrophenyl substitution) surface antigens. Similarly, Bevan (1975) has shown that killing directed against non-H–2 histocompatibility antigens also requires *H–2K* or *D* sharing between sensitizing and target cells.

Two hypotheses have been advanced to explain these findings (Fig. 4). One is that viruses or chemicals alter the H–2 antigens, and that these are recognized as foreign and the cell is killed—i.e., altered self (Zinkernagel and Doherty, 1974). This has been further expanded to suggest that the function of the *H–2K* and *D* recognition receptors is precisely to recognize altered self, either as virus or pathogen modification or, perhaps, by tumorigenesis (Burnett, 1973; Doherty and Zinkernagel, 1975).

The other hypothesis is that there is a dual recognition process, one set of receptors recognizing *K* or *D*, and other receptors recognizing the virus.

Most of the experimental evidence favors the dual receptor hypothesis (Zinkernagel and Doherty, 1977). There is no real evidence in favor of the extrapolation that this is the whole function of the *H–2K* and *D* system. Attempts have been made to provide a unifying hypo-

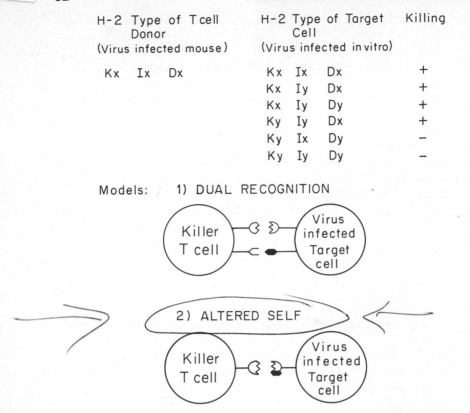

H-2 Type of T cell Donor (Virus infected mouse)			H-2 Type of Target Cell (Virus infected in vitro)			Killing
Kx	Ix	Dx	Kx	Ix	Dx	+
			Kx	Iy	Dx	+
			Kx	Iy	Dy	+
			Ky	Iy	Dx	+
			Ky	Ix	Dy	−
			Ky	Iy	Dy	−

Models: 1) DUAL RECOGNITION

2) ALTERED SELF

◆ Virus antigen   H-2 Self recognition molecules

Figure 4. The Blanden-Doherty-Zinkernagel experiments with the two alternative explanations: dual recognition and altered self.

thesis for the function of the whole MHC (e.g., Nabholz and Miggiano, 1976). They generally propose that alteration of cell surface antigenicity by viruses, bacteria, or foreign cells is the function of *H–2K* or *D*. Soluble antigen may modify Ia antigens, which are similarly recognized as foreign and stimulate helper or suppressor T cells. An extension of this hypothesis suggests that the *I* region products are glycosyl transferases and that antigen may be modified or recognized by these enzymes acting as receptors for sugar residues (Blanden et al., 1976).

Nonimmunological Functions of the MHC. A small amount of data suggests that the MHC might be involved in nonimmunological functions. Meruelo and Edidin (1975) showed that cyclic AMP levels in mouse livers were affected over a two-fold range by H–2 type. Linkage with H–2 was shown in breeding studies and by the use of congenic mice. There was some evidence that the levels were affected by two or more genes, mapping at both the K and D ends.

Ivanyi and coworkers (1972a, b) have shown that testosterone levels and testes weight are influenced by H–2 type. Both these experiments suggest that H–2 associated molecules may affect hormone binding with receptors. How these functions integrate with other MHC functions is not certain.

THE MHC IN MAN

The MHC in the mouse has been described in some detail because it has become apparent that all mammals and probably all vertebrates possess an equivalent system. The similarities between mouse and man will become apparent in the following section and they allow certain predictions to be made in analyzing the HLA system and in assessing the biological role of this genetic complex. It should be emphasized that the study of HLA antigens has proceeded in parallel with the mouse work, and in some notable instances major advances have occurred first in the human. For example, in 1971, Yunis and Amos showed that the mixed lymphocyte reaction (MLR) was controlled by a locus distinct from the human equivalent of K and D. In population studies, the occurrence of strong linkage disequilibrium and striking disease associations as first recognized in man.

The Regions

HLA–A, B, and C. Interest in histocompatibility antigens in humans was first aroused by early experience in therapeutic transplantation of kidneys. The serological methods developed in the mouse seemed appropriate to use, but extensive cross-immunization experiments could not be performed for ethical reasons. However, multiply transfused patients were shown to have antileukocyte antibodies (Dausset, 1954). Payne and Rolfs (1958) and van Rood et al. (1958) showed that during pregnancy mothers were frequently immunized against paternal HLA antigens, probably by transplacental passage of fetal lymphocytes. A pioneering group of laboratories therefore started extensive screening programs to find pregnancy

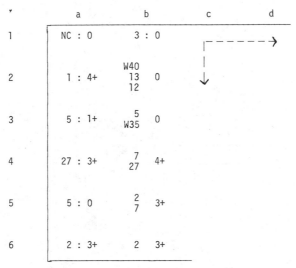

HLA SEROLOGICAL TYPING   CELL DONOR: HLA 1,2,27,8

Figure 5. HLA serological typing. Schematic representation of a tissue typing tray showing the results of the cell donor (HLA-1,2,7,8) after incubation with anti-HLA sera and complement. In each well is shown the specificity of the antisera and the degree of cytotoxicity: 0 <20%, 1+ <40%, 2+ <40%, 3+ <80%, and 4+ >80% killing. NC: normal control serum. Antisera a 1-6 and b6 are monospecific; b 2-5 are poly-specific. In a normal typing approximately 80 sera are tested.

sera of restricted specificity and with high cytotoxic titers. They exchanged sera and methods in a unique series of international workshops and in 12 years developed a sophisticated and highly reproducible method of HLA typing. Peripheral blood lymphocytes are separated from the donor's blood and tested in microtiter trays with a panel of antisera. There are normally 4 to 5 antisera representing each specificity. After incubation and addition of complement, the dead cells are counted for each well. The checkerboard pattern of re-actions can then be analyzed to assign HLA type (Fig. 5). Typing by this method has progressed to the point at which in many labora-tories it is routine procedure offered as a clinical service.

In the early work, two allelic series of antigens were clearly defined, the LA system of Payne et al. (1964) and the Four series of van Rood (1962). In 1967, Bodmer et al. proposed that the two series were controlled by different genetic loci, and this distinction was confirmed by the findings of the 1967 Histocompatibility Testing Workshop (Cepellini et al., 1967). All subsequent data have been in agreement with this theory, and a recombination distance of 0.8 to 1.0 percent between A and B has been found (Biijnen et al., 1976). Some confusion has been aroused by the changing terminology in this field, but the present terms are permanent. The first locus defined, *LA*, is now *A*, and the second, *Four,* is *B* (WHO–IUIS Terminology Committee, 1975) (Fig. 6).

Multiple alleles have been found at each locus, and further subdivision of some antigens, which are probably cross-reacting groups, is to be expected. This applies particularly to those antigens with a provisional "w" (Workshop) designation. In 1975 a third locus, *C,* was clearly defined (Bodmer, 1975). This followed observations by several laboratories (van Rood and Eernisse, 1968; Walford et al., 1969; Dausset et al., 1969; Thorsby, 1974) of antigens that seemed to be distinct from the recognized *A* and *B* series. *A* and *B* are thought to be direct analogues of the mouse *D* and *K* loci; no mouse equivalent for *C* is known. Very recent work by Goodfellow and Payne (1976) suggests that in Japanese this *C* locus can be split into two. Thus whereas Cw1 and Cw3 behave as alleles in Caucasians, they are inherited as a haplotype (Payne et al., 1975) in Asians. The inference of these data is that the *C* locus has duplicated into two loci in Japanese, at least.

Chemical analysis has shown that A, B, and C antigens are glycoproteins of 45,000 molecular weight, are associated with B_2 microglobulin, and show sequence homology (Terhorst et al., 1976; Bridgen et al., 1976; Snary et al., 1977).

The D Region. In 1971, Yunis and Amos showed in a recombinant family that the mixed lymphocyte reaction (the proliferative response of lymphocytes of two individuals when mixed in vitro) was controlled by a locus distinct from A and B. Previously, it had been thought that the reaction reflected differences in A and B antigens. This finding, essentially that occasionally A–B identical siblings react in the MLR, has been repeatedly confirmed. The *D* locus has been mapped outside *A* and *B*, closer to *B* at a recombination distance of 1 per cent. It is probable that this locus *(D)* is the strongest MLR locus and that others exist. A second weak MLR locus in the MHC has been proposed (Thorsby, 1974), and others outside the MHC probably exist.

Because of the extreme rarity of finding two unrelated individuals mutually nonstimulatory in the MLR, a method for studying polymorphism in this system was sought. Bradley et al. (1973) and Mempel et al. (1973) proposed a method of doing this. It is possible to *make* the MLR a one-way reaction by irradiation, or treating with mitomycin, one lymphocyte population. These lymphocytes are then

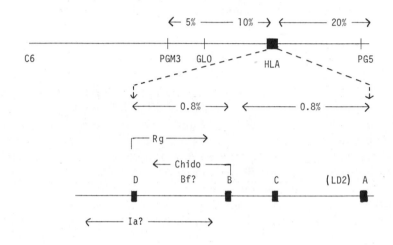

Disease Association	++	++	+	+
MLR Stimulation	++	-	-	+ -
Antigens expressed on:				
All nucleated cells	-	+	+	+
T lymphocytes	?-	+	+	+
B lymphocytes	+	+	+	+
Molecular weight	33,000	45,000	45,000	45,000
Associated chain	25,000	12,000	12,000	12,000
		(β_2m)	(β_2m)	(β_2m)

Figure 6. Chromosome map of the HLA complex. The known properties of each component are listed. GLO: red cell glyoxylase. PGM3: phosphoglucomutase 3. Rg: Rodgers blood group 1. Chido: Chido blood group. Bf: properdin factor B.

HOMOZYGOUS STIMULATING CELLS (IRRADIATED)

RESPONDING CELLS (UNIRRADIATED)	Dw1	Dw1	Dw2	Dw2 - - - - - - -> Dw6		Heterozygous 1	2	Controls 3	No added cells
1 (Dw2/-)	62	49	3	7	40	96	52	37	1
2 (Dw1/Dw6)	4	11	47	75	6	81	47	49	3
3 -/-	94	71	49	84	78	67	71	55	5

Figure 7. Typing by the MLR reaction. This illustration shows the results of a typing experiment. The figures shown are the mean (of triplicates) thymidine incorporation as counts per minute $\times 10^{-3}$ for each combination. Various ways exist for handling the data (see Thorsby and Piazza, 1975), but in this instance it is clear that counts of less than 10×10^3 represent nonstimulation ("typing responses").

unable to proliferate, and any reaction, usually measured by incorporation of ^{3}H thymidine into DNA, is due to the nonirradiated cell population. Because of the phenomenon of self-tolerance, an individual's cells will not respond in the MLR to cells that share his MLR (D locus) type either as an identical heterozygote or, if homozygous, for one of his D types. Therefore, by the use of cells from $HLA–D$ homozygous persons, it is possible to type for D specificities (Fig. 7).

Interest in this laborious method of defining an HLA locus was greatly provoked by the finding (Meo et al., 1973; Widmer et al., 1973; Fathman et al., 1974; Lonai and McDevitt, 1974b) that in the mouse the MLR was also predominantly controlled by one locus ($I–A$) and that it mapped in the I region. The theoretical possibility that study of the human D locus might yield information about human Ir genes was immediately recognized by all workers in this field.

Several laboratories therefore searched for families with members homozygous for $HLA–D$ determinants, and submitted these cells in a series of international exchanges culminating in the VIth International Histocompatibility Workshop (Thorsby and Piazza, 1975). Homozygotes either were identified as the $HLA–A$ and B homozygous offspring of cousin or incest matings, or were sought in outbred families, usually among A and B homozygotes, on the assumption that there would be linkage disequilibrium between alleles of the B and D loci. In both instances, MLRs were carried out within the families to prove homozygosity. An $HLA–D$ homozygote should stimulate neither parent, no offspring, and no sibling who shares an HLA haplotype.

Fifteen laboratories typed a panel of random responders with the available MLR typing cells, and the results were analyzed at the VIth International Histocompatibility Testing Workshop.

Based on cluster analyses six specificities were clearly identified in Caucasians, Dw1–6. Two additional provisional specificities were less clearly defined and were given the provisional designations *HLA–D* LD 107 and 108 (see Table 1) (Thorsby and Piazza, 1975). These eight specificities probably represent about 50 percent of the *D* locus genome in Caucasians. Since the workshop, several new types have been found. In our laboratory, we have clearly identified two new specificities primarily found in Japanese (Sasazuki et al., 1976a) and one type, provisionally labeled LD–MA, which is rare in Caucasians but is in strong linkage disequilibrium with Bw17. These findings have been confirmed by other workers (Sasazuki et al., 1976; Terasaki and Opelz, 1976; Grosse-Wilde, 1976). Other laboratories also have similar new specificities. These will be analyzed at the VIIth Histocompatibility Workshop in 1977, and it is therefore probable that more of the *D* genome will be accounted for.

This method, however, will always remain cumbersome, especially because of the need to find and repeatedly bleed homozygotes. Although it is easy to transform human peripheral blood B lymphocytes into B cell lines, these do not seem to work well for MLR typing and give apparently discrepant results (Gatti et al., 1976). Sheehy et al. (1975) have developed an alternative method whereby one population of cells is mixed with a stimulating cell, the reaction is allowed to go beyond the peak of the MLR, and the responder is rechallenged with the cells to be typed. If these stimulator cells share a *D* specificity with the initial stimulator cells, there is greater stimulation than if they do not. This typing method obviates the need for homozygous cells and is currently under assessment in several laboratories.

Methods of *D* locus typing that depend on the MLR beg questions about the reaction itself. Its biological meaning is unknown, and anomalous reactions are fairly frequent. It is not certain whether the types so far defined represent the products of a single *D* locus or a cluster of loci—i.e., the *D* region. Serological analysis could answer this question.

Based on the finding in the mouse that MLC stimulating determinants mapped in the Ia region of the MHC, and that most Ia antigens are predominantly expressed on B lymphocytes, human alloantigens have been sought using B lymphocytes or B cell lines as target cells in the cytotoxicity test.

Transformed B cell lines seem to express alloantigens on the surface normally. They have been used extensively by Bodmer's group to screen pregnancy sera for anti-B cell activity. These sera may then be tested against B cells from panels of donors. Peripheral blood lymphocytes are only 10 to 25 percent B cells and must be purified prior to testing. This presents problems, but a method of removing T cells based on the phenomenon that they bind to sheep red blood cells is widely used and seems adequate.

Based on these methods, several groups are defining series of antigenic specificities that are apparently allelic (van Rood et al., 1975; Ting et al., 1976; Barnstable et al., 1976; Winchester et al., 1976; Mann et al., 1976). The series described by Ting et al. appear to define two loci. Some correlation between the MLR defined *D* specificities exists (e.g., Barnstable et al., 1976). It is therefore possible that the antigens are those that provoke the MLR. Alternatively, they may simply be in linkage disequilibrium.

An exciting experiment is now in progress for the VIIth International Histocompatibility Workshop. In approximately twenty laboratories, panels of 50 to 60 blood donors are being typed by standardized homozygous typing cells in the MLR, and their B cells are being typed serologically. This should greatly clarify the relationship between the *D* specificities defined by the two methods. It is possible that new loci in the *D* region will be found if the *D* region is the equivalent of the mouse *I* region.

The chemistry of human B cell alloantigens is relatively far advanced. Snary et al. (1977) have shown that there are two polypeptide chain structures of 33,000 and 25,000 molecular weight. The latter chain is controlled by a separate chromosome from the rest of the MHC and appears to show no polymorphism (Barnstable et al., 1976). The structure is thus analogous to Ia in guinea pigs (Schwartz and Cullen 1976) and that proposed in mice. This finding, together with the tissue distribution of the antigens and the fact that allogeneic and xenogeneic anti-Ia sera block the MLR, justifies the use of the term "Ia" for the human B cell alloantigens.

Complement Genes. Detailed studies have been made of the human complement system and are reviewed elsewhere (e.g., Müller-Eberhard, 1975). Complement is an essential part of the body's defense mechanism, acting in conjunction with the immune system. Some classes of immunoglobulins bind complement, as do subpopulations of lymphocytes. Complement components are thus brought into contact with foreign materials. They appear to be particularly active in lysing cell membranes—e.g., bacteria, allogeneic or xenogeneic cells. They also bind to immune antibody-antigenic complexes and may then be harmful. The complement system consists of a series of enzymes and substrates that react in an ordered sequence of reactions. This cascade may be activated by two pathways; the classic one involving components C1, C4, and C2, and the alternative pathway through properdin factor B (also known as Bf, and glycine rich glycopeptide, GBG). The two pathways both act on C3 and share a common sequence from there on.

As has been already described, the mouse *H–2* type influences C3 levels (Ferreira and Nussenzweig, 1975) and Ss may be part of C4. In man it was shown by Allen (1974) that properdin factor B (Bf, GBG) was linked to the *HLA* system. Electrophoretic variants are known; and although linked to HLA, the exact map position of Bf is uncertain. It has also been shown that C2 deficiency is *HLA* linked (Fu et al., 1974; Friend et al., 1975) and that C4 levels are *HLA* linked (Rittner et al., 1975b). C1 was not linked (Day et al., 1975).

Taking the mouse and human data together, it is clear that the MHC genetically controls the complement system and that this control is exerted on the components involved in the early cell binding phase of the complement cascade. The common feature of cell recognition of these and other MHC components is apparent, as is the common function of defense against pathogens.

Genetics of the HLA System. GENETIC MAPPING. Four regions of the human *HLA* system are therefore defined and may have equivalents in the mouse: *A* and *B* equivalent to *D* and *K* respectively, the human *D* locus region equivalent to the mouse *I* region, and the possible equivalence of the complement controlling genes with the mouse *S* region. The human *C* locus, however, seems to have no mouse equivalent. The map data are shown in Figure 6. *A* and *B* are separated by a recombination distance of 0.8 percent. *HLA–D* maps outside *A* and *B* (Yunis and Amos, 1971) and is closer to *B* with a recombination frequency of 1 percent (Thorsby, 1974). *HLA–C* maps between *A* and *D* and is closer to *B* (Löw et al., 1974). Human Ia specificities have not been mapped, although they are assumed to be close to *D*. Ting et al. (1976) have evidence that there are two loci controlling *B* cell alloantigens.

The positions of the complement controlling loci are also not well defined. Bf maps between *A* and *D* and probably between *B* and *D* (Rittner et al., 1975a; Olaisen et al., 1975; Lamm et al., 1976; Biijnen et al., 1976). The positions of C2 and C4 are less certain.

The *HLA* complex is on chromosome 6. This was demonstrated by Lamm et al. (1974), who showed that a chromosome 6 pericentric inversion segregated in a family with *HLA* haplotype. Jongsma et al. (1973), van Someren et al. (1974), and Jones et al. (1976) have also shown that in human–hamster cell or human–mouse cell hybrids the expression of HLA antigens is controlled by chromosome 6. This expression also requires β_2 microglobulin, controlled by chromosome 15 (Jones et al., 1976). The position of the centromere is uncertain.

Some other human genetic markers map on chromosome 6. These are the blood groups Chido (Ch[a]), Rodgers (Rg[a]), PGM3, white cell enzyme phosphoglucomatose-3, and red cell glyoxylase. Recombination data show their map positions as in Figure 6 (Biijnen et al., 1976). Negative linkage results have been found for several other markers, including ABO blood groups and immunoglobulin allotypes.

Balner has reported a series of studies on the rhesus monkey with some interesting findings that may be relevant to the human MHC (Roger et al., 1976). The relative positions of the "A", "B", and "D" loci are the same as in humans. Recombination data provisionally map Bf, two Ia loci, and two Ir loci, as shown in Figure 8. The positions of the Bf and one of the Ia loci to the right of "A" are unexpected and do not coincide with the available human data. Confirmation of these results must await the finding of more recombinant families and further characterization of the Ia specificities.

Map data in the mouse are well established (Figs. 1 and 8). It is interesting that the mouse MLR stimulating locus is between K and D, whereas the human D locus is outside A and B. This implies that there has been an inversion in the mouse or human ancestor, or that the H–2 HLA pairs I–D, K–B, and D–A are not really homologous.

MHC map data in other species are less complete. In guinea pigs the I region was defined first and a serological search for A and

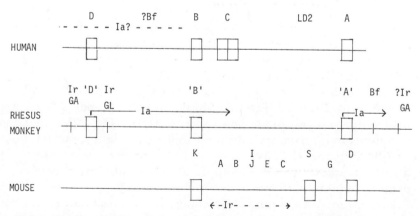

Figure 8. Comparison of the chromosome maps of the MHCs of the mouse, rhesus monkey, and man.

B followed. In the dog the *D* locus equivalent appears to map outside the *A–B* equivalents (van den Tweel et al., 1974).

POLYMORPHISM. The MHC's of all animals studied are highly polymorphic. The human is the best studied outbred population and shows polymorphism at all loci studied. Table 1 shows the identified alleles at the *A*, *B*, *C*, and *D* loci and the gene frequencies. The two loci, *C* and *D*, with the highest "blank" gene frequencies have only recently been defined, and it is anticipated that the presently defined alleles are the common ones, that they may be split, and that many rare alleles will shortly be found. Based on the present data in Caucasians, over 12,000 haplotypes are possible.

Table 1 also shows that there are striking racial differences in antigen frequencies. Certain antigens are thus completely absent in certain populations but common in others; e.g., *HLA–B8* is common in Caucasians and rare in other populations.

The degree of HLA polymorphism in the whole human species is therefore extreme and exceeds any other genetic system so far studied, with the special exception of immunoglobulin variable regions.

LINKAGE DISEQUILIBRIUM. Striking linkage disequilibria are observed for pairs of *HLA* alleles in all populations investigated. As an example, *HLA–A1* and *B8*, with respective gene frequencies of 0.14 and 0.1, should occur together at frequency of 0.014 but actually occur at a frequency of 0.064. This gives a Δ value of 0.05 (i.e., 0.064 − 0.014). As the maximum possible Δ value is 0.10 (the frequency of *HLA8*) minus 0.014:0.086, this represents very significant disequilibrium. In fact, for this haplotype the linkage disequilibrium extends into the *D* region: HLA–A1–B8–Dw3 occurs with a frequency of 0.024 compared to the expected frequency of 0.001.

The most significant Δ values are shown in Table 2. Differences in racial groups are shown where data are available. It is clear that in addition to different gene frequencies in different populations, different linkage disequilibria occur.

How Equivalent Are the Mouse and Human MHC's? Before proceeding to discuss functional studies on the human MHC, it is worth comparing the human and mouse MHC (Fig. 8). Functional experiments in humans are extremely difficult, and there is a tendency to clarify confusing data by reference to the mouse system. Thus, for instance, diseases associated with the *D* locus antigen are commonly explained as being due to specific immune response genes.

There is obvious chemical homology between D and K antigens in the mouse and human A and B antigens. They have the same molecular weight, and sequence data show strong homology (Silver and Hood, 1976). Similarly, human and mouse Ia antigens seem similar

Table 1.   Polymorphism of the HLA System: Percent Antigen Frequencies in 3 Racial Groups[*]

Locus	Specificity	European Caucasians	African Blacks	Japanese
A	1	29	9	2
	W36	0	5	0
	2	39	23	54
	28	12	23	2
	3	26	9	2
	11	18	21	21
	9[†]	17	15	54
	10[†]	7	10	9
	W43	0	5	0
	W19	23	50	13
B	5	7	3	24
	W35	16	6	19
	HR	< 1	4	0
	B18	9	10	0
	7	23	24	10
	W42	0	3	0
	W22	6	0	10
	W22J	0	0	4.5
	8	25	8	0
	12	23	13	10
	TT	3	4	2
	13	4	4	3
	W40	10	3	20
	W41	1	1	0
	14	6	8	0
	W15	9	2	13
	W16[†]	5	2	7
	W17	13	32	3
	W21	3	2	0
	27	6	1	1
	W37	2	0	2
C	W1	5	0	32
	W2	6	16	< 1
	W4	11	21	4
	W5	10	1	< 1
D	W1	19	nt	24[§]
	W2	15	nt	8[§]
	W3	16	nt	0[§]
	W4	16	nt	15[§]
	W5	15	nt	nt
	W6	10	nt	nt
	LD107	10	nt	nt
	LD108	8	nt	nt
	LD MA[‡]	5	nt	nt
	LD HO[§]	0	nt	17
	LD YT[§]	0	nt	19

[*] Modified from Bodmer, 1975, and Thorsby and Piazza, 1975.
[†] These specificities are now split.
[‡] Unpublished data from this laboratory.
[§] Sasazuki et al., 1977a.

Table 2. Linkage Disequilibria in the HLA System in
Caucasians and Japanese[*]

	A	B	C	D	Percentage Haplotype Frequency	Δ
Caucasians:	1	8			6.7	0.05
	3	7			4.0	0.03
	W29	12			2.5	0.02
		27	W1		1.2	0.01
		27	W2		2.1	0.02
		W40	W3		4.0	0.04
		W15	W3		4.2	0.04
		W35	W4		8.0	0.07
		B12	W5		6.3	0.05
		W35		W1	3.0	0.02
		B7		W2	4.1	0.03
		B8		W3	5.5	0.04
		W15		W4	2.0	0.02
		W16		W5	1.5	0.01
		W16		W6	0.8	0.01
Japanese	2	W40			10.6	0.04
	11	W22			2.3	0.02
	W19.6	12			4.5	0.03
	10	W10			7.3	0.04
		W22	Cw1		5.0	0.04
		W40	Cw3		7.9	0.04
		W15	Cw3		4.8	0.03
		W35	Cw3		5.1	0.03
		W15	Cw4		2.1	0.02
		Bw35		LD HO	12.3	0.05
		Bw22J		LD YT	9.0	0.05

[*]Data derived from Joint Report Histocompatibility Testing, 1970, 1972, and 1975. Caucasian A-B linkage disequilibria are shown only when present in the majority of European Caucasian populations. The Japanese data are derived from American Japanese populations, except for B-C associations, Joint Report, 1972, 1975, Sasazuki et al., 1977a.

Linkage disequilibrium (Δ) is calculated from the formula $\Delta = (p\,AB) - (pA \times pB)$ where p AB, pA, pB are the observed haplotype or gene frequencies of haplotype AB and genes A, B, respectively. Only Δ values greater than 0.01 are recorded.

chemically and appear to function similarly in the MLR. There are differences, however, particularly in regard to chromosomal mapping.

Hood (personal communication) has pointed out, however, that A is more analogous to B and D to K than either A is to D or B to K. Although based on limited sequence data, this has important implications. It may mean that the A–B and D–K duplications occurred relatively recently and independently in the ancestors of the two species. If this is true, the exactness of homology between mouse and man may not be very great. There is some evidence for this. The human D locus maps outside A and B, whereas Ia maps between D and K. The mouse has no C region as yet defined, which may mean that C represents an extra duplication of the A–B series. Furthermore, the evidence for two C loci found in Japanese and not in Caucasians by Goodfellow and Payne (1976) could mean that there are different amounts of duplication within a species.* Although very preliminary, the map data for complement components in man, and Ia antigens and Ir genes in rhesus monkeys, suggest that there may be further dissimilarities.

Other explanations exist. Marsh (1977) has suggested that the true equivalents of A and B might be K and D respectively. The weak MLR stimulating locus between A and B would thus be equivalent to the I region. Ir genes would be expected to map close to A, and a mouse equivalent of D to the right of H–$2D$ would thus be predicted.

Barnstable et al. (1977) have proposed that the sequence data may be explained by there having been selection for likeness between A and B and D and K, respectively.

Overall the similarity between the two systems is such that similar functions must be expected. The role in control of the complement system is already apparent in both species. The data concerning other functions will now be discussed.

Functional Studies on the HLA System

Ir genes have not been clearly defined in humans. Levine et al. (1972) published a small number of family pedigrees indicating that ragweed hypersensitivity to ragweed allergen E was linked to an HLA haplotype. This was apparently confirmed by Blumenthal et al. (1974), who estimated a recombination distance of 20 units between the Ir gene and the HLA–B locus. These papers have been criticized by Bias and Marsh (1975), who pointed out the methodological pitfalls in their studies and who have also reported a failure to confirm

---

*There is at least one precedent for differing degrees of duplication in different mammals. Immunoglobulin λ chains represent varying proportions of the light chain components of immunoglobulins in different species; in mice the λ chain is found on less than 5 percent of immunoglobulin, and appears to have a single linked associated variable region. In man, λ gene products are found on 40 percent of immunoglobulin molecules and probably are associated with multiple variable region gene products. The degree of duplication in the Vλ genes therefore appears to be quite different in the two species.

the haplotype association in a much larger series of families. Marsh et al. (1974) have shown that the serum IgE level may be under the control of an autosomal recessive gene, and it is possible that the pedigrees of Levine and Blumenthal may have reflected segregation of this gene. Marsh et al. (1974) proposed that high serum IgE levels may convert low responders into hypersensitivity patients by an unknown mechanism, and that a search for *Ir* genes for allergens is only permissible in individuals with a low IgE phenotype. Marsh (1976) has shown that sensitivity to the grass allergens Ra5 (ragweed) and rye 1 are associated with possession of *HLA–B7* and *B8*, respectively. Family studies have recently been performed, but no clear segregation of immune responsiveness with HLA haplotype could be demonstrated (Black et al., 1976).

In another study, Marsh (1976) has shown that sensitivity to the ragweed antigen Ra3 in persons with the low IgE phenotype is associated with the *A* locus antigen A2. Therefore, although family studies have not been decisive, the immune response to various grass antigens is associated with particular *HLA* types. This could indicate that these responses are controlled by *Ir* genes, although other explanations, such as *HLA* associated variation in absorption of the allergens through the nasal mucosa, are possible. Marsh has proposed that there are two *Ir* gene loci, one close to *B* and one close to *A*.

Other evidence for an association between immune response and HLA comes from Greenberg et al. (1975), who showed that the T cell proliferative response to streptococcal antigens was associated with *HLA–B5* in Caucasians and American Indians. This assay probably measures T cell recognition of antigens and is therefore appropriate for study of immune response genes (Shevach et al., 1972; Lonai and McDevitt, 1974a). A criticism of Greenberg's study, however, is that distinction between high and low responsiveness for an individual is somewhat arbitrary, but the association seems valid, and is with a *B* locus antigen. This study does, however, depend on environmental exposure, and the *HLA–B* association could reflect susceptibility to repeated streptococcal infection and thus hyperimmunization.

Spencer et al. (1976) showed that after immunization with live influenza virus, individuals with HLA-Bw16 had a lower antibody titer than individuals with other *HLA* types. Again, this could reflect an *HLA* association with infectivity. The authors attempted to explain the results by a dominant *Ir* gene determining responsiveness so that antibody and cell mediated immunity would block viral replication before sufficient virus had been produced to give a strong antigenic stimulus.

Definitive demonstration of human *Ir* genes will probably come only from studies involving deliberate immunization with new antigens. Ethical restrictions limit this approach to very cautious protocols. Scher et al. (1975) immunized 60 volunteers with the synthetic peptide (Glu, Lys, Tyr) (GLT) known to be under *Ir* gene control in guinea pigs and mice. Responsiveness was measured by antibody levels, by antigen stimulated T cell proliferation in vitro, and by skin testing. No association with *HLA* could be demonstrated. However, as this would be apparent only if linkage disequilibrium existed, family studies would now be appropriate.

We have undertaken a study of the human immune response to a series of protein antigens in families. A single immunization only was given and the antigen stimulated T cell proliferative response measured. The first antigen studied, diphtheria toxoid, revealed a significant proportion of low responders. Responsiveness in this assay, however, could not be linked to *HLA*, and examples were found of *HLA–A–B–D* identical siblings differing in their responsiveness (McMichael et al., 1977a). In a second study the response to purified influenza hemagglutinin was measured in the same way. Polymorphism in the response was found, but again no clear *HLA* linkage was demonstrated (McMichael et al., 1977b). In a preliminary study 14 randomly chosen unrelated volunteers have been immunized with 100 μg (T,G)–A--L 1383 in saline. No responders were found in the proliferative assay in vitro, suggesting that the restrictions on the use of the synthetic antigens (limited dose, no adjuvant, and a single injection) may be too limiting, or that responsiveness is a rare phenotype.

An unusual approach has been tried by Taussig and Cepellini (1976). Taussig and Munro (1975) have shown that a T cell soluble factor can be generated by incubation of mouse T lymphocytes with (T, G)–A--L or (Phe,G)-A--L. This factor can replace T cells, when mixed with mouse B cells in vivo, and generate an antibody response to (T,G)–A--L. In mice the ability to generate and to accept this factor seems to be controlled by *I* region genes. Some human lymphocytes can absorb out this activity, and the polymorphism in preliminary experiments was linked to the *HLA* system.

However human *Ir* genes are defined, their map position will be critical to an understanding of the *HLA* and disease associations. Some possible evidence on the map position comes from studies in the rhesus monkey by Roger et al. (1976). Two *Ir* genes were identified in several monkey families (Fig. 8). In two families there were apparent recombinants, although these have not been progeny tested yet. The *Ir* and *Ia* genes appeared to map in both the *D* region and the A region. One *Ir* gene mapped between *D* and *B*, the other outside the *A–D* region. There is thus some evidence that there may be two *Ia* and *Ir* regions in primates. This would be consistent with the finding of Marsh (1976) of an *HLA–A* and *B* region association with ragweed allergy. Further support comes from some human families, where there is stimulation in the MLR mapping close to the *HLA–A* locus (Thorsby, 1974). This led Marsh (1976) to propose that *HLA–A* and *H–2K* are homologous instead of the usually accepted pairing of *HLA–B* and *H–2K*.

Information concerning other functions of the human *I* region is scanty. *Ir* genes have been proposed to explain the specific lack of responsiveness sometimes found in mixed lymphocyte reactions. This would be easily testable because nonresponsiveness to a particular homozygous typing cell should be recessive, in contrast to the codominant expression of a *D* locus specificity. This has not been reported.

No data have been presented on *I* region control of suppressor T cells in humans. Similarly, no reports of *HLA* associated control of cellular cytotoxicity to virus or chemically modified lymphocytes are known to these authors.

Finally, no studies on the effect of HLA on hormone function are known. It has, however, been reported that chlorpromazine could specifically block absorption of anti-*HLA–A1* activity in typing sera by *HLA–A1* positive cells, suggesting that the drug binds to this *HLA* molecule (Smeraldi and Scorza-Smeraldi, 1976).

MHC AND DISEASE ASSOCIATIONS

Animal Studies

In mice susceptibility to Gross and Friend virus leukemogenesis was found to be linked to the *H–2* system (Lilly, 1966, 1971). Thus *H–2K* mice were susceptible to Gross virus (Gv) leukemia. Resistance was found to be dominant, and this gene, *Rgv–1*, may function as an *Ir* gene controlling the immune response to a leukemia antigen. Gv leukemia is also under the control of at least one other gene, *Rgv–2*, which segregates independently of *H–2* (Lilly, 1971).

Friend virus leukemogenesis is also *H–2* linked. Again, more than one gene is probably operative (Lilly, 1970). It is interesting that susceptibility maps to the *D* end of the *H–2* complex and is thus unlikely to be under *Ir* gene control. Recently Meruelo and McDevitt (1976) have shown that susceptibility to radiation virus leukemia is also *H–2* linked, and again this maps to the *D* end of *H–2*.

In another study, Vladitiu and Rose (1971) showed that autoimmune thyroiditis in mice could be induced by immunization with thyroglobulin in Freund's complete adjuvant. Susceptibility to the thyroiditis was *H-2* linked and appeared to be due to the direct effect of an *Ir* gene.

Also in mice, Oldstone et al. (1973) showed that susceptibility to the naturally occurring disease lymphocytic choriomeningitis was controlled by an *Ir* gene. In this instance, the disease has an autoimmune component such that T cell mediated immunity to the virus under *Ir* control leads to tissue damage which is harmful to the host.

Human Studies

In man, the detailed knowledge of naturally occurring disease is much more extensive. In the past, correlations of disease with other genetic systems have previously been sought, particularly ABO and MN blood groups, hemoglobulin variants, haptoglobin types, and immunoglobin allotypes. The most significant findings were the associations of hemoglobin S, thalassemia, and red cell glucose-6-phosphate dehydrogenase (G6PD) deficiency with malaria resistance (Allison, 1954; Cepellini, 1955; Siniscalco et al., 1966). In areas where malaria is endemic, there is a relatively high frequency of these diseases. This may be because these genes confer some resistance to malaria infection and thus offer advantages to the heterozygote while being potentially lethal in the homozygote. Disease associations with the other polymorphisms have been of low significance and disappointing.

The *HLA* system is therefore unique in that it shows significant association with an enormous variety of diseases. In some instances the degree of association is extremely high.

There is an extraordinary wealth of data on association with disease in Caucasians, increasing information on Japanese, and minimal data on other racial groups. Table 3 summarizes the known associations as reported to the HLA and Disease Registry (Ryder and Svejgaard, 1976), as submitted in abstract form to the First International Congress on HLA and Disease, or as published but missed by the Registry. Table 4 gives a list of equally important negative associations that have been reported. In some instances a disease appears in both tables, which may indicate a different racial group or subpopulation or simply conflicting data.

Some general points should be made first. Whereas *HLA* typing is now a precise measurement, in some instances the diagnosis of a

Table 3. HLA and Disease Associations*

Type of Disease	Disease	HLA Type	Racial Group	Antigen Frequency Patients	Antigen Frequency Controls	Relative Risk	P Value	Number of Study	References†
Joint disease	Ankylosing spondylitis	B27	Caucasian	89.8	8.0	87.8	1×10^{-10}	17	
		B27	Japanese	66.7	0.0	305.7	1×10^{-10}	1	
		B27	Haida Indians	100.0	50	34.4	1.7×10^{-5}	1	
		B27	Bella Coola Indians	100.0	20.2	20.2	1.9×10^{-2}	1	
		B27	Pima Indians	36.0	18.0	2.6	1.0×10^{-3}	1	1
	Reiter's disease	B27	Caucasian	78.2	8.4	35.9	1.0×10^{-10}	8	
	Yersinia arthritis	B27	Caucasian	79.4	9.4	24.3	1.0×10^{-10}	2	
	Salmonella arthritis	B27	Caucasian	66.7	8.6	17.6	3.6×10^{-10}	2	
	Psoriatic arthritis	B13	Caucasian	19.8	5.5	4.8	9.6×10^{-10}	5	
	Central joints	B27		40.2	8.7	8.6	1.0×10^{-4}	5	
		Bw17		11.6	5.5	2.5	4.6×10^{-3}	5	
		Bw38		22.7	2.9	9.1	5.6×10^{-6}	5	
	Peripheral joints	B13	Caucasian	9.9	5.5	2.3	9.5×10^{-3}	5	
		B27		15.5	8.7	2.5	3.5×10^{-4}	5	
		Bw17		24.8	5.5	5.8	1.0×10^{-10}	5	
		Bw38		12.6	2.9	4.5	3.2×10^{-4}	5	
	Juvenile rheumatoid arthritis	B27	Caucasian	26.4	8.5	4.7	1.0×10^{-10}	7	
	Rheumatoid arthritis	Dw4	Caucasian	42.2	15.7	3.0	1×10^{-5}	2	2,3
		Cw3	Caucasian	30.0	17.0	2.7	1×10^{-2}	1	3
	Sjögren's syndrome	B8	Caucasian	50.6	24.0	3.2	1.0×10^{-7}	1	
		Dw3	Caucasian	53.0	17.0	5.2	1×10^{-3}	1	4
Neurological disease	Multiple sclerosis	A3	Caucasian	35.6	25.5	1.51	9.4×10^{-9}	6	
		B7	Caucasian	34.3	24.2	1.57	7.6×10^{-10}	6	
		Dw2	Caucasian	60.0	15.0	8.5	1.0×10^{-9}	3	
	Myasthenia gravis	A1	Caucasian	44.6	26.3	2.45	1.0×10^{-10}	5	
		B8	Caucasian	57.7	22.9	4.40	1.0×10^{-10}	5	
		Dw3	Caucasian	43.0	17.0	3.5	1.0×10^{-4}	2	
	Paralytic poliomyelitis	B7	Caucasian	37.8	19.0	2.6	6.5×10^{-4}	2	5,6
	Schizophrenia	A28	Caucasian	18.9	6.3	3.48	2.8×10^{-6}	2	
				4.3	7.0	0.73	n.s.	2	
	Manic depression	Bw16	Caucasian	12.6	5.2	2.37	7.9×10^{-3}	2	

Category	Disease	Race	Antigen	Patients %	Controls %	Relative risk	p	n	Ref.
Endocrine glands Thyroid	Graves' disease	Caucasian	B8	36.7	21.7	2.13	1.0×10^{-6}	6	
			Dw3	50.0	21.7	4.0	1.0×10^{-4}	3	7,8,9
Adrenal	deQuervain's thyroiditis	Japanese	Bw35	56.8	20.5	4.97	4.6×10^{-5}	1	10
	Addison's disease	Caucasian	Bw35	76.9	12.5	22.2	1.0×10^{-10}	2	
			B8	50.0	22.7	3.9	7.3×10^{-6}	2	7
			Dw3	70.0	21.7	10.5	1.0×10^{-3}	1	
Pancreas	Diabetes	Caucasian	B8	36.7	21.8	2.1	1.0×10^{-10}	8	
	Juvenile onset diabetes		Bw15	22.8	14.9	2.1	1.0×10^{-10}	8	7
			Dw3	50.0	4.7	4.5	1.0×10^{-3}	1	7
Gastrointestinal tract	Chronic active hepatitis	Caucasian	A1	41.6	28.4	1.8	6.4×10^{-5}	5	
			B8	44.2	20.3	3.0	1.0×10^{-10}	5	11
			Dw3	60.0	21.7	7.2	1.0×10^{-3}	2	12
				25.0	21.7	1.3	n.s.		
	Celiac disease (gluten enteropathy)	Caucasian	A1	63.7	29.5	4.2	1.0×10^{-10}	7	
			B8	71.2	23.1	8.8	1.0×10^{-10}	9	
			Dw3	98.0	15.0	278	1.0×10^{-5}	1	13
	Hemochromatosis	Caucasian	A3	78.4	27.0	9.5	2.1×10^{-11}	2	
			B14	25.5	3.4	9.23	5.3×10^{-6}	2	
	Ulcerative colitis	Japanese	B5	80.0	30.8	9.3	1.0×10^{-3}	1	14
	Pernicious anemia	Caucasian	B7	35.8	22.1	2.2	1.2×10^{-4}	3	
Skin	Psoriasis	Caucasian	B13	19.7	4.5	4.65	1.0×10^{-10}	6	
			Bw17	26.2	7.8	4.7	1.0×10^{-10}	6	
			Bw37	7.7	1.4	5.4	1.0×10^{-10}	3	
			D-LD MA	36.0	5.0	10.2	1.0×10^{-3}	2	15
	Dermatitis herpetiformis	Caucasian	A1	69.0	30.1	4.4	1.0×10^{-10}	5	
			B8	77.0	24.7	9.2	1.0×10^{-10}	6	
	Pemphigus vulgaris	Caucasian	A10	39.3	12.7	3.1	1.2×10^{-4}	3	
	Behçet's disease	Caucasian	B5	35.1	11.1	4.3	8.1×10^{-5}	3	
		Japanese	B5	75.0	30.8	6.5	2.4×10^{-6}	1	
	Herpes labialis	Caucasian	A1	55.6	25.1	3.7	1.3×10^{-6}	1	
			B8	33.3	16.8	2.5	3.5×10^{-4}	1	
Eye disease	Anterior uveitis	Caucasian	B27	56.8	7.7	15.4	1.0×10^{-4}	2	16
	Vogt-Koyanagi-Harada disease	Japanese	B22J	42.9	13.2	4.5	2.0×10^{-2}	1	16
			D-LDYT	66.6	16.0	11.2	1.0×10^{-4}	1	

Table continued on following page.

Table 3. HLA and Disease Associations – *Continued*

Type of Disease	Disease	Racial Group	HLA Type	Antigen Frequency		Relative Risk	P Value	Number of Study	References†
				Patients	Controls				
Congenital malformation	Congenital heart disease	Caucasian	A2	80.0	43.9	4.9	1.3×10^{-6}		1
Malignant disease	Hodgkin's disease	Caucasian	A1	31.1	39	1.4	1×10^{-6}		17
			B5	10.6	16	1.6	1×10^{-6}		17
			B8	23.7	29	1.3	1×10^{-4}		17
			Bw18	7.1	13	1.9	1×10^{-6}		17
	Acute lymphatic leukemia	Caucasian	A2	60.0	53.6	1.3	1×10^{-2}		10
			B8	29.0	23.7	1.3	1×10^{-2}		10
			Bw18	29.0	25.2	1.3	1×10^{-2}		10
	Retinoblastoma	Caucasian	Bw35	25.4	11.0	2.75	3.8×10^{-4}		1
	Nasopharyngeal cancer	Chinese	Sia2	44.0	21.0	1.9	1.0×10^{-3}		17

*Data taken from Ryder and Svejgaard (1976), unless otherwise referenced.

†All references may be found in Ryder and Svejgaard (1976), except the following:

1. Calin, et al. 1976.
2. Stastny, 1976.
3. McMichael et al., 1977c.
4. Ivanyi et al., 1976a.
5. Möller et al. 1975.
6. Kaakinen et al., 1975.
7. Thomsen et al., 1975.
8. McMichael et al., 1975.
9. Thorsby et al., 1975.
10. Grumet, et al., 1975.
11. Opelz et al., 1976.
12. Page et al., 1975.
13. Keuning et al., 1976.
14. Tsuchiya et al., 1976.
15. McMichael et al., unpublished data; Grosse-Wilde, personal communication.
16. Yakura et al., 1976.
17. Simons et al., 1975.

Table 4.   Diseases Studied Which Show No HLA Association °

Type of Disease	Disease	Racial Group	Number of Studies
Infectious	Mononucleosis	Caucasian	2
	Congenital rubella	Caucasian	1
	Leprosy	Varied	6
Malignancy	Multiple myeloma	Caucasian	4
	Burkitt's lymphoma	African blacks	3
	Melanoma	Caucasian	5
	Carcinoma of breast	Caucasian	7
	Trophoblastic carcinoma	Caucasian	2
Other	Hashimoto's disease	Caucasian	4
	Ulcerative colitis	Caucasian	4
	Crohn's disease	Caucasian	5
	Maturity onset diabetes	Caucasian	3
	Scleroderma	Caucasian	1
	Spina bifida	Caucasian	1
	Cystic fibrosis	Caucasian	1
	Down's syndrome	Caucasian	1
	Asbestosis	Caucasian	1

° Data taken from Ryder and Svejgaard, 1976.

disease is not. For instance, the diagnosis of schizophrenia varies significantly between countries and between physicians within a country, which may account for the variable *HLA* findings in this disease. Also, in some instances the "disease" may reflect the end result of a variety of pathogenetic processes. There have, for instance, been reports of association between thyrotoxicosis and HLA (Thorsby et al., 1975); thyrotoxicosis is a syndrome resulting from overactivity of the thyroid gland, which may be due to an autoimmune disease (Graves' disease) or thyroxin secretion by a thyroid adenoma. Other studies showed that the HLA association was with Graves' disease (Thomsen et al., 1975; McMichael et al., 1975)

In most cases, associations have been made within a teaching hospital inpatient and clinic population. This may not be representative of the whole disease population and, although not invalidating the results, may indicate that severity, not initiation of the disease, is associated with the *HLA* system. This may be the case for rheumatoid arthritis, mild forms of which may affect as much as 1 to 2 per cent of the population. Conversely, in fatal disease the apparent association may be with prolonged survival rather than susceptibility.

In many diseases, the *HLA* system has been only partially typed, usually only for the *HLA–A* and *B* loci. Figure 9 therefore shows diseases in which the *HLA* system has been typed for the *A, B,* and

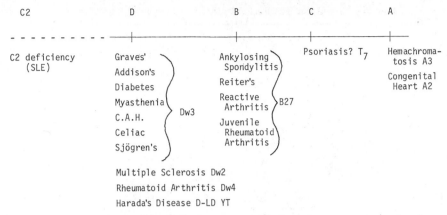

Figure 9. Diseases for which the region with the primary association has been assigned (on the basis of highest relative risk). C.A.H.: chronic active hepatitis.

D loci (and in a few instances the *C* locus). This should indicate at which locus the association is strongest. Because of the linkage disequilibria that are known to exist, an apparent association may be found for a locus that is not primarily involved. A good example is multiple sclerosis, which was historically first associated with an *A* locus antigen A3 (Naito et al., 1972), relative risk (1.51); then with B7 (Jersild et al., 1973b), relative risk (5.7); then Dw2 (Jersild et al., 1973a), relative risk (8.5); and now very strong association with a B cell alloantigen (Winchester et al., 1976). Also shown in this figure are diseases that are clearly associated with an *A* locus antigen even though they have not been *D* locus typed, namely idiopathic hemochromatosis (Bomford et al., 1976; Fauchet et al., 1976), recurrent herpes simplex infection (Russell, 1976), and congenital heart disease (Buc et al., 1975). Because there is no known linkage disequilibrium between *A* and *D* that is not secondary to *A–B* and *B–D* linkage disequilibrium, it is unlikely that these diseases will be shown in the future to be more closely associated with a *D* allele.

CHD

A few instances are known in which a disease is associated with a particular haplotype. These are shown in Table 5. The best example is deficiency of the complement component C2 which is associated with the very rare haplotype A10–Bw18–Dw2 (Fu et al., 1974). In most examples the haplotype association is secondary to a previously known linkage disequilibrium (e.g., Graves' disease with 1,8,Dw3). In a provocative paper, Terasaki and Mickey (1975) examined computed haplotypes in 32 different diseases. Although reservations must be made about the validity of these haplotype assignments in the absence of family studies, some interesting findings

Table 5. Diseases Associated with Particular HLA Haplotypes

Disease	A	B	C	D	Significant Linkage Disequilibrium in Control Population
C2 deficiency[1]	10	W18		W2	—
Hemochromatosis[2]	3	14			—
Graves' disease,[3] etc.	1	8		W3	+
Graves' disease[4] (Japan)		W35		LD HO	+
Multiple sclerosis[5]	3	7		W2	+
Vogt-Koyanaga-Harada disease[6] (Japan)		22J		LD YT	+
Aplastic anemia[7]	2	12			—
Reiter's disease, ankylosing spondylitis[7]	2	27			—
Reiter's disease[7]	3	27			—

References:
[1]Fu et al., 1974.
[2]Fauchet et al., 1976
[3]For references see Table 3.
[4]Sasazuki, personal communication.
[5]Jersild et al., 1973a.
[6]Yakura et al., 1976.
[7]Terasaki and Mickey, 1975.

emerged. In ankylosing spondylitis and Reiter's disease, there is a very high association with B27–antigen frequencies of 95 and 85 percent, respectively, compared to 5 percent in normals. It was found, however, that there were marked differences in A–B haplotypes in the two diseases; the frequency of A3–B27 was 0.5 percent for ankylosing spondylitis (AS) and 13.7 percent for Reiter's disease (RD), and the frequency of A11–B27 was 0.9 per cent in AS and 12.1 percent in RD; Aw32–B27 was 2.3 percent in AS and 0 in RD. These findings suggest that the MHC linked genetic factors involved in the two diseases are different.

Very few reports have commented on the frequency of homozygosity in their series. Page et al. (1975) found an increased frequency of B8 homozygotes in chronic active hepatitis, but this was not found by Opelz et al. (1976). It would seem therefore that in most of the examples cited susceptibility is dominant.

All the aforementioned associations are with susceptibility. There has been very little comment on resistance to disease. These studies are harder to perform statistically, but are of great importance if it is true that the present genetic features of HLA system reflect selection of haplotypes that confer resistance to infectious disease. It is perhaps notable that no clear *HLA* association has been reported for susceptibility to any major infectious disease.

If these associations are primarily with genes linked to the *HLA* system but not the *HLA–A, B, C,* and *D* antigens themselves, the finding of an association is dependent on the existence of linkage disequilibrium for that antigen with a recognizable allele. A negative *HLA* association therefore does not mean that an MHC gene is not involved in the disease process. The existence of different linkage disequilibria in different populations could prove to be very useful in finding these "silent" diseases. An example is ulcerative colitis, which has been shown in several studies to show no *HLA* association in Caucasians (e.g., Gleeson et al., 1972; Asquith et al., 1974). In Japanese, however, 85 percent of patients have *HLA–B5,* compared to 40 percent of controls (Tsuchiya et al., 1976). The *B5* complex antigens (B5 and Bw35) are in strong linkage disequilibrium with LD HO in Japanese (Sasazuki et al., 1977b), but are only in weak disequilibrium with Dw1 in Caucasians (Thorsby and Piazza, 1975).

It is not possible to discuss each disease association in any detail; the following comments will be confirmed to the associations that have excited the most interest. Prime of these is the association of HLA–B27 with ankylosing spondylitis (AS), first recognized by Caffrey and James (1973) and later analyzed in detail by Schlosstein et al. (1973) and Brewerton et al. (1973). This disease affects primarily the sacroiliac joints and, later, joints of the spine and hip and sometimes peripheral joints. It is an inflammation of tendon and ligament insertions, and these joints may be involved because they are weight bearing. The originally described male:female sex ratio of 10:1 now appears to be a myth. Calin and Fries (1975) showed that, when questioned, 20 percent of B27 positive individuals, male or female, had back pain and, when x-rayed, showed evidence of AS. Reiter's disease overlaps with AS but follows infection of the urinary tract, usually urethritis, or bowel (Shigella, Salmonella, or Yersinia). After Shigella dysentery 20 percent of B27 positive patients go on to develop Reiter's disease (RD) (Calin and Fries, 1976). It affects the same joints as AS but with a higher frequency of peripheral joint involvement. In both AS and RD, uveitis and aortic valve involvement may occur; in RD, characteristic skin and mucocutaneous membrane lesions may be seen.

The very strong association of both diseases with B27 is shown in Table 3. Three hypotheses have been described for this association: that B27 alone is directly involved in the disease as a single gene; that B27 itself interacts with at least one other gene on another chromosome; and that the association is due to a gene in linkage disequilibrium with B27. Against the first hypothesis is the fact that 80 percent of individuals with B27 never develop AS or RD (Calin and Fries, 1975). This seems to be true even when they are clearly exposed to the presumed pathogen, as has happened in outbreaks of Shigella, Salmonella, or Yersinia infections (Aho et al., 1975). Also, apparently identical disease does occur in the absence of B27 in a few cases. One family study has shown possible crossover between B27 and a disease susceptibility gene (Dick et al., 1974), and another suggests a requirement of at least one non-MHC gene (van der Linden et al., 1974). The linked gene hypothesis is most consistent with the data, particularly the apparent recombination and the haplotype data of Terasaki and Mickey (1975). Data from different racial groups is confusing. In Japan, B27 and AS are very rare but the two occur together in 60 percent of cases (Sonozaki et al., 1975), strongly suggesting a role for B27 itself. In Bella Coola and Haida Indians in North America, the B27 gene frequency is very high and is clearly associated with AS (Gofton et al., 1975; Mills et al., 1975). However, in Pima Indians the association between the two is not very great, and in females the frequency of B27 in AS patients was normal (Calin et al., 1976). This may mean that the disease is different in Pimas, that the B27 glycoprotein is functionally different although serologically similar, or that a different linkage disequilibrium exists in this population.

One way to resolve the question of whether B27 or a linked gene causes the disease would be to ascertain the disease incidence in relatives of B27 positive AS patients and B27 positive normals. The frequency of B27 in both groups should be identical; but if disease is due to a linked disease susceptibility gene, the incidence of disease should be quite different. Alternatively, if B27 itself is involved, it may be relatively easy to find an animal model, given the homology between mammalian MHC. The problem would then be amenable to direct experimentation. This is, of course tantalizing, because in the case of Reiter's disease Shigella and Yersinia have been long identified as organisms that trigger the disease.

It seems likely, as new serological markers are found for other diseases with very high association — e.g., the B cell alloantigen described by Winchester et al. (1976) for multiple sclerosis, and Dw3 for gluten enteropathy — that the same questions of whether the gene identified is the disease susceptibility gene itself will be raised.

Another interesting group of associations are the diseases associated with HLA–8. Table 6 describes the features of the associations. One group, Graves' disease, juvenile onset diabetes, and Ad-

Table 6.   Diseases Associated with the HLA-A1-B8-Dw3 Haplotype

Disease	Primary Association°	Target Organ	Organ-Specific Autoantibodies
Graves' disease†	Dw3	Thyroid (overactive)	Long acting thyroid stimulator Anti-microsomal Anti-thyroglobulin
Addison's disease†	Dw3	Adrenal	Anti-adrenal antibodies
Juvenile onset diabetes†	Dw3	Islets of Langerhans, pancreas	
Chronic active hepatitis‡	B8/Dw3§	Liver	Anti-nuclear antibody Rheumatoid factor
Celiac disease¶	Dw3	Intestinal mucosa	? To skin
Dermatitis herpetiformis¶			
Myasthenia gravis	Dw3	Neuromuscular junction	Anti-nuclear Anti-endplate Anti-muscle
Sjögren's syndrome	Dw3	Salivary glands	Rheumatoid factor Anti-nuclear antibody Anti-thyroglobulin

°Primary association based on HLA component with highest relative risk value (Table 3).

†Diseases in this group and pernicious anemia occur together at a higher than expected frequency.

‡Frequency of HLA-B8 seems to be inversely associated with the presence of hepatitis-associated antigen (HAA). Possible increased frequency of HLA homozygosity.

§Conflicting data (see Table 3).

¶Disease process triggered by gluten.

dison's disease (in two of three studies), has the strongest association with HLA–Dw3 (Thomsen et al., 1975; McMichael et al., 1975; Thorsby et al., 1975) and a relatively high incidence of the haplotype A1–B8–Dw3. These three diseases had been clustered before the demonstration of the HLA association because of the frequent presence of organ-specific autoantibodies, because of their occasional occurrence together, and because their targets are the main nonreproductive endocrine glands. It has also been shown that myasthenia gravis has a high association with HLA–Dw3 (Möller et al., 1975; Pirskanen and Tiilikainen, 1976), and that Sjögren's disease has an HLA–B8–Dw3 association (Ivanyi et al., 1976a; Opelz et al., 1976). Both of these also show organ-specific autoantibodies, although these are said to be less frequent in HLA–B8–Dw3 positive patients with myasthenia gravis than in other patients with these diseases (Pirskanen and Tiilikainen, 1976). Chronic active hepatitis also can show autoantibodies, and these are more frequent in HLA–B8 positive patients (Mackay and Morris, 1972; Galbraith et al., 1974; Bach et al., 1975). This disease, however, is probably triggered by a virus infection (Eddleston and Williams, 1974). Finally, gluten enteropathy, which has a 95 percent association with Dw3 (Keuning et al., 1976), and the related disease dermatitis herpetiformis show evidence of autoantibodies in the skin (Seah et al., 1972).

There is thus a very impressive association of the HLA–B8–Dw3 haplotype in diseases which show organ-specific autoantibodies. It has been suggested that this haplotype is associated with generalized hyperimmune responsiveness (Eddleston et al., 1976), although the evidence is unconvincing. Nonspecific hyper-responsiveness in mice is under multigenic control, but no direct linkage to the H–2 system has been demonstrated (Biozzi et al., 1972). It is tempting to speculate on a common mechanism that would correlate these findings with the remarkable linkage disequilibrium that exists between A1, B8, and Dw3 and the high frequency of this haplotype. Again, it is likely that linked genes are implicated because, in Japanese, Graves' disease at least is associated with Bw35, which in turn is in strong linkage disequilibrium with LD HO (Sasazuki et al., 1976a). Although B8 and Dw3 appear to be completely absent in Japanese, most of these diseases occur with a frequency comparable to that in Caucasians. Recently, Sasazuki (personal communication) has shown that LD HO is more strongly associated with Graves' disease in Japanese than is Bw35. This raises the possibility that the B8–Dw3 and Bw35 LD HO haplotype share common linked genes that can cause autoimmune disease.

Chronic active hepatitis is of interest, because many cases are probably initiated by infection with a virus for which a marker exists, Australia antigen or hepatitis associated antigen (HAA). Reported differences in the frequency of HLA-B8 in this disease of 30 to 80 percent correlate well with the presence or absence of HAA positive patients (Mackay and Morris, 1972; Bertrams et al., 1974). A study by Bach et al. (1975) showed that in renal dialysis units, where for unknown reasons HAA infection of patients is relatively frequent, HLA–B8 positive patients rapidly became HAA negative. The presence of HLA–B8 could thus be associated with the rapid elimination of this virus, although the subsequent development of the chronic disease may be facilitated in some way.

Gluten enteropathy has the highest known association with the *HLA* system: 98 percent of patients have Dw3, defined both by MLR typing and by B cell specific alloantisera (Keuning et al., 1976). Mann et al. (1976) have also shown that there is a second B cell specific antigen that is not HLA linked and that appears to bind the wheat protein gliadin which is known to initiate the disease. This antigen was detectable only in patients, and further analysis of this antigen will be of interest.

The diseases associated with B27 and B8–Dw3 are relatively rare and can be broadly described as having an immune process play some role in etiology. This is true of some others, such as multiple sclerosis, and is consistent with the MHC having a function in immune regulation. Attention should be drawn to diseases in which to date no immune process has been considered to be part of the mechanism — namely, idiopathic hemochromatosis (increased absorption of iron from the gut), congenital heart malformations, and possibly schizophrenia (Ivanyi et al., 1976b). There has probably been a bias in searching for association in "immune disease," including autoimmune disease, infections, and malignancies. HLA products may be implicated in a wider variety of diseases.

Mechanisms of Disease Associations

Association with an HLA allele is taken to indicate that an HLA linked product is in some way involved in the disease process. This may be in the initiating pathological event, in determining the course of the disease, or in determining the response to therapy. Almost all associations are for susceptibility rather than resistance, and the effect is dominant. In no instance, with the exception of C2 deficiency, does the *HLA* type associated with disease confer a 100 percent probability of contracting the disease. Thus, although 95 percent of patients with ankylosing spondylitis have HLA–B27, only 20 percent of B27 positive individuals develop AS (Calin and Fries, 1975). This may indicate that the actual disease susceptibility gene, although absolutely associated with the disease, is present in only 20 percent of B27 positive haplotypes. More probably, there is a multifactorial etiology for the disease; B27 or a closely linked gene is mandatory, and interacts with other factors, genetic or environmental. Similar considerations obviously apply to all disease associations with the *HLA* complex, except C2 deficiency, in which the simple genetic defect can be mapped to the *HLA* complex.

The hypotheses that could explain the association of HLA antigens with disease are shown in Table 7. Two types of mechanisms are possible: those dependent on the function of a linked gene such as an *Ir* gene, and those in which the HLA antigen itself is involved. Demonstration of an HLA antigen association with a linked gene in a

Table 7. Explanations for HLA and Disease Association

	Mechanism	Strongest Association Expected
Direct effect of HLA antigen	Molecular mimicry	A, B, C, D, Bf, etc.
	Virus or pathogen receptor or toxin receptor	A, B, C
	Incorporation into pathogen	A, B, C, D
	Complement deficiency	Complement genes
Linked genes	*Ir* genes	D
	Is genes	D
	Other linked genes	A, B, C, D

population is dependent on the existence of linkage disequilibrium between the two.

The Ir Gene Hypothesis.   It is widely assumed that *Ir* genes in the human will map close to the *HLA–D* locus because of their functional interrelationship with Ia antigens (pages 46 to 50). Thus the finding that many diseases have a primary association with a *D* locus antigen was predicted (McDevitt and Bodmer, 1974) and may indicate an *Ir* gene role in pathogenesis. The assumption that the majority of diseases would have strong correlation with *D* region products is not yet proved, because typing for this region is still cumbersome and can be performed at only a relatively few laboratories. Certain diseases do not clearly associate with the *D* region, notably the "nonimmune" diseases hemochromatosis and congenital heart malformations, as well as ankylosing spondylitis and Reiter's disease (Sachs et al., 1975).

Because *Ir* genes have not been clearly defined in humans, this explanation for *D* locus associated diseases remains unproved. However, because *Ir* genes have been found in several species, they must exist in humans, and appear to be strong candidates to explain involvement of the MHC in disease.

Ir genes are dominant and so is susceptibility to all the diseases shown in Table 3. This implies that an *Ir* gene effect would be harmful, possibly through the formation of antigen-antibody complexes or cell mediated immunity leading to inflammation and tissue damage. The finding that almost all autoimmune diseases, defined as such prior to the development of *HLA* typing, have *HLA* associations may therefore be significant.

One caution remains, however. Demonstration of *Ir* genes in experimental animals requires careful control of experimental condi-

tions. Synthetic peptides, low dose antigens, or antigens with minimal differences from host proteins must be used. The concept that *Ir*
genes may control the immune response to proliferating pathogens
when there is a high dose of antigen may be incorrect. However, in
situations in which low dose exposure to infectious agents occurs,
they would be expected to exert a major effect. It might be improba-
ble that an *Ir* gene to Shigella is solely responsible for the development of Reiter's disease after Shigella dysentery. It is more likely
that an *Ir* gene would be involved in the humoral immune response
to slow virus infections, or to altered self proteins, or to antigen
expressed in small amounts in Shigella, such as bacteriophage antigens.

   Immune Suppressor Genes.   Antigen specific suppressor factors
mapping in the *HLA* region have not yet been demonstrated in man.
They could play a role in disease. One problem in assigning this
mechanism to known HLA–disease associations is that if the mechanism involved lack of suppression and heightened immune response,
as might occur in autoimmune disease, the association should be
recessive. Weak immune response to pathogens, however, would be
dominantly associated and could therefore predispose to infectious
disease. The absence of any demonstrable association of an HLA antigen with any major infectious disease does not eliminate this mechanism. The prevalence of most infectious diseases has changed very
dramatically in the last 50 years with the introduction of vaccination
schedules and antibiotics, and with unexplained alterations in bacterial pathogenicity. It is therefore almost impossible to determine the
susceptibility of Caucasians with particular HLA types to, say, malaria, schistosomiasis, or even tuberculosis. Studies on indigenous African, Asian, or South American populations may yet reveal dramatic
associations.

   Pathogen Interaction with HLA Gene Products.   Blanden et al.
(1976) and Zinkernagel and Doherty (1974) have elegantly shown
that *H-2K* or *H-2D* compatibility is required for antigen specific
killer T cells to lyse virus infected targets. This has been shown for
several naturally occurring virus infections and one bacterial infection in mice (Table 8). In some cases sharing of one antigen (e.g.,
H-2D) is more important than compatibility for the other. *D* or *K* end
antigens may dominate.

   Such a mechanism could play a part in human disease, particularly when the association is primarily with an A or B antigen, e.g.,
herpes simplex, hemochromatosis, or ankylosing spondylitis. However, the requirement for *HLA–A* and *B* compatibility for cytolysis of
virus infected cells has not yet been shown.

Table 8. Pathogens for Which *H-2D* or *K* Involvement in Generation of
Cytotoxic T Cells Has Been Demonstrated

Lymphocytic choriomeningitis virus	Zinkernagel and Doherty, 1974
Ectromelia virus	Gardner et al., 1974
Leukovirus	Lavrin et al., 1973
Sendai virus	Doherty, quoted by Blanden et al., 1976
Rous sarcoma virus (in chicken)	Wainberg et al., 1974
Listeria monocytogenes	Zinkernagel, 1974

A criticism of this mechanism is that it remains to be shown that one allele at *H–2K* or *D* is more effective in generating killer T cells than other alleles at the same locus. This would be an integral part of any disease-HLA mechanism proposed along the lines of these experiments (Doherty and Zinkernagel, 1975). The postulate would be that particular *HLA* types fail to interact with certain viruses, and this would lead to a failure of T cell immunity toward that virus. However, this would mean that resistance and not susceptibility would be dominant.

Complement.   Complement is the third major component of the MHC that could be included in disease pathogenesis. In man, C2 and C4 and properdin B are linked to the *HLA* system. Of these, C2 deficiency is clearly associated with disease (Day et al., 1975).

Individuals homozygous for C2 deficiency may be healthy and normal. However, there appears to be a high frequency of lupus-like disease in these individuals (Stern et al., 1976). The mechanism is not understood. SLE (systemic lupus erythematosus) is characterized by serum antibodies to nuclear antigens. These can form immune complexes which can result in damage to renal glomeruli, skin, small blood vessels, and other tissues. The damage caused by complexes is mediated by complement, but how C2 deficiency plays a role in this process is not understood.

An extraordinary association has been found between the rare haplotype A10-Bw18-Dw2 and C2 deficiency. This haplotype has been found in families both in the Eastern United States and in Germany and Scandinavia. An estimated gene frequency for C2 deficiency is 0.005, and it is probably therefore associated with many other HLA haplotypes. It is possible that some C2 deficiency genes have a common and relatively recent family origin on the aforementioned haplotype.

Heterozygotes for C2 deficiency are usually normal but do have a higher frequency of intrinsic asthma (Mowbray, 1976). C4 and properdin factor B (GBG) deficiency have not been described. Electrophoretic variations of GBG are known, but diseases have not been associated with these. If further polymorphisms are found for the complement components, disease association may be found. The complement pathways are clearly involved in inflammatory processes subsequent to immune reactions. Subtle variations could clearly result in variation in response, although the specificity implicit in immune reactions would be lacking.

Other Functions of the MHC. It has been suggested that the MHC products act as cell surface hormone receptors (Svejgaard and Ryder, 1976), or could interact with hormone receptors. The level of cyclic AMP in hepatocytes was shown by Meruelo and Edidin (1975) to be *H–2* linked. Similarly, Ivanyi et al. (1972b) have shown that testosterone levels in mice are influenced by *H–2* type. It has been suggested that HLA antigens are distinct from those hormone receptors but interact sterically. This could be extended to antigen binding and could thus explain the relationship between Ia antigens and *Ir* genes. These hypotheses are potentially testable because antibody to the HLA antigens should affect receptor activity.

The cluster of endocrine diseases that are associated with HLA–Dw3 and B8 could possibly have a hormonal mechanism. HLA associated receptors for inhibitory hormones, HLA molecules affecting feedback control, or receptors accepting pathological "hormones" such as *long acting thyroid stimulator* (LATS) are possibilities that could be tested.

Psoriatic skin lesion may show abnormal levels of cyclic AMP (Mui et al., 1975), and the association with *HLA* is therefore exciting. Other possible mechanisms exist for this disease, however, including viral infection.

It is also possible, of course, that there are simply linked genes specific for each disease that are in no way related to known functions of the MHC. Thus certain enzymes might be controlled by loci on chromosome 6 and abnormalities of these might cause specific diseases. However, the linkage disequilibrium would have to be very strong for genes outside the MHC. This could be possible if there is a T/t-like system which suppresses crossing-over beyond the MHC. The known functions linked to the MHC—namely, immune regulation, complement regulation, and possibly interaction with hormone receptors—seem at present to be much more likely candidates to explain these disease associations.

Antigenic Mimicry. The previously described mechanisms have implicated known functions of the MHC. Other possibilities exist. The simplest is that pathogens possess molecules that are antigenically similar to HLA antigens. Because of self-tolerance the host is unable to mount a T cell or B cell immune response to these pathogens.

One example of this is clearly documented. Streptococcal antigens cross-react immunologically with heart muscle antigens (Kaplan and Meyeserian, 1962), which may be important in the etiology of rheumatic fever.

An interesting approach to the study of B27 related disease was made by Ebringer et al. (1976). Antisera to human B27 positive lymphocytes made in rabbits were cross-reactive with *Klebsiella aerogenes* and anti-Klebsiella made in rabbits recognized B27 positive lymphocytes. One explanation of this finding is antigen mimicry, although rigorous testing will be required to show that it is B27 itself that cross-reacts with Klebsiella.

Incorporation of MHC Antigens in Pathogens.   A few examples are known. In experiments on infection of mice with Schistosoma, it was found by Clegg et al. (1975) that the parasite acquired host red cell antigens. No relationship between the MHC and susceptibility has been demonstrated.

In a preliminary report, Lilly (1976) has shown that mouse Friend virus induced tumor lines excrete virus at different rates according to their *H–2* type. *H–2*^{b} mice excrete virus for several months; *H–2*^{d} mice do not. Analysis of viral lysates showed that *H–2D*^{b} antigens had been incorporated by the budding virus. If this exciting finding is confirmed, it indicates that HLA or *H–2* antigens can directly affect the rate of proliferation of a virus. This would clearly be a mechanism for disease susceptibility.

Other Mechanisms.   Bodmer and coworkers (Bodmer, 1972; Barnstable et al., 1976) have alluded to nonimmunological intercell recognition as a function of the MHC. They cite the Blanden-Zinkernagel-Doherty results as evidence and also suggest that the sequence homologies between *A* and *B* and between *D* and *K* may indicate that there was pressure to select for likeness between these two linked products.

This hypothesis would add a new dimension to the subject because, unlike the other mechanisms for a role of MHC products in responsiveness, it offers no explanation for the polymorphism. Very few of the diseases listed in Table 1 could be attributed to faults in this process, with the exception of the association of congenital heart disease with HLA–A2 (Buc et al., 1975).

It has also been suggested that the defects of embryogenesis coded for by the *T/t* system in the mouse might correspond to congenital neural tube defects (spina bifida and anencephaly) in the human. The *T/t* system, although about 15 crossover units from the *H–2* system, has a profound effect on *H–2* because of suppression of crossing-over (Artzt and Bennett, 1975). The prediction that when several family members were afflicted by a neural tube defect they should share HLA haplotypes was tested by Bobrow et al. (1975). No association was found. Amos et al. (1975), however, using more sensitive diagnostic criteria to define abnormality, found an association in a large kindred.

Congenital malformations account for a relatively small amount of adult disease. However, they are not rare. An estimated 25 percent of all human pregnancies end in spontaneous abortion, and a high percentage of aborted fetuses have lethal malformations. The possible association of the MHC with control of embryogenesis has far ranging implications.

The possible explanations for HLA-disease association are thus numerous and varied. It is likely that several of the described mechanisms could be involved in different diseases.

CONCLUSIONS

Several attempts have been made to provide a unifying hypothesis to encompass most of the known functions of the major histocompatibility system (e.g., Blanden et al., 1976; Nabholz and Miggiano, 1976). Although these are probably overspeculative, it is possible to make some comment on the nature of the polymorphism and the linkage disequilibria in relation to disease association (Bodmer, 1972).

The *HLA* system and its mammalian counterparts appear to be the most polymorphic genetic systems known. Although 30 percent of all genes may be polymorphic, most show fewer alleles. If a polymorphism is not accepted as such until an allele reaches a gene frequency of 1 percent (Ford, 1966), recent mutations should be excluded. In the *HLA* system, all alleles described occur at or above this frequency, implying that there must have been some degree of selection in the population to attain these relatively high frequencies. This is true whether one accepts the conventional view that there are a small number (*A, B, C,* and *D*) of highly polymorphic loci or the possibility raised by Bodmer (1972) that there are multiple loci each with a smaller number of alleles.

The latter hypothesis would mean that the *HLA* structural gene loci are not abnormally polymorphic and that a separate genetic mechanism controls which loci are expressed. Possible evidence for this view comes from the experiments of Festenstein (1976), who found new H–2 antigens appearing on tumor cell lines, and from the finding that CW1 and CW3 are inherited as a haplotype in Japanese (Payne et al., 1975).

An allele can be selected for either by an increased frequency of fertilization of the ovum by sperm carrying that gene, or by causing greater fitness. The T/t system has been shown to cause segregation distortion and because of suppression of crossing-over, which extends into H–2, particular H–2 types might therefore be selected for as a consequence. A neutral mutation occurring in H–2 could actually achieve a high frequency by this mechanism. However, all HLA alleles at all loci have been found to obey Mendelian laws, and this mechanism seems unlikely to have played a role in establishing the HLA polymorphism.

Selection for heterozygotes, favoring the polymorphism, could occur at the fetal stage of life. A known example of this is rhesus incompatibility, in which feto-maternal rhesus blood group differences may result in harmful maternal antibodies directed against fetal red cells. This immunization occurs only if fetus and mother are ABO compatible. The ABO polymorphism is thus advantageous in protecting against the effects of another polymorphism. Contrary to expectations, feto-maternal HLA incompatibility is not harmful, and there is evidence that MHC incompatibility can result in increased placental weight, which could be advantageous (James, 1967). Homozygous fetuses have not been found to be at a disadvantage in a number of surveys. It may be important, however, that such studies were carried out in populations in which fetal and perinatal mortality rates are low, in contrast to the very high death rates that occur in underprivileged populations and that occurred in all peoples in the recent past. Although this sort of mechanism can be envisaged as being important in mammals, it is obviously unimportant in egg-laying vertebrates in which the polymorphic major histocompatibility systems evolved.

Selection by disease is a real possibility, in view of the multiple associations known between HLA and disease. The selection could operate through closely linked genes, such as Is or Ir genes, or directly through the HLA antigens themselves. It is worth considering the effects of the different mechanisms described previously on generating the polymorphism.

Immune response genes are dominantly expressed HLA linked genes and may confer disease resistance. Heterozygotes would be favored if there are multiple Ir genes in the human I region that arose by gene duplication and mutation to generate new Ir gene specificities. Recent history has numerous examples of catastrophic disease epidemics with extremely high mortalities in afflicted populations. These could obviously have exerted dramatic selective effects on previously rare Ir gene mutations. The fact that some antigens are under the control of paired Ir genes may also account for the linkage disequilibrium seen in the *HLA* system. Neutral *HLA–A*, *B*, and *C* mutations might be favorably selected by being present on the same haplotype as an advantageous pair of *Ir* genes. This effect would be most profound if the *Ir* genes map across the whole human MHC as Ia antigens appear to do in the monkey (Roger et al., 1976).

Immune suppression genes present problems. As stated previously, lack of suppression may be advantageous in offering vigorous immune responses to infection. This would mean that homozygotes would be favored so that this mechanism of disease association could not favor a polymorphism.

Mechanisms of association involving direct effects on *HLA* genes may also explain the polymorphism. Molecular mimicry is probably not a common mechanism for HLA and disease association. However, if it were, mutation of the HLA antigens as a mechanism of evading pathogens might occur. New mutations would have an immediate advantage of disease resistance. However, this would probably be short lived, because the extremely high replication rate of pathogens compared to vertebrates would give ample opportunity to select new virulent mutants.

Incorporation of HLA antigens into pathogens could have two effects. First, particular *HLA* types may favor virus replication; and second, cross-infection might be prevented because of the presence of these MHC antigens in the pathogen. Both could favor generation of the polymorphism.

Self-recognition, as occurs in the cell mediated cytolysis of virus infected cells would favor generation of polymorphism if the altered self hypothesis is true. The assumption would have to be made that interaction with individual viruses is specific for particular HLA antigens. The more HLA antigens an individual possesses, the greater would be its ability to resist infection. Gene duplication and polymorphism in the MHC would thus be advantageous.

It is probable that most of the polymorphism and linkage disequilibria seen now are relics of previous selective events. Some evidence comes from the admixture of African Blacks and Caucasians seen in the American Black. In the seven or eight generations since this began, the African Black linkage disequilibria have been lost and the gene frequencies have changed (Payne et al., 1977). A similar phenomenon has been seen in the frequency of the hemoglobin S trait, which has become less frequent in a malaria-free environment.

Most of the diseases listed in Table 3 can exert very little selective pressure, as they occur late in life. The hypothesis that diseases have shaped the features of the *HLA* system depends upon the prediction that there will be strong associations between *HLA* and major infectious diseases. Piazza et al. (1972) have shown that HLA antigen frequencies differ in Sardinian mountain and valley dwellers, possibly because the latter lived, until recently, in an endemic malaria area. Study of populations currently exposed to disease such as malaria, schistosomiasis, trypanosomiasis, and tuberculosis is urgently needed.

PROSPECTS

·The *Ir* gene hypothesis remains the most attractive mechanism for explaining *HLA* and disease associations. It is logically the most satisfying because the presumed function of the immune system is to combat disease processes such as those initiated by pathogens. It is most easily resolvable with the polymorphism, and the recently found *Ir* gene interactions could explain the linkage disequilibria. Direct typing for *Ir* genes should reveal stronger disease associations, assuming that *Ir* genes will be clustered together on the chromosome and in linkage disequilibrium. Functional methods of finding *Ir* genes in humans are still not available, however, and will probably require methodological advances in establishing primary and secondary immune responses in vitro with human peripheral blood lymphocytes.

If Ia antigens are the *Ir* gene products, it may not be necessary to show by functional assays that *Ir* genes cause disease. As discussed previously, *Ia* and *Ir* are genetically inseparable in the mouse *H-2* complex. Functional studies show *Ia* to be involved in lymphoid cell interactions. Helper and suppressor factors carry Ia determinants. *Ir* and *Ia* must therefore be closely related. The search for disease associations with Ia antigens should therefore be fruitful. Already, celiac disease and multiple sclerosis have been found to have nearly 100 percent association with serologically defined human Ia antigens. More associations should follow.

References

Aho, K., P. Ahvonen, P. Alkio, A. Lassus, E. Saivanen, K. Sievers, and A. Tiilikainen. 1975. HLA 27 in reactive arthritis following infection. Ann. Rheum. Dis. (suppl.) 34:29.

Allen, F. H. 1974. Linkage of HL-A and GBG. Vox Sang. 27:382.

Allison, A. C. 1954. Protection afforded by sickle cell trait against subtertian malarial infection. Brit. Med. J. 1:290.

Allison, A. C., and D. F. Clyde. 1961. Malaria in African children with deficient glucose-6-phosphate dehydrogenase. Brit. Med. J. 1:1346.

Alter, B. J., D. J. Schendel, M. L. Bach, F. H. Bach, J. Klein, and J. H. Stimpfling. 1973. Cell mediated lympholysis. Importance of serologically defined H-2 regions. J. Exp. Med. 137:1303.

Amos, D. B., R. Ruderman, N. R. Mendell, and A. H. Johnson. 1975. Linkage between HLA and spinal development. Transpl. Proc. (suppl.) 7:93.

Artzt, K., and D. Bennett, 1975. Analogies between embryonic (T/t) antigens and adult major histocompatibility (H–2) antigens. Nature 256:545.

Asquith, P., P. Mackintosh, P. L. Stokes, G. K. T. Holmes, and W. T. Cooke. 1974. Histocompatibility antigens in patients with inflammatory bowel disease. Lancet 1:113.

Bach, F. H., and K. Hirschhorn. 1964. Lymphocyte interaction: A potential histocompatibility test in vitro. Science 142:813.

Bach, F. H., M. B. Widmer, M. L. Bach, and J. Klein. 1972. Serologically defined and lymphocyte defined components of the major histocompatibility complex in the mouse. J. Exp. Med. 136:1430.

Bach, J. F., J. Zingraff, B. Descamps, C. Naret, and P. Jungers. 1975. HLA 1,8 phenotype and HB antigenemia in haemodialysis patients. Lancet 2:707.

Bain, B., M. R. Vas, and L. Löwenstein. 1964. The development of large immature mononuclear cells in mixed leucocyte cultures. Blood 23:108.

Baker, P. J., P. W. Stashak, D. F. Amsbaugh, and B. Prescott. 1974. Regulation of the antibody response to type III pneumococcal polysaccharide. IV. Role of suppressor T cells in the development of low dose paralysis. J. Immunol. 112:2020.

Barnstable, C. J., E. A. Jones, W. F. Bodmer, J. G. Bodmer, B. Arce-Gomez, D. Snary, and M. Crumpton. 1977. Genetics and serology of HLA linked human Ia antigens. Cold Spring Harbor Symp. Quant. Biol. In press.

Basten, A., and J. G. Howard. 1973. Thymus independence. Contr. Topics Immunobiol. 2:265.

Benacerraf, B., and M. Dorf. 1976. The Nature and Function of Specific H-Linked Immune Response Genes and Immune Suppression Genes. In The Role of Products of the Histocompatibility Gene Complex in Immune Responses, Katz, D. H., and B. Benacerraf (Eds.), pp. 225–248. New York, Academic Press.

Benacerraf, B., and H. O. McDevitt. 1972. Histocompatibility linked immune response genes. Science 175:273.

Bennett, D. 1975. The T-locus of the mouse—review. Cell 6:441.

Bertrams, J., Reis, H. E., Kuwert, E., and Selmaier, H. 1975. Hepatitis associated antigen (HAA), HLA antigens and auto lymphocytotoxins (CoCoCy) in chronic aggressive and chronic persistent hepatitis. Z. Immun. Forsch. Bd. 146S:300.

Bevan, M. 1975. The major histocompatibility complex determines susceptibility to cytotoxic T cells directed against minor histocompatibility antigens. J. Exp. Med. 142:1349.

Bias, W. B., and D. G. Marsh. 1975. HLA linked antigen E immune response genes: An unproved hypothesis. Science 188:375.

Biijnen, A. B., I. Schroeder, P. Meera, F. H. Allen, C. M. Giles, W. R. T. Los, W. S. Volkers, and J. J. van Rood. 1976. Linkage relationships of the loci of the major histocompatibility complex in families with a recombination in the HLA region. J. Immunogenet. 3:171.

Biozzi, G., R. Asofsky, R. Lieberman, C. Stiffel, D. Morton, and B. Benacerraf. 1972. Serum concentrations and allotypes of immunoglobulins in two lines of mice genetically selected for high- and low-antibody synthesis. J. Exp. Med. 132:752.

Black, P. L., D. G. Marsh, E. Jarrett, G. J. Delespesse, and W. B. Bias. 1976. Family studies of association between HLA and specific immune responses to highly purified pollen allergens. Immunogenetics 3:349.

Blanden, R. V., P. C. Doherty, M. B. C. Dunlop, I. D. Gardner, R. M. Zinkernagel, and C. S. David. 1975. Genes required for cytotoxicity against virus infected target cells in K and D regions of H-2 complex. Nature 254:269.

Blanden, R. V., A. J. Hapel, and D. C. Jackson. 1976. Speculations: Mode of action of Ir genes and the nature of T cell receptors for antigens. Immunochemistry 13:179.

Blumenthal, M. N., D. B. Amos, H. Noreen, N. Y. Mendell, and E. J. Yunis. 1974. Genetic mapping of Ir locus in man: Linkage to second locus of HLA. Science 184:1301.

Bobrow, M., J. G. Bodmer, W. F. Bodmer, H. O. McDevitt, J. Lorber, and P. Swift. 1975. The search for a human equivalent of the mouse T-locus—negative results from a study of HLA types in spina bifida. Tissue Antigens 5:234.
Bodmer, J. 1975. The ABC of HLA. In Joint Report on Serology of the VIth Histocompatibility Testing Workshop, J. Bodmer, (Ed.). Histocompatibility Testing 1975, pp. 21–114. Copenhagen, Munksgaard.
Bodmer, W. F. 1972. Evolutionary significance of the HLA system. Nature 237:139.
Bodmer, W. F., J. Bodmer, S. Adler, R. Payne, and J. Bialek. 1966. Genetics of '4' and 'LA' human leucocyte groups. Ann. N.Y. Acad. Sci. 129:473.
Bomford, A., A. L. W. F. Eddleston, R. Williams, L. Kennedy, and J. R. Batchelor. 1976 (Abs.). HLA-A3 and Idiopathic Haemochromatosis. In HLA and Disease Abstracts, p. 153. Paris, Inserm.
Bradley, B. A., J. M. Edwards, and D. Franks. 1973. Histocompatibility phenotyping by the mixed lymphocyte reaction. Tissue Antigens 3:340.
Bretscher, O., and M. Cohn. 1970. A theory of self-nonself discrimination. Science 169:1042.
Brewerton, D. A., M. Caffrey, F. D. Hart, D. C. D. James, A. Nicholls, and R. D. Sturrock. 1973. Ankylosing spondylitis and HL-A 27. Lancet 1:907.
Bridgen, J., D. Snary, M. J. Crumption, C. Barnstable, P. Goodfellow, and W. F. Bodmer. 1976. Isolation and N-terminal amino acid sequence of membrane bound human HLA-A and HLA-B antigens. Nature 261:200.
Buc, M., S. Nyulassy, J. Stefanovic, J. Jacubcova, and M. Benedekova. 1975. HLA–2 and congenital heart malformations. Tissue Antigens 5:128.
Burnett, F. M. 1959. The Conal Selection Theory of Acquired Immunity. Cambridge, Cambridge University Press.
Burnett, F. M. 1973. Multiple polymorphism in relation to histocompatibility antigens. Nature 245:359.
Caffrey, M. F. P., and D. C. O. James. 1973. Human lymphocyte antigen association in ankylosing spondylitis. Nature 242:121.
Calin, A., P. H. Bennett, J. Jupiter, and P. I. Terasaki. 1976 (Abs). HLA B27 and Sacroiliitis in Pima Indians. In HLA and Disease Abstracts. Paris, Inserm.
Calin, A., and J. F. Fries. 1975. The striking prevalence of ankylosing spondylitis in "healthy" W27 positive males and females. A controlled study. New Eng. J. Med. 293:835.
Calin, A., and J. F. Fries. 1976. An "experimental" epidemic of Reiter's syndrome revisited. Follow-up evidence on genetic and environmental factors. Ann. Intern. Med. 84:584.
Cantor, H., and E. Boyse. 1975. Functional subclasses of T lymphocytes bearing different Ly antigens. I. The generation of functionally distinct T cell subclasses is a differentiative process independent of antigen. J. Exp. Med. 141:1376.
Capkova, J., and P. Demant. 1974. Genetic studies of the H–2 associated complement gene. Folia Biol. 20:101.
Cepellini, R. 1955. Negative correlation between altitude above sea level and incidence of thalassemia in four Sardinian villages. Cold Spring Harbor Symp. Quant. Biol. 20:252.
Cepellini, R., E. S. Curtoni, P. L. Mattiuz, V. Miggiano, G. Scudeller, and A. Serra. 1967. Genetics of Leucocyte Antigens. A Family Study of Segregation and Linkage. In Histocompatibility Testing 1967, p. 149. Copenhagen, Munksgaard.
Claman, H. N., E. A. Chaperon, and R. F. Triplett. 1966. Thymus–marrow cell combinations. Synergism in antibody production. Proc. Soc. Exp. Biol. Med. 122:1167.
Clegg, J. A., S. R. Smithers, and R. J. Terry, 1975. Acquisition of human antigens by Schistosoma mansoni during cultivation in vitro. Parasitology 70:67.
Colombani, J., M. Colombani, D. C. Shreffler, and C. S. David. 1976. Separation of anti-Ia (I region associated antigens) from anti-H-2 antibodies in complex sera by absorption on blood platelets. Description of the new specificities. Tissue Antigens 7:74.
Crumpton, M. J., and D. Snary. 1977. Isolation and structure of human histocompatibility (HLA) antigens. Current Topics Immunochem. In press.

Cullen, S. E., J. H. Freed, P. H. Atkinson, and S. J. Nathenson. 1975. Evidence that protein determines Ia antigenic specificity. Transpl. Proc. 7:237.

Cunningham, B. A., and I. Berggard. 1974. Structure, evolution and significance of β_2 microglobulin. Transpl. Rev. 21:3.

Dausset, J. 1954. Leuco-agglutinins. IV. Leuco-agglutinins and blood transfusion. Vox Sang. 4:190.

Dausset, J., J. Colombani, L. Legrand, and N. Feingold. 1969. Les sub loci du système HLA. Le système principal d'histocompatibilité de l'homme. Presse Med. 77:849.

David, C. S., D. C. Shreffler, and J. Frelinger. 1973. New lymphocyte antigen system (Lna) controlled by the *Ir* region of the mouse *H–2* complex. Proc. Nat. Acad. Sci. 70:2509.

Day, N. K., P. Rubenstein, M. de Brauo, B. Moncoda, J. A. Hansen, B. Dupont, M. Thomsen, A. Svejgaard, and C. Jersild. 1975. Hereditary Cl_r Deficiency: Lack of Linkage to the HL-A Region in Two Families. In Histocompatibility Testing 1975, p. 960. Copenhagen, Munksgaard.

Demant, P., J. Capkova, E. Hinzova, and B. Voracova. 1973. The role of histocompatibility-2-linked Ss-Slp region in the control of mouse complement. Proc. Nat. Acad. Sci. 70:863.

Dick, H. M., R. D. Sturrock, W. C. Dick, and W. W. Buchanan. 1974. Inheritance of ankylosing spondylitis and HLA antigen W27. Lancet 2:24.

Doherty, P. C., and R. M. Zinkernagel. 1975. A biologic role for the major histocompatibility antigens. Lancet 1:1406.

Dorf, M. E., J. H. Stimpfling, and B. Benacerraf. 1975. Requirement for two *H-2* complex *Ir* genes for the immune response to the L-Glu, L-Lys, L-Phe terpolymer. J. Exp. Med. 141:1459.

Ebringer, A., P. Cowling, N. Ngwa Suh, D. C. D. James, and R. W. Ebringer. 1976. Cross Reactivity Between *Klebsiella aerogenes* Species and B27 Lymphocyte Antigens as an Aetiological Factor in Ankylosing Spondylitis (Abs.). In HLA and Disease, p. 27. Paris, Inserm.

Eddleston, A. L. W. F., R. M. Galbraith, R. Williams, J. Pattison, D. Doniadu, L. A. Kennedy, and J. R. Batchelor. 1976. HLA B8 and B12 and Enhanced Antibody Responses in Chronic Active Hepatitis. In HLA and Disease, p. 156. Paris, Inserm.

Eddleston, A. L. W. F., and R. Williams. 1974. Inadequate antibody response to HBAg or suppressor T cell defect in development of active chronic hepatitis. Lancet 2:1543.

Eichmann, K., and K. Rajewsky. 1975. Induction of T and B cell immunity by anti-idiotypic antibody. Eur. J. Immunol. 5:661.

Eisen, H. N., and G. W. Siskind. 1964. Variations in affinities of antibodies during the immune response. Biochemistry 3:996.

Eisjvoogel, V. P., R. du Bois, C. J. M. Meleif, W. P. Zeylemaker, L. Koning, and L. de Groot-Kooy. 1973. Lymphocyte activation and destruction in vitro in relation to MLC and HLA. Transpl. Proc. 5:415.

Ellman, L., I. Green, J. Martin, and B. Benacerraf. 1970. Linkage between the poly-L-lysine gene and the locus controlling the major histocompatibility antigens in strain 2 guinea pigs. Proc. Nat. Acad. Sci. 66:322.

Fathman, C. G., B. S. Handwerger, and D. H. Sachs. 1974. Evidence for a role of *Ir*-associated alloantigens in mixed lymphocyte culture stimulation. J. Exp. Med. 140:853.

Fauchet, R., M. Simon, M. Bourd, B. Genetet, N. Genetet, and J. L. Alexandre. 1976 (Abs.). Idiopathic Haemochromatosis and HLA Antigens. In HLA and Disease Abstracts. Paris, Inserm.

Ferreira, A., and V. Nussenzweig. 1975. Genetic linkage between serum levels of the third component of complement and the *H-2* complex. J. Exp. Med. 141:513.

Festenstein, H. 1976. Paper presented at HLA and Disease meeting. In HLA and Disease. Dausset, J. (Ed.). Paris, Inserm, in press.

Ford, E. B. 1966. Genetic polymorphism. Proc. Roy. Soc. Biol. 164:350.

Friend, P., Y. Kim, B. Handwerger, N. Reinsmoen, A. Michael, and E. Yunis. 1975. C2 Deficiency in Man. Relationship, Including Probable Genetic Mapping, to the Mixed Lymphocyte Reaction Stimulator (S or LD) Determinant Short 7a. In Histocompatibility Testing 1975, p. 928. Copenhagen, Munksgaard.

Fu, S. M., H. G. Kunkel, H. P. Brusman, F. H. Allen, and M. Fotino. 1974. Evidence for linkage between HLA histocompatibility genes and those involved in the synthesis of the second component of complement. J. Exp. Med. 140:1108.

Galbraith, R. M., A. L. Eddleston, M. G. Smith, R. Williams, R. N. McSween, G. Watkinson, H. Dick, L. A. Kennedy, and J. R. Batchelor, 1974. Histocompatibility antigens in active chronic hepatitis and primary biliary cirrhosis. Brit. Med. J. 3:604.

Gally, J. A., and G. M. Edelman. 1972. The genetic control of immunoglobulin synthesis. Ann. Rev. Genet. 6:1.

Gardner, I., N. A. Bowern, and R. V. Blanden, 1974. Cell mediated cytotoxicity against ectromelia virus infected target cells. Eur. J. Immunol. 4:68.

Gatti, R. A., E. A. Svedmyr, and W. Leibold. 1976. Evidence for a second MLR locus on chromosome 6 (Abs). Fed. Proc. 35:353.

Gershon, R. K., and K. Kondo. 1971. Infectious immunological tolerance. Immunology 21:903.

Gleeson, M. H., J. S. Walker, J. Wentzell, J. A. Chapman, and R. Harris. 1972. Human leucocyte antigens in Crohn's disease and ulcerative colitis. Gut 13:438.

Gofton, J. P., A. Chalmers, G. E. Price, and C. E. Reeve. 1975. HLA 27 and ankylosing spondylitis in B.C. Indians. J. Rheum. 2:314.

Goodfellow, P., E. Jones, V. van Heymingers, E. Solomon, M. Bobrow, V. Miggiano, and W. F. Bodmer. 1975. The β_2 microglobulin gene is on chromosome 15 and not in the HLA region. Nature 254:267.

Goodfellow, P. N., and R. O. Payne, 1976. Personal communication.

Gorer, P. A. 1937. The genetic and antigenic basis of tumour transplantation. J. Path. Bact. 44:691.

Gorer, P. A., and P. O'Gorman. 1956. The cytotoxic activity of isoantibodies in mice. Transpl. Bull. 3:142.

Götze, D., F. A. Reisfeld, and J. Klein. 1973. Serological evidence for antigens controlled by the *Ir* region in mice. J. Exp. Med. 138:1003.

Greenberg, L. J., E. D. Gray, and E. J. Yunis. 1975. Association of HLA5 and immune responsiveness in vitro to streptococcal antigens. J. Exp. Med. 141:935.

Grosse-Wilde, H. 1976. Personal communication.

Grumet, F. C., R. O. Payne, I. Konishi, T. Moni, and J. P. Kriss. 1975. HLA antigens in Japanese patients with Graves' disease. Tissue Antigens 6:347.

Haldane, J. B. S. 1933. The genetics of cancer. Nature 132:265.

Hämmerling, G. J., B. D. Deak, G. Mauve, U. Hämmerling, and H. O. McDevitt. 1974. B lymphocyte alloantigens controlled by the *I*-region of the major histocompatibility complex in mice. Immunogenetics 1:68.

Hansen, T. H., H. S. Shin, and D. C. Shreffler. 1975. Evidence for the involvement of the Ss protein of the mouse in the hemolytic complement system. J. Exp. Med. *141*:1216.

Hauptfeld, V., D. Klein, and J. Klein. 1973. Serological identification of an *Ir* region product. Science 181:167.

Hayry, P., and V. Defendi. 1970. Mixed lymphocyte cultures produce effector cells. Model in vitro for allograft rejection. Science 108:133.

Herzenberg, L. A., K. Okumura, and C. M. Metzler. 1975. Regulation of immunoglobulin and antibody production by allotype suppressor T cells in mice. Transpl. Rev. 27:57.

Hinzova, E., P. Demant, and P. Ivanyi. 1972. Genetic control of haemolytic complement in mice: Association with H–2. Folia Biol. 18:237.

Hood, L. 1972. Two genes: One polypeptide chain—fact or fiction? Fed. Proc. 31:177.

Ivanyi, P., S. Gregorova, and M. Mickova. 1972a. Genetic differences in thymus, lymph node, testes, and vesicular gland weights among inbred mouse strains: Association with major histocompatibility (H–2) system. Folia Biol. 18:81.

Ivanyi, P., R. Hampl, L. Starka, and M. Mickova. 1972b. Genetic association between *H-2* gene and testosterone metabolism in mice. Nature–New Biol. 238:280.

Ivanyi, D., E. Hinzova, K. Sula, I. Drizhal, E. Erbenova, H. Macunova, C. Dostal, J. Horezs, and J. Balik. 1976a. Increased Frequency of HLA-B8 and HLA-Dw3 in Sjögren's Syndrome (SS) (abs.). In HLA and Disease Abstracts. Paris, Inserm.

Ivanyi, D. P. Zemek, and P. Ivanyi. 1976b. HLA antigens in Schizophrenia (abs.). In HLA and Disease Abstracts, p. 69. Paris, Inserm.

James, D. A. 1967. Some effects of immunological factors on gestation in mice. J. Reprod. Fert. 14:265.

Jersild, C., T. Fog, G. S. Hansen, J. Thomsen, A. Svejgaard, and B. Dupont, 1973a. Histocompatibility determinants in multiple sclerosis with special reference to the clinical course. Lancet 2:1221.

Jersild, C., A. Svejgaard, T. Fog, and U. T. Amnitzbo. 1973b. HLA antigens and disease. I. Multiple sclersosis. Tissue Antigens 3:243.

Jones, E. A., P. Goodfellow, R. H. Kennett, and W. F. Bodmer. 1976. The independent expression of HLA and β_2 microglobulin on human-mouse hybrids. Somatic Cell Genet. In press.

Jones, P. 1976. Personal communication.

Jongsma, A., H. van Someren, A. Westerveld, A. Hogenmyer, and P. Pearson. 1973. Localization of genes on human chromosomes using human–Chinese hamster somatic cell hybrids. Assignment of PGM3 to chromosome G6 and ragweed mapping of the PGD, PGM and Pep-C genes on chromosome C1. Humangenetik 20:195.

Kaakinen, A., R. Pirskanen, and A. Tiilikainen. 1975. LD antigens associated with HLA8 and myasthenia gravis. Tissue Antigens 6:175.

Kaplan, M. H., and M. Meyeserian. 1962. An immunological cross reaction between group A streptococcal cells and human heart tissue. Lancet 1:706.

Kapp, J. A., C. W. Pierce, S. Schlossman, and B. Benacerraf. 1974. Genetic control of immune responses in vitro. V. Stimulation of suppressor T cells in nonresponder mice by the terpolymer l-glutamic acid[60]-l-alanine[30]-l-tyrosine[10] (GAT). J. Exp. Med. 140:648.

Katz, D. H. 1972. The allogenic effect on immune responses: Model for regulatory influences of T lymphocytes on the immune system. Transpl. Proc. 12:141.

Katz, D. H., and B. Benacerraf. 1976a. Genetic Control of Lymphocyte Interactions and Differentiation. In The Role of Products of the Histocompatibility Complex in Immune Response, Katz, D. H., and B. Benacerraf (Eds.), pp. 355–385. New York, Academic Press.

Katz, D. H., and B. Benacerraf (Eds.). 1976b. The Role of the Histocompatibility Gene Complex in the Immune Response. New York, Academic Press.

Keuning, J. J., A. S. Pena, A. van Leeuwen, J. P., van Hooff, and J. J. van Rood. 1976. HLA-Dw3 associated with coeliac disease. Lancet 1:506.

Klein, J. 1975. Biology of the Mouse Histocompatibility-2 Complex. New York, Springer-Verlag.

Klein, J., and D. C. Shreffler. 1971. The H-2 model for major histocompatibility systems. Transpl. Rev. 6:3.

Kreth, H. W., and A. R. Williamson. 1971. Cell surveillance model for lymphocyte cooperation. Nature 234:454.

Lamm, L. U., U. Friedrich, G. B. Petersen, F. Jorgensen, J. Nielsen, A. J. Therkelesen, and F. Kissmeyer-Nielsen. 1974. Assignment of the major histocompatibility complex to chromosome 6 in a family with a peri-centric inversion. Hum. Hered. 24:273.

Lamm, L. U., F. Jorgensen, and F. Kissmeyer-Nielsen. 1976. Bf maps between the HLA-A and D loci. Tissue Antigens 7:122.

Lavrin, D. H., R. B. Herberman, M. Nunn, and M. Soaves. 1973. In vitro cytotoxicity studies of murine sarcoma virus-induced immunity in mice. J. Nat. Cancer Inst. 51:1497.

Levine, B. B., R. H. Stember, and M. Fotino. 1972. Ragweed hayfever: Genetic control and linkage to HLA haplotypes. Science 178:1201.

Lightbody, J., D. Bernoco, V. C. Miggiano, and R. Cepellini. 1971. Cell mediated lympholysis in man after sensitization of effector lymphocytes through mixed leukocyte culture. G. Batt. Virol. Immunol. 64:243.

Lilly, F. 1966. The inheritance of susceptibility to the Gross leukemia virus in mice. Genetics 53:529.

Lilly, F. 1970. Fv-2: Identification and location of a second gene governing the spleen locus response to Friend leukemia virus in mice. J. Nat. Cancer Inst. 45:163.

Lilly, F. 1971. The influence of H-2 type on Gross virus leukemogenesis in mice. Transpl. Proc. 3:1239.

Lilly, F. 1976. Communication at HLA and Disease Meeting, Paris.

Lonai, P., and H. O. McDevitt. 1974a. Genetic control of the immune response: In vitro stimulation of lymphocytes by (T,G)-A--L, (H,G)-A--L, and (Phe,G)-A--L. J. Exp. Med. 140:977.

Lonai, P. and H. O. McDevitt, 1974b. I-region genes are expressed on T and B lymphocytes: Studies of the mixed lymphocyte reaction (MLR). J. Exp. Med. 140:1317.

Löw, B., L. Messeter, S. Mansson, and T. Lindholm. 1974. Crossing over between the SD-2 (FOUR) and SD-3 (AJ) loci of the human major histocompatibility chromosome region (abs.). Tissue Antigens 4:405.

Mackay, I. R., and P. J. Morris. 1972. Association of autoimmune active chronic hepatitis with HLA-1,8. Lancet 2:793.

Mann, D. L., D. L. Nelson, S. I. Katz, L. D. Abelson, and W. Strober. 1976. Specific B cell alloantigens associated with gluten sensitive enteropathy and dermatitis herpetiformis. Lancet 2:110.

Marchialonis, J. J. 1974. Molecular and Functional Properties of Lymphocyte Surface Immunoglobulins. In The Immune System, Genes, Receptors, Signals, Sercarz, E. E., A. R. Williamson, and C. F. Fox (Eds.), p. 141. New York, Academic Press.

Marsh, D. G. 1977. Allergy: A model for studying the genetics of human immune response. Nobel Symposium No. 33, "Molecular and Biological Aspects of the Acute Allergic Reactions," Stockholm, March 1976, Johanssen, S. G. O., K. Strandberg, and B. Uvrias (Eds.). London, Plenum Press, in press.

Marsh, D. G., W. B. Bias, and K. Ishizaka. 1974. Genetic control of basal serum immunoglobulin E level and its effect on specific reaginic sensitivity. Proc. Nat. Acad. Sci. U.S.A. 71:3588.

McDevitt, H. O., and B. Benacerraf. 1969. Genetic control of specific immune responses. Adv. Immunol. 11:31.

McDevitt, H. O., and W. F. Bodmer, 1974. HLA immune response genes and disease. Lancet 1:1269.

McDevitt, H. O., B. D. Deak, D. C. Shreffler, J. Klein, J. H. Stimpfling, and G. D. Snell, 1972. Genetic control of the immune response. Mapping of the Ir-1 locus. J. Exp. Med. 135:1259.

McDevitt, H. O., and M. Sela. 1965. Genetic control of the antibody response. J. Exp. Med. 122:517.

McMichael, A. J., and T. Sasazuki, 1977. A suppressor T cell in the human mixed lymphocyte reaction. Submitted for publication.

McMichael, A. J., T. Sasazuki, and H. O. McDevitt, 1977a. The human immune response to diphtheria toxoid. Transpl. Proc., In press.

McMichael, A. J., T. Sasazuki, H. O. McDevitt, and J. Skehel. 1977b. The human immune response to influenza hemogglutinins. Manuscript in preparation.

McMichael, A. J., T. Sasazuki, R. Payne, F. C. Grumet, H. O. McDevitt, and J. Kriss. 1975. An HLA8 Associated LD Antigen in Patients with Graves' Disease. In Histocompatibility Testing 1975, p. 769. Copenhagen, Munksgaard.

McMichael, A. J., T. Sasazuki, R. Payne, and H. O. McDevitt. 1977c. Increased frequency of HLA Cw3 and Cw4 in rheumatoid arthritis. Arthritis and Rheumatism, in press.

Medawar, P. B. 1944. The behavior and fate of skin autografts and skin homografts in rabbits. J. Anat. 78:176.

Melchers, I., and K. Rajewsky. 1975. Specific control of responsiveness by two complementary Ir loci in the H-2 complex. Eur. J. Immunol. 5:753.

Mempel, W., H. Grosse-Wilde, P. Baumann, B. Netzel, I. Steinbauer-Rosenthal, S. Scholz, J. Bertrams, and E. D. Albert. 1973. Population genetics of the MLC response: Typing for MLC determinants using homozygous and heterozygous reference cells. Transpl. Proc. 5:1529.

Meo, T., C. S. David, M. Nabholz, V. Miggiano, and D. C. Shreffler. 1973. A major role for the *Ir-1* region of the mouse *H-2* complex in the mixed lymphocyte reaction. Transpl. Proc. 5:377.

Meo, T., T. Krasteff, and D. C. Shreffler, 1975. Immunochemical characterization of murine *H-2* controlled Ss (serum substance) protein through identification of its human homologue as the fourth component of complement. Proc. Nat. Acad. Sci. U.S.A. 72:4536.

Meruelo, D., and M. Edidin. 1975. Association of mouse liver adenosine 3'5'-cyclic monophosphate (cyclic AMP) levels with histocompatibility-2-genotype. Proc. Nat. Acad. Sci. 72:2644.

Meruelo, D., and H. O. McDevitt. 1976. Unpublished data.

Miller, J. F. A. P., and G. F. Mitchell. 1969. Thymus and antigen-reactive cells. Transpl. Rev. 1:3.

Miller, J. F. A. P., M. A. Vada, A. Whitelaw, and J. Gamble. 1976. *H-2* Linked *Ir* Gene Regulation of Delayed-Type Hypersensitivity in Mice. In The Role of Products of the Histocompatibility Complex in Immune Responses, Katz, D. H., and B. Benacerraf. (Eds.), pp. 403–415. New York, Academic Press.

Mills, D. M., Y. Arai, and R. C. Gupta. 1975. HLA antigens and sacroiliitis. J.A.M.A. 231:268.

Mitchison, N. A. 1971a. The carrier effect in the secondary response to hapten protein conjugates. I. Measurement of the effect with transferred cells and objections to the local environment hypothesis. Eur. J. Immunol. 1:10.

Mitchison, N. A. 1971b. The carrier effect in the secondary response to hapten protein conjugates. II. Cellular cooperation. Eur. J. Immunol. 1:18.

Möller, E., H. Link, G. Matell, B. Olhagen, and L. Stendhal. 1975. LD Alleles in Ankylosing Spondylitis, Myasthenia Gravis, Multiple Sclerosis, and Optic Neuritis. In Histocompatibility Testing 1975, p. 778. Copenhagen, Munksgaard.

Mowbray, J. F. 1976. Association of Heterozygous C2 Deficiency with Both Disease and HLA (Abs.). In HLA and Disease. Paris, Inserm.

Mui, M. M., S. L. Hsai, and K. M. Halprin. 1975. Further studies on adenyl cyclase in psoriasis. Brit. J. Derm. 92:255.

Müller-Eberhard, H. J. 1975 Complement. Ann. Rev. Biochem. 44:697.

Munro, A. J., and M. J. Taussig. 1975. Two genes in the major histocompatibility complex control immune response. Nature 256:103.

Murphy, D. B., L. A. Herzenberg, K. Okumura, L. A. Herzenberg, and H. O. McDevitt. 1976. A new subregion (*I-J*) marked by a locus (*Ia-4*) controlling surface determinants on suppressor T lymphocytes. J. Exp. Med. 144:699.

Nabholz, M., and V. Miggiano. 1976. The Biological Significance of the Mixed Leukocyte Reaction. In B and T Cells in Immune Recognition, Loor, F., and G. Roelants (Eds.)., Chichester, England, Wiley & Sons, International Publishing Company.

Naito, S., N. Namerow, M. R. Mickey, and P. Terasaki. 1972. Multiple sclerosis: Association with HLA 3. Tissue Antigens 2:1.

Nathenson, S. G., and Cullen, S. E. 1974. Biochemical properties and immunochemical-genetic relationships of mouse H-2 alloantigens. Biochim. Biophys. Acta 344:1.

Olaisen, B., P. Teisberg, T. Gedde-Dahl, and E. Thorsby. 1975. The Bf locus in the HLA region of chromosome 6: Linkage and association studies. Humangenetik 30:291.

Oldstone, M. B. A., F. J. Dixon, G. F. Mitchell, and H. O. McDevitt. 1973. Histocompatibility linked genetic control of disease susceptibility. Murine lymphocytic choriomeningitis virus infection. J. Exp. Med. 137:1201.

Opelz, G., P. Terasaki, A. Vogten, S. Schlam, W. Summerskill, S. Kasson, T. Chused, and K. Fye. 1976. Association of HLA-Dw3 with chronic active liver disease and Sjögren's disease (abs.). In HLA and Disease Abstracts, p. 167. Paris, Inserm.

Page, A. R., H. L. Sharp, L. J. Greenberg, and E. J. Yunis. 1975. Genetic analysis of patients with chronic active hepatitis. J. Clin. Inv. 56:530, 1975.

Payne, R., M. Feldman, H. Cann, and J. G. Bodmer. 1977. Comparison of HLA data of the North American Black with the African Black and North American Caucasoid population. Tissue Antigens. In press.

Payne, R., R. Radvany, F. C. Grumet, M. Felman, and H. Cann. 1975. Two Third Series Antigens Transmitted Together—A Possible Fourth SD Locus? In Histocompatibility Testing 1975, pp. 343–347. Copenhagen, Munksgaard.

Payne, R., and M. R. Rolfs, 1958. Fetomaternal leukocyte incompatibility. J. Clin. Invest., 37:1756.

Payne, R., M. Tripp, J. Weigle, W. Bodmer, and J. Bodmer. 1964. A new leukocyte isoantigen system in man. Cold Spring Harbor Symp. Quant. Biol. 29:285.

Piazza, A., M. C. Belvedere, D. Bernoco, C. Conighi, L. Contu, E. S. Curtoni, P. L. Mattiuz, W. Mayr, P. Richiardi, G. Schudeller, and R. Cepellini. 1972. HLA Variation in Four Sardinian Villages Under Differential Selective Pressure by Malaria. In Histocompatibility Testing 1972, Dausset, J., and J. Colombani (Eds.), pp. 73–84. Copenhagen, Munksgaard.

Pirskanen, R., and A. Tiilikainen. 1976. Myasthenia Gravis and HLA (abs.). In HLA and Disease Abstracts, p. 79. Paris, Inserm.

Rittner, C., H. Grosse-Wilde, B. Rittner, B. Netzel, S. Scholz, H. Lorenz, and E. D. Albert. 1975a. Linkage group HLA-MLC-Bf (properdin factor B). The site of Bf locus at the immunogenetic linkage group on chromosome 6. Humangenetik 27:173.

Rittner, C., G. Hauptmann, H. Grosse-Wilde, E. Grosshaus, M. M. Tongio, and S. Mayer. 1975b. Linkage Between HLA (Major Histocompatibility Gene Complex) and Genes controlling the Synthesis of the Fourth Component of Complement. In Histocompatibility Testing 1975, p. 945. Copenhagen, Munksgaard.

Roger, J. H., W. van Vreeswijk, M. E. Dorf, and H. Balner. 1976. The major histocompatibility complex of rhesus monkeys. VI. Serology and genetics of Ia-like antigens. Tissue Antigens 8:67.

Russell, A. S. 1976. HLA and Herpes Simplex Virus Type 1 (abs.). In HLA and Disease Abstracts, p. 116. Paris, Inserm.

Ryder, L. P., and A. Svejgaard. 1976. Associations Between HLA and Disease. In Report from the HLA and Disease Registry of Copenhagen 1976. Copenhagen, published by the authors.

Sachs, D. H., and J. L. Cone. 1973. A mouse B-cell alloantigen determined by gene(s) linked to the major histocompatibility complex. J. Exp. Med. 138:1289.

Sachs, J. A., S. Sterioff, S. Robinette, E. Wolf, L. F. Curry, and H. Festenstein. 1975. Ankylosing spondylitis and the major histocompatibility system. Tissue Antigens 5:120.

Sasazuki, T., A. J. McMichael, R. Payne, and H. O. McDevitt. 1977a. HLA haplotype differences between Japanese and Caucasians. Tissue Antigens, in press.

Sasazuki, T., A. McMichael, R. Payne, H. O. McDevitt, H. Yakura, A. Wakisaka, M. Aizawa, and K. Itakara. 1977b. An HLA-D specificity in the Japanese population. Tissue Antigens 9:62.

Scher, I., A. K. Berning, D. M. Strong, and I. Green. 1975. The immune response to a synthetic amino acid terpolymer in man: Relationship to HLA type. J. Immunol. 115:36.

Schlosstein, L., P. I. Terasaki, R. Bluestone, and C. M. Pearson, 1973. High association of an HLA antigen W27 with ankylosing spondylitis. New Eng. J. Med. 288:704.

Schmitt-Verhulst, A., and G. M. Shearer. 1975. Bifunctional major histocompatibility linked genetic regulation of cell-mediated lympholysis to trinitrophenyl modified autologous lymphocytes. J. Exp. Med. 142:914.

Schwartz, B. D., and S. E. Cullen. 1976. The Chemistry of Mouse and Guinea Pig Ia Antigens. In The Role of Products of the Histocompatibility Gene Complex in Immune Responses, Katz, D. H., and B. Benacerraf (Eds.), pp. 691–701. New York, Academic Press.

Schwartz, R. H., M. E. Dorf. B. Benacerraf, and W. E. Paul. 1976. The requirement for two complementary $Ir\text{-}Gl\emptyset$ immune response genes in the T lymphocyte proliferative response to poly ($Glu^{53}Lys^{36}Phe^{11}$). J. Exp. Med. 143:897.

Seah, P. P., L. Fry, J. S. Steward, B. L. Chapman, A. V. Hoffbrand, and E. J. Holbor-row. 1972. Immunoglobulins in the skin in dermatitis herpetiformis and coeliac disease. Lancet 1:611.

Seaver, S. S., A. Brown, G. Hämmerling, and H. O. McDevitt, 1976. Genetic control of the immune response: Ability of antigen of defined amino acid sequence to be recognized by the *Ir-1* gene system. Eur. J. Immunol. 6:502.

Shearer, G. M., T. G. Rehn, and C. A. Gartarin. 1975. Cell mediated lympholysis of trinitrophenyl-modified lymphocytes. J. Exp. Med. 141:1348.

Sheehy, M. J., P. M. Sondel, F. H. Bach, M. L. Sapori, and M. J. Bach. 1975. Rapid Detection of LD Determinants: The PLT Assay. In Histocompatibility Testing 1975, p. 569. Copenhagen, Munksgaard.

Shevach, E., W. E. Paul, and I. Green. 1972. Histocompatibility-linked immune response gene function in guinea pigs. Specific inhibition of antigen-induced lymphocyte proliferation by alloantisera. J.Exp. Med. 136:1207.

Shreffler, D. C., and C. S. David. 1972. Studies on recombination within the mouse *H–2* complex. 1. Three recombinants which position the *Ss* locus within the complex. Tissue Antigens 2:232.

Silver, J., and L. Hood. 1976. Genetic and Evolutionary Implications of the Partial Amino Acid Sequences of H–2K and H–2D Alloantigens. In The Role of Genes of the Major Histocompatibility Complex in Immune Responses, Katz, D. H., and B. Benacerraf (Eds.), p. 677, New York, Academic Press.

Simons, M. J., S. H. Chan, J. H. C. Ho, O. W. Chan, N. E. Day, and G. B. de The. 1975. A Singapore 2 Associated LD Antigen in Chinese Patients with Naso-pharyngeal Carcinoma. In Histocompatability Testing 1975, p. 809. Copenhagen, Munksgaard.

Siniscalco, M., L. Bernini, G. Filippi, B. Latte, P. Meera Kahn, S. Piomelli, and M. Rattazzi. 1966. Population genetics of hemoglobulin variants, thalassemia and glucose 6 phosphate dehydrogenase deficiency with particular reference to the malaria hypothesis. Bull. WHO 34:379.

Smeraldi, E., and R. Scorza-Smeraldi. 1976. Interference between anti-HLA an-tibodies and chlorpromazine. Nature 260:532.

Snary, D., C. J. Barnstable, P. Goodfellow, W. F. Bodmer, and M. J. Crumptom. 1977. Cold Spring Harbor Symp. Quant. Biol. In press.

Snell, G. D. 1948. Methods for the study of histocompatibility genes. J. Genet. 49:87.

Snell, G. D. 1974. Immunogenetics: Retrospect and prospect. Immunogenetics 1:1.

Solliday, S., and F. H. Bach. 1970. Cytotoxicity: Specificity after in vitro sensitization. Science 170:1406.

Sonozaki, H., H. Seki, S. Chang, M. Okuyama, and T. Juji. 1975. Human lymphocyte antigen HLA 27 in Japanese patients with ankylosing spondylitis. Tissue Antigens 5:131.

Spencer, M. J., J. O. Cherry, and P. I. Terasaki. 1976. HLA antigens and antibody response after influenza A vaccination. New Eng. J. Med. 294:13.

Stastny, P. 1976. Mixed lymphocyte cultures in rheumatoid arthritis. J. Clin. Invest. 57:1148.

Stern, R., S. M. Fu, M. Fotino, V. Agnello, and H. G. Kunkel. 1976. Hereditary C2 deficiency: Association with skin lesions resembling the discoid lesions of sys-temic lupus erythematosus. Arth. Rheum. 19:517.

Strober, S. 1970. Effect of mineral adjuvant on lymphocyte cooperation in the second-ary antibody response to a hapten protein conjugate. Nature 228:1324.

Svejgaard, A., and L. P. Ryder. 1976. Interaction of HLA molecules with non-im-munological lysands as an explanation of HLA and disease associations. Lancet 2:547.

Tada, T., M. Taniguchi, and C. S. David. 1976. Properties of antigen specific suppres-sor T cell factors in the regulation of antibody response of the mouse. IV. Specific subregion assignment of the gene(s) that codes for the suppressive T cell factor in the *H–2* histocompatibility complex. J. Exp. Med. *144*:713.

Taussig, M., and R. Cepellini. 1976. Communicated at the 1st International Congress on HLA and Disease, Paris.

Taussig, M. J., and A. J. Munro. 1975. Antigen Specific T Cell Factor in Cell Cooperation and Genetic Control of the Immune Response. In Immune Recognition,
Rosenthal, A. S. (Ed.), p. 791. New York, Academic Press.
Terasaki, P., and M. R. Mickey. 1975. HLA haplotypes of 32 diseases. Transpl. Rev.
22:105.
Terasaki, P., and G. Opelz. 1976. Personal communication.
Terhorst, C., P. Dorham, D. L. Mann, and J. L. Strominger. 1976. Structure of HLA an-
tigens: Amino acid and carbohydrate compositions and N-terminal sequences of
four antigen preparations. Proc. Nat. Acad. Sci. U.S.A. 73:910.
Thomsen, M., P. Platz, O. O. Anderson, M. Christy, J. Lyngsøe, J. Nemp, K. Rasmussen,
L. P. Ryder, L. Staub-Nielsen, and A. Svejgaard. 1975. MLC typing in juvenile
diabetes mellitus and idiopathic Addison's disease. Transpl. Rev. 22:125.
Thorsby, E. 1974. The human major histocompatibility complex. Transpl. Rev. 18:52.
Thorsby, E., and A. Piazza. 1975. Joint Report from the Sixth International Histocom-
patibility Testing Workshop. II. Typing for HLA-D (LD-1 or MLC) Determi-
nants. In Histocompatibility Testing 1975. Copenhagen, Munksgaard.
Thorsby, E., E. Svejgaard, J. H. Soleus, and L. Dornstad. 1975. The frequency of major
histocompatability antigens SD and LD in thyrotoxicosis. Tissue Antigens 6:54.
Ting, A., M. R. Mickey, and P. Terasaki. 1976. B lymphocyte alloantigens in caucasians. J. Exp. Med. 143:981.
Tsuchiya, M., T. Yoshida, Y. Mizano, K. Kanta, T. Hibi, and K. Tsuji. 1976. HLA Antigens and Ulcerative Colitis in Japan. In HLA and Disease Abstracts, p. 169.
Paris, Inserm.
van den Tweel, J. G., H. M. Vriesendrop, A. Termijtelen, D. L. Westbroek, M. L. Bach,
and J. J. van Rood. 1974. Genetic aspects of canine mixed leucocyte cultures. J.
Exp. Med. 140:825.
van der Linden, J. M. J. P., J. J. Keuning, J. H. C. Wuisman, A. Cats, J. J. van Rood,
and A. A. Pena. 1974. HLA 27 and ankylosing spondylitis: A family study. Lancet
1:520.
van Rood, J. J. 1962. Leucocyte Grouping, Thesis, Leiden.
van Rood, J. J., and J. G. Eernisse. 1968. The detection of transplantation antigens in
leukocytes. Semin. Hematol., 5:187.
van Rood, J. J., J. G. Eernisse, and A. van Leeuwen. 1958. Leukocyte antibodies in
sera of pregnant women. Nature 181:1735.
van Rood, J. J., A. van Leeuwen, A. Parleveit, A. Termijtelen, and J. J. Keuning. 1975.
LD Typing by Serology. IV. Description of a New Locus with Three Alleles. In
Histocompatibility Testing 1975. p. 629. Copenhagen, Munksgaard.
van Someren, H., A. Westerfield, A. Hayenmeyer, J. R. Mees, P. Meera Khan, and O. B.
Zaalberg. 1974. Human antigen and enzyme markers in man–Chinese hamster
somatic cell hybrids: Evidence for synteny between HLA, PGM, 1ME₁ and IPO-B
loci. Proc. Nat. Acad. Sci. U.S.A. 71:962.
Vaz, N. M., J. M. Philips-Quagliata, B. B. Levine, and E. Vaz. 1971. H–2 linked ge-
netic control of immune responsiveness to ovalbumin and ovamucoid. J. Exp.
Med. 134:1335.
Vitetta, E. S., C. Bianco, V. Nussenzweig, and J. W. Uhr. 1972. Cell surface Ig. IV.
Distribution among thymocytes, bone marrow cells and their derived populations.
J. Exp. Med. 136:81.
Vladitiu, A. O., and N. R. Rose. 1971. Autoimmune murine thyroiditis: Relationship to
histocompatibility (H–2) type. Science 168:852.
Wainberg, M. A., Y. Marksin, D. W. Weiss, and F. Doljanski. 1974. Cellular immunity
against Rous sarcomas of chickens. Preferential reactivity against autochthonous
target cells as determined by lymphocyte adherence and cytotoxicity in vitro.
Proc. Nat. Acad. Sci. U.S.A. 71:3565.
Waldmann, T. A., M. Durm, S. Broder, M. Blackman, R. M. Blaese, and W. Strober.
1974. Role of suppressor T cells in pathogenesis of common variable hypogam-
maglobulinaemia. Lancet 2:609.
Walford, R. L., S. Finkelstein, C. Hanna, and Z. Collins. 1969. Third sublocus in the
HLA human transplantation system. Nature 224:74.

WHO-IUIS terminology Committee. 1975. Histocompatibility Testing. p. 5. Copen-
    hagen, Munksgaard.
Widmer, M. B., C. Omodei-Zonni, M. L. Bach, F. H. Bach, and J. Klein. 1973. Impor-
    tance of different regions of H–2 for MLC stimulation. Tissue Antigens 3:309.
Wigzell, H., and H. Binz. 1976. Idiotypic Receptors for Antigen on T Lymphocytes. In
    The Role of Products of the Major Histocompatibility Complex in Immune
    Response, Katz, D. H., and B. Benacerraf (Eds.), pp. 461–475. New York, Aca-
    demic Press.
Winchester, R. J., G. Ebers, S. M. Fu, L. Espinosa, J. Zabinskie, and H. G. Kunkel.
    1972. B cell alloantigens Ag 7a in multiple sclerosis. Lancet 2:814.
Yakura, H., A. Wakisaka, M. Aizawa, K. Hakama, Y. Tagawa, and S. Suguira. 1976.
    HLA-D antigen of Japanese origin (LD-Wa) and its association with Vogt-
    Koyanagi-Harada syndrome. Tissue Antigens 3:35.
Yunis, E. Y., and D. B. Amos. 1971. Three closely linked genetic systems relevant to
    transplantation. Proc. Nat. Acad. Sci. 68:3031.
Zembala, M., and G. L. Asherson. 1973. Depression of the T cell phenomenon of con-
    tact sensitivity by T cells from unresponsive mice. Nature 244:227.
Zinkernagel, R. M. 1974. Restriction by H–2 gene complex of transfer of cell mediated
    immunity to Listeria monocytogenes. Nature 251:230.
Zinkernagel, R. M., and P. C. Doherty, 1974. Immunological surveillance against al-
    tered self components by sensitised T lymphocytes in lymphocytic choriomen-
    ingitis. Nature 251:547.
Zinkernagel, R. M., and P. C. Doherty. 1977. The concept that surveillance of self is
    mediated via the same set of genes that determines recognition of allogeneic cells.
    Cold Spring Harbor Symp. Quant. Biol. In press.

3

Genetic Studies and Biologic Strategies in the Affective Disorders

ELLIOT S. GERSHON
STEVEN D. TARGUM
LINDA R. KESSLER
CAROLYN M. MAZURE
WILLIAM E. BUNNEY, JR.

Dr. Gershon is Unit Chief, Section on Psychogenetics; Dr. Targum, Dr. Kessler, and Ms. Mazure are in the Section on Psychogenetics, Adult Psychiatry Branch, National Institute of Mental Health, Bldg. 10, Room 3N218, Bethesda, Maryland 20014. Dr. Bunney is Chief, Adult Psychiatry Branch, National Institute of Mental Health.

INTRODUCTION

During the past two decades there have been parallel advances in the biology and pharmacology of the affective disorders (mania and depression), and in genetic and family studies of these disorders, but relatively few studies have attempted to identify biologic factors that are inherited in these disorders. In this paper, we will briefly review the evidence for genetic and biologic factors in affective illness, paying particular attention to those questions that remain unresolved, and then discuss appropriate strategies for testing biologic-genetic hypotheses in relation to recently reported studies and in areas which appear promising to us for future studies.

Typology of Affective Illness

Before reviewing the current evidence on genetic factors in affective illness, it is necessary to consider some issues in the typology of affective illness.

The two types of major psychiatric illness, affective disorders and schizophrenia, have largely distinct clinical features and can be reliably differentiated from each other on this basis. Further evidence that these two classes of disorders are distinct from each other is found in the specific effectiveness of antidepressant drugs and lithium carbonate in the treatment of affective disorders but not in schizophrenia (Davis and Cole, 1976; Fieve, 1976). No combination of strictly defined schizophrenia and affective disorder was found in a series of monozygotic (MZ) twin pairs (Tsuang, 1975; Mitsuda, 1967; Asano, 1967), and family studies (Stendstedt, 1952; Goetzl et al., 1974; Wimmer, 1922; Winokur, 1972; Cohen et al., 1972) have shown few schizophrenic relatives of affectively ill patients (probands) or the converse. However, there are some overlapping clinical, biochemical, and pharmacologic features between the affective illnesses and schizophrenia (Carpenter et al., 1973; Mitsuda, 1967; Goodwin and Post, 1975).

The importance of precision of classification within the affective disorders for the analysis of genetic hypotheses is clear. Kendell (1976) has reviewed numerous proposed typologies which attempt to define homogeneous subgroups within the affective disorders. Typologies based on present clinical features and past history distinguish patients on neurotic/psychotic or endogenous/reactive continuums, and have been supported by factor analytic studies, cluster analysis, and other multivariate techniques. The genetic validity of these approaches remains essentially untested.

From a genetic viewpoint, a typology is of interest only if it separates out transmissible forms of illness. The question of familial transmission has been studied for all primary affective disorders taken together, and for the unipolar (UP) and bipolar (BP) forms of primary affective disorder.

Primary affective disorder (Feighner, et al., 1972; Robins and Guze, 1972) (defined as an affective illness occurring in the absence of previously existing diagnosable, non-affective psychiatric illness) is characterized by episodic or chronic mood states of depression or mania severe enough to cause impairment in normal social functioning. In the reported genetic studies, the probands with affective illness had all been impaired enough to require hospitalization.

The affective syndromes may be further described as follows:

1. *Depression* is a dysphoric mood characterized by despondency, hopelessness, worry, and five of the following eight symptoms: poor appetite or weight loss, sleep difficulty, fatigability or malaise, agitation or retardation, loss of interest in usual activities, feelings of self-reproach or guilt, complaints of slowed-up thoughts or diminished ability to concentrate, and suicidal ideation.

2. *Mania* is characterized by a mood of euphoria or of a paranoid-angry state and three of the following six symptom categories: hyperactivity, pressured style of speech, racing thoughts, grandiosity, decreased need for sleep, and easy distractability. Those patients with peculiar alterations of perceptions and thinking as a major manifestation of their illness in the absence of prominent mood symptoms would not be included.

Evidence for a Genetic Factor

Strategies to develop evidence for a genetic factor in affective illness include (1) twin and family studies, (2) adoption studies, (3) chromosomal linkage markers, and (4) transmission of physiologic-biochemical deficits.

In a genetically transmitted disorder, the concordance rate should be higher in MZ twins than in dizygotic (DZ) twins because of the greater genetic similarity in MZ twins. Twin data for affective disorder in six studies were reviewed by Gershon et al. (1976), who noted an overall concordance rate for MZ twins of 69.2 percent, compared to 13.3 percent of DZ twins ($p < 0.001$). Assuming that the intrapair differences of environment are the same for MZ and DZ twins, the higher concordance rate for MZ twins indicates that affective disorder is heritable. Price (1968) reviewed 12 MZ twin pairs who were reared apart and found a concordance rate for affective illness of 67 percent, implying that the MZ twin concordance is not due to shared environment. The presence of discordant twin pairs suggests that other than genetic factors influence the probability that the disorder will be manifest, such as variable penetrance, phenocopies, or age of onset.

Family studies of affective illness have consistently reported significantly higher incidence of affective illness in first degree relatives of ill probands compared to the general population. The morbid risk for affective illness in first degree relatives (parents, sibs, and children) of affectively ill probands varied from 5.9 to 18.4 percent in male relatives and 7.1 to 31.9 percent in female relatives in eight studies reviewed by Gershon et al. (1976). These figures are significantly higher than the 0.6 to 3.3 percent general population prevalence for affective illness (Fremming, 1951; Helgassen, 1964; Gershon and Liebowitz, 1975) that have been reported. Parenthetically, it may be noted that in most studies these prevalences are much lower than the mendelian ratios expected for single major locus inheritance, implying either that there is reduced penetrance or that the genetic inheritance is by a more complex mechanism.

Adoption studies can be utilized to distinguish between postnatal environmental and genetic factors in several ways: by comparing morbidity risks for illness in natural biologic versus adoptive relatives of affectively ill probands, by studying the incidence of affective illness in the adopted-away offspring of affectively ill parents vs. well parents, or by studying adopted children of ill adoptive parents vs. well adoptive parents (Rosenthal, 1970). In alcoholism, sociopathy, and schizophrenia, adoption studies suggest a prenatal transmission as recently reviewed by Crowe (1975). Adoption studies in affective illness have not yet been reported. Chromosomal linkage markers and biologic findings in affective disorder as evidence for a genetic factor are discussed below.

CLINICAL SUBGROUPS WITHIN THE AFFECTIVE DISORDERS

Unipolar and Bipolar Illness

Primary affective disorders can be subdivided into unipolar (UP) and bipolar (BP) illness, as proposed by Leonhard (1957) and Leonhard et al. (1962), in which UP patients have had depression but never mania, and BP patients have had mania or hypomania and depression (although patients with mania only are now included in this grouping, based on data of Perris [1966]). In their initial descriptions of UP and BP illness, Leonhard (1957) and Leonhard et al. (1962) noted that the prevalence of endogenous psychoses was different in the relatives of each type of patient, and suggested that these represented genetically distinct entities. This hypothesis has been central to much of the genetic and biologic research in affective illness for the past 15 years, and it is now timely to review the biologic and genetic evidence on the relation between BP and UP affective illness.

Twin and Family Studies of UP and BP Illness. The separation of UP and BP illness into distinct genotypic entities requires that the transmission of these subtypes be independent of each other. Twin data collated by Zerbin-Rudin (1969) and reviewed by Perris (1974b) reveal an 81 percent concordance for type of illness among MZ twin pairs who were concordant for affective illness (70 percent of the sample).

The prevalence for type of affective illness varies according to the population studied. Gershon et al. (1975b) have reported a BP:UP prevalence ratio approaching 1:1 in Israel, whereas Perris' (1966) Scandinavian data approaches 1:4. If polarity in an ill-co-twin were determined by chance alone, the expected MZ twin concordance for polarity of illness, using these ratios as a range, would be between 50 and 68 percent. The MZ twin concordance observed for polarity (81 percent) is significantly higher ($p < .05$) than would be expected by chance alone. The possibility that BP and UP illness are merely random phenotypic manifestations of the same genotype is therefore ruled out.

Perris' (1974b) review shows 19 percent *discordance* for polarity of affective illness, and 30 percent discordance for presence of illness in MZ twin pairs. Assuming these are not phenocopies, the data imply that the same genotype may be phenotypically manifested as either UP or BP or as no illness at all in a MZ co-twin. The question remains how distinct these entities are when randomly sampled in a population.

The family data do not resolve this issue (Table 1). All family studies (Angst, 1966; Perris, 1966; Winokur and Clayton, 1967; Goetzl et al., 1974; Helzer and Winokur, 1974; Gershon et al., 1975b; James and Chapman, 1975) have shown that relatives of bipolar probands have a greater morbidity risk for the development of affective illness than the relatives of unipolar probands. However, all investigators but Perris (1966) found both UP and BP illness in the relatives of BP probands. Perris' study differs from the others because of his stricter criteria for UP illness, which required three depressive

Table 1. Affective Illness in First-Degree Relatives

Bipolar Probands		Number at Risk	Morbid Risk (%)	
			BP	UP
James and Chapman, 1975		239	6.4	13.2
Gershon et al., 1975b		341	3.8	6.8
Goetzl et al., 1974		212	2.8	13.7
Helzer and Winokur, 1974		151	4.6	10.6
Winokur and Clayton, 1967		167	10.2	20.4
Perris, 1966		627	10.2	0.5
Angst, 1966		161	4.3	13.0
	Totals	1898	6.8	8.3
Unipolar Probands				
Angst, 1966		811	0.3	5.1
Perris, 1966		684	0.3	6.4
Gershon et al., 1975b		96	2.1	11.5
	Totals	1591	0.4	6.0

episodes, rather than one as used by other investigators. Perris defines another group of relatives as "other depressions and suicide," which other workers might diagnose as UP illness, and finds this group more prevalent in relatives of BP probands (8.6 percent) than in the relatives of UP probands (6.8 percent). Thus Perris' data may not be at variance with the other studies. Even though there are few BP relatives of UP probands, the consistent finding that BP illness does not "breed true" implies that at least some UP illness is genetically related to BP. Specific genetic hypotheses on this relationship are considered below in the discussions of genetic models and chromosomal linkage. The hypothesis that BP illness is transmitted by a single major locus X-chromosome dominant gene has been of particular interest, in view of the findings in some studies of high rate of mother-son and virtually absent father-son transmission (Winokur and Clayton, 1967; Helzer and Winokur, 1974), although other family studies have not found this (Stendstedt, 1952; Goetzl, 1974; Mendlewicz and Rainer, 1974; Gershon et al., 1975a).

Biologic and Pharmacologic Studies of UP and BP Illness. Twin and family studies suggest that UP and BP are both genetically transmitted, but do not reveal if they are genetically distinct. Clear biologic or pharmacologic distinctions between the two types of patients would suggest a genetic difference that could be studied in pedigrees (Childs, 1976; Stewart and Elston, 1973). There is a considerable literature comparing the two types of patients, which is summarized in Tables 2 and 3.

Table 2. Unipolar-Bipolar Illness: Biologic Comparisons

Studies of monoamine metabolites in depression:

Urinary MHPG	BP < Controls < UP*	Goodwin and Beckmann, 1975
	BP = UP < Controls	Maas et al., 1968
	BP < UP*	Schildkraut, 1973
CSF 5-HIAA (Baseline)	BP = Controls > UP*	Ashcroft et al., 1973
	BP = UP	van Praag et al., 1973
(Accumulation)	BP < UP < Controls	van Praag et al., 1973
	BP < UP* = Controls	Bowers, 1974
	BP = UP < Controls	Goodwin and Post, 1975
CSF HVA (Baseline)	BP = UP	Goodwin and Post, 1975
	BP = Controls > UP*	Ashcroft et al., 1973
	BP = UP = Controls	van Praag et al., 1973
(Accumulation)	BP = UP < Controls	van Praag et al., 1973
	BP < Controls < UP*	Bowers, 1974
	BP = UP < Controls	Goodwin and Post, 1975

Monamine enzyme studies:

Platelet MAO	BP > Controls	Nies, 1971, 1974 (personal communication)
	BP < UP = Controls*	Murphy and Weiss, 1972
	BP < Controls < UP*	Landowski et al., 1975
	BP < Controls	Leckman et al., (unpublished data)
	BP > Controls	Belmaker et al., 1976
Erythrocyte COMT	UP ♀ < BP ♀ < Controls	Dunner et al., 1971
	UP ♂ = BP ♂ = Controls	
	UP = BP = Controls	Mattson et al., 1974
	UP = BP > Controls	Gershon and Jonas, 1975

Neuroendocrine studies in depression:

Abnormal dexamethasone suppression	BP > UP > Controls	Carroll et al., 1976
L-Dopa stimulation of growth hormone	BP > UP = Controls*	Gold et al. (unpublished data a)
	BP = UP = Controls	Sachar et al., 1975
L-Dopa suppression of prolactin	BP > UP = Controls*	Gold et al. (unpublished data a)
	BP = UP = Controls	Sachar et al., 1975
Insulin stimulation of growth hormone	BP = Controls > UP*	Sachar et al., 1973
THR stimulation of TSH	BP > Controls > UP*	Gold et al. (unpublished data b)
Glucocorticoids in urine	BP < UP < Controls	Dunner et al., 1972
	BP = UP	Gold et al. (unpublished data b)

Table continued on opposite page

Table 2.   Unipolar-Bipolar Illness: Biologic Comparisons — *Continued*

Sleep studies in depression:		
Hypersomnia	BP < UP	Detre et al., 1972
REM latency	BP = UP < Controls	Kupfer, 1976

Neurophysiologic studies in depression:		
Augmentation of evoked		
response	BP > Controls > UP	Buchsbaum et al., 1971
	♂: BP > Controls > UP°	Buchsbaum et al., 1973
	♀: BP = UP > Controls	
	BP = UP > Controls	Gershon and Buchsbaum, 1976

°Reported UP-BH differences are statistically significant for at least p < .05.

Table 3.   Unipolar-Bipolar Illness: Pharmacologic Comparisons

Lithium studies:		
Response in acute depression	BP > UP	Goodwin et al., 1972
	BP > UP	Noyes et al., 1974
	BP > UP	Mendels, 1974
	BP > UP	Baron et al., 1975
	BP = UP	Rybakowski et al., 1974b
Prophylaxis	BP = UP	Prien et al., 1973
	BP = UP	Fieve et al., 1976
	BP = UP	Coppen et al., 1976b
RBC: Plasma ratio	BP > UP	Mendels and Frazer, 1973
	BP > UP°	Cazzullo et al., 1975
	BP > UP°	Ramsey et al., 1976
	BP > UP°	Knorring et al., 1976
	BP = UP	Rybakowski et al., 1974a
	BP = UP	Leckman et al. (unpublished data b)
	BP = UP	Elizur et al., 1972

Induction of hypomania or mania:		
L-Dopa	BP > UP°	Murphy et al., 1971
Tricyclics	BP > UP	Bunney et al., 1970a
	BP > UP	Prien et al., 1973
	BP > UP	Coppen et al., 1976a

Antidepressant response:		
L-Tryptophan	BP > UP	Murphy et al., 1974
L-Dopa	BPII > UP	Gershon et al., 1971a
Amphetamine	BP = UP	Fawcett et al., 1972

°Reported UP-BP differences are statistically significant for at least p < .05.

Catecholamine and indoleamine metabolites in the urine and cerebrospinal fluid (CSF) have been widely studied, including urinary 3-methoxy-4-hydroxyphenylglycol (MHPG, a metabolite of norepinephrine), CSF homovanillic acid (HVA, a metabolite of dopamine), and CSF 5-hydroxyindoleacetic acid (5-HIAA, a metabolite of serotonin).

Goodwin and Post (1975) and Schildkraut et al. (1973) found urinary MHPG to be reduced in BP patients compared to UP patients, but Maas et al. (1968) could find no UP-BP difference. Coppen et al. (1972a) found reduced CSF 5-HIAA in BP patients, whereas Ashcroft et al. (1973) found CSF 5-HIAA and HVA reduced in UP patients, and others have found no UP-BP difference (van Praag et al., 1973; Goodwin and Post, 1975). The administration of probenecid inhibits the transport of these metabolites out of the CSF, and accumulation over time is thought to reflect rate of synthesis in the brain. Bowers (1974) reported reduced accumulation of CSF 5-HIAA and HVA in BP patients. Van Praag et al. (1973) could replicate this for 5-HIAA only, and Goodwin and Post (1975) found no significant UP-BP difference for either 5-HIAA or HVA accumulation in the largest sample that has been reported.

Platelet monoamine oxidase (MAO) and erythrocyte catechol-O-methyl transferase (COMT) have been reported to be reduced in depressed patients compared to controls (Murphy and Weiss, 1972; Leckman et al., unpublished data a; Dunner et al., 1971), but other investigators have not confirmed these findings (Nies et al., 1971; Belmaker et al., 1976; Gershon et al., 1975b). Two studies (Murphy and Weiss, 1972; Landowski et al., 1975) found platelet MAO activity reduced in BP patients only, but Nies et al. (1971) found no UP-BP difference in a large heterogeneous sample. Dunner et al. (1971) found COMT activity lower in UP females than in other depressed patients, but later studies have not replicated this finding (Mattson et al., 1974; Gershon et al., 1975b; Dunner et al., in press).

Neuroendocrine differences have also been reported. Sachar et al. (1973) found in an early report that BP patients show greater stimulation of growth hormone and greater suppression of prolactin after L-dopa administration than do UP patients, but this finding did not hold up when they corrected for patient-control sample differences in the number of postmenopausal women (Sachar et al., 1975). Gold et al. (unpublished data a) make the correction and still find a UP-BP difference. It has recently been found (Gold et al., unpublished data b) that TSH response to TRH was blunted in ten UP patients as compared to controls, but enhanced in BP patients. Carroll et al. (1976) report that BP patients resist dexamethasone suppression more than UP patients, but the difference is not statistically significant.

In neurophysiologic studies, Buchsbaum et al. (1971) initially reported that BP patients had a greater augmentation of evoked response than UP patients, but in a later sample this was true of BP males only (Buchsbaum et al., 1973), and recently no UP-BP difference was found at all (Gershon and Buchsbaum, 1976). Sleep studies by Detre et al. (1972) and Kupfer (1976) report more hypersomnia and shortened REM sleep latencies in BP compared to UP patients.

An antidepressant response to L-dopa or L-tryptophan in BP but not UP patients has been reported in one study by Goodwin et al. (1970), but not in other investigations (Bowers, 1970; Dunner and Fieve, 1975). There have also been reports that only depressed UP patients improve on L-tryptophan (Broadhurst, 1970; Coppen et al., 1972b) or L-dopa (Matussek, 1971; Nahunek et al., 1972), but other studies report failure of UP's to respond to either (Gayford et al., 1973; Carroll et al., 1970; Bowers, 1970; Murphy et al., 1973). These conflicting findings with amine precursors in depression weaken the reported UP-BP differences.

Lithium carbonate has been thought to be a specific pharmacologic treatment for bipolar patients. If its effect were limited to BP patients, a unique physiologic disorder would be suggested. More BP patients than UP patients show positive response to lithium when acutely depressed (Goodwin et al., 1972; Noyes et al., 1974; Mendels, 1974; Baron et al., 1975), but both BP and UP groups respond to lithium prophylaxis (Prien et al., 1973; Fieve et al., 1976; Coppen et al., 1976b). Four studies (Mendels and Frazer, 1973; Cazzullo et al., 1975; Ramsey et al., 1976; Knorring et al., 1976) have reported significantly higher RBC : plasma lithium ratios in BP compared to UP patients, but three studies have not (Elizur et al., 1972; Rybakowski et al., 1974a; and Leckman et al., unpublished data a). Recently, Lee et al. (1975) found that the RBC : plasma lithium ratio depended on the absolute plasma lithium value, and that this relation was variable from one subject to another. This finding suggests that the measurement of this ratio may not be a sound predictor of lithium response in depression or be suitable to differentiate subgroups. Nevertheless, recent reports (Casper et al., 1976; Mendels, 1976) continue to find that lithium responders have significantly higher RBC : plasma lithium ratios than lithium nonresponders. Lithium response in acute depression may reveal a true difference among affectively ill groups, and may be a more reliable indicator of subtypes than the UP-BP dichotomy, as suggested by Mendels (1976).

The provocation of mania or hypomania by L-dopa or tricyclic antidepressants has been consistently found more often in BP than in UP patients (Murphy et al., 1971; Bunney et al., 1970a; Prien et al., 1973; Coppen et al., 1976b). The conclusion that this is an underly-

ing UP-BP difference depends on demonstrating that the mania in
the BP patients is not a spontaneous eruption of the previously existing disorder; for tricyclics, such evidence is offered by Prien et al.
(1973), who have an untreated bipolar control group. However, since a
substantial proportion of UP patients can be provoked into mania or
hypomania with tricyclics, the hypothesis that the vulnerability to
manic states is present only in BP patients is not supported, as
reviewed elsewhere (Bunney, personal communication).

To summarize, the biologic data reveal largely nonreplicable differences between bipolar and unipolar patients. Clinical pharmacologic response data show more reproducible differences, but the
degree of BP-UP overlap in lithium response and provocation of
mania by tricyclics suggests that if there is an underlying bio-
logic/pharmacologic dichotomy, it does not coincide well with the
UP/BP clinical dichotomy. Much of the biologic and pharmacologic
data summarized in Tables 2 and 3 are most consistent in the BP vs.
controls findings, whereas the findings on UP patients are more variable, suggesting that BP illness may be a more homogeneous entity
than UP. No unique biologic or pharmacologic characteristic is as-
signable to one but not the other type of illness.

Strategies to Elucidate Biologic Basis of BP/UP Differences.
Let us consider two general classes of hypothesis which might account for phenotypic overlap of UP and BP illness. A common genetic diathesis for both UP and BP illness, in which BP illness occurs
in individuals with a greater genetic and environmental load, is one
possibility. In this case, biologic and pharmacologic differences would
be greatest between BP patients and controls, with UP patients falling
in between any given variable. An alternative hypothesis of at least
two distinct genotypes, one of which could be phenotypically variable
(manifest as either BP or UP illness), allowing for UP-BP heterogeneity in twin pairs and families, could also be considered. In this case,
there would be no a priori expectations on the biologic differences between UP and BP illness; however, we would anticipate at least two
kinds of UP persons—one of whom is genetically (and biologically)
related to BP illness, and others who are not. In either case we could
predict biologic and pharmacologic variables which distinguish between subtypes.

Several investigators (Winokur, 1972; Fieve, 1973; Kupfer et al.,
1975; Mendels, 1976) have suggested that a subgroup of UP patients
may be genetically and biologically related to BP patients. The
presence of mania in the family history of UP patients may be a distinguishing characteristic between UP patient subgroups. This hypothesis has not been adequately tested. Kupfer et al. (1975) have

reported on two groups of UP patients, one of which they state is related to BP patients in terms of positive response to lithium carbonate, personality variables, and family history features (history of mood swings in relatives). The authors did not interview relatives directly, and the nature of the mood swings they report is uncertain. More rigorous biologic and pharmacologic investigations of UP illness in BP families vs. UP illness in families with no history of mania are required.

Other Subdivisions of UP Illness.   Another variable which may be a transmitted factor in affective illness is the age of onset. A younger age of onset (before 40 years of age) is associated with an increased morbid risk for affective illness in first degree relatives of UP and BP patients, as reviewed by Gershon et al. (1976). Winokur (1974) and Winokur et al. (1971) have used age of onset to define two subgroups of UP illness.

Winokur et al. (1971) exclude UP probands with BP illness in their families from their analyses and by so doing assume they belong to a different genotypic grouping. They describe a "depression spectrum disease" in early onset probands, and pure depressive disease in late onset probands. The former is characterized by a female with early onset of illness, alcoholism among primary male relatives, and more depression in female than male relatives. The latter is characterized by a late onset male with no familial increase of alcoholism and equal amounts of depression in male and female relatives.

The finding of high prevalence of alcoholism and sociopathy and greater morbid risk for affective illness in relatives of early onset probands compared to relatives of late onset probands has been reported in studies of 1255 probands (Cadoret, 1976).

Shields (1975) has reanalyzed clinical-genetic material collected by Slater in 1938 and finds that within the unipolar group the number of relatives with alcoholism, sociopathy, or hysteria was similar for male and female probands (0.27 and 0.32, respectively) and for those with onset before and after age 40 (0.31 cases per proband). These data, collected in Berlin before World War II, suggest that the American studies may be defining cultural rather than genetic factors.

In order to prove that early onset in the proband can delineate a genetic entity, it would be necessary to show that ill relatives also had early onset. Neither Winokur et al. (1975) nor Gershon et al. (1975b) could find this relationship. However, Winokur did find a statistically significant association of late onset of illness in relatives of late onset probands. Thus the findings so far reported are inconclusive and cannot support a hypothesis that depression spectrum disease and pure depressive disease are separable genotypes. The finding of alcoholism associated with early onset unipolar depression is of interest and suggests an underlying relationship between these disorders, as discussed below.

Subdivisions of BP Illness.   The presence of bipolar subgroups further complicates the biologic studies of UP and BP disorders. Dunner et al. (1976) describe two BP types: BPI (evidence of mania) and BPII (evidence of hypomania). This group reported differential responses to L-dopa and differences in platelet MAO and 17-OH corticosteroid excretion between BPI and BPII groups. BPII patients had significantly higher suicide rates. The age of onset for BPII illness is between the younger onset of BPI and the later onset UP illness. Gershon et al. (1971b) noted that the antidepressant response to L-dopa previously reported had occurred in BPII (n = 5) patients only. Family studies have not as yet been applied to this subdivision of bipolar patients.

Further subdivisions of the UP-BP dichotomy have been proposed (Fieve, 1973; Mendels, 1976), but controlled biochemical or pharmacologic studies to support them have not yet been reported. The possibility of developing other subgroups of affectively ill patients based on clinical (severity, age of onset, personality variables), biochemical (neurotransmitter metabolite or enzyme differences), or pharmacologic (lithium or other drug responsiveness) criteria is promising, as is discussed later in this review.

Although the UP-BP dichotomy appears not to define two distinct genetic entities, polarity is a transmitted characteristic of affective illness, and some UP patients share the same transmitted vulnerability as some BP patients. Subdivisions of UP and BP illness do not appear as firmly established.

Is There a Genetic Spectrum of Affective Illnesses? — Clinical Evidence

It has been repeatedly shown that certain specific psychiatric disorders occur with greater frequency in the families of patients with affective disorders or schizophrenia than in the families of controls (Schulsinger, 1976; Gershon et al., 1971b; Winokur et al., 1975). From a genetic viewpoint we are interested in whether a whole spectrum of clinical pathologies is transmitted within families of patients with affective illness and whether this accounts for the apparent reduced penetrance in the affective disorders. To demonstrate that a spectrum of illnesses is transmitted along with a given type of major affective illness, it is required that the same type of major affective illness be seen in the relatives and that each proposed entity in the spectrum also be more frequent. Let us call a disorder within the spectrum a related disorder. Transmission of related disorders within families, rather than clinical or phenomenologic similarity, is the criterion for defining related disorders within a spectrum, although transmission of biologic and pharmacologic variables is also of interest.

Disorders found in the co-twin of monozygotic twin pairs with affective illness are clearly related to the same genetic predisposition, assuming there is one. Enough unipolar-bipolar monozygotic twin pairs have been demonstrated to infer that these disorders are related in at least some cases (Perris, 1974b), as noted above.

Alcoholism was found to be increased in relatives of early-onset unipolar patients as compared with late onset, in studies by Winokur and his colleagues in St. Louis (Winokur, 1974). However, elsewhere in the United States, Dunner et al. (1976) found no increased alcoholism in families of bipolar or unipolar patients as compared with control families, although there was an increase in families of bipolar II patients. Helzer and Winokur (1974) found an increase in alcoholism in relatives of male bipolar probands, but Morrison (1975) found no increase in alcoholism in families of bipolar patients unless the patient was himself alcoholic. Gershon (1975b) reported no increase in alcoholism in families of unipolar or bipolar patients in Israel.

In studying affective disorder in the relatives of alcoholics, Winokur et al. (1970) reported on morbid risk for affective disorder of 14 percent in first degree relatives of 259 alcoholic probands. However, as their Table 1 (p. 107) illustrates, only 176 of the 259 had a primary diagnosis of alcoholism. Schuckit et al. (1969) found that affective disorder was frequently found in the first degree relatives of alcoholics. However, when relatives of 39 primary alcoholics were compared to 19 alcoholic probands with a pre-existing affective illness, there was a significantly larger number of affective illness in the relatives of this latter group (17.1 percent) than in the relatives of index cases with primary alcoholism (6.5 percent, p <.01). The population prevalence of affective disorder reported by these investigators is 2.7 percent (Winokur and Pitts, 1965).

In addition to the apparent role of alcoholism as part of the spectrum of affective disorder, these data suggest that alcoholism in families of patients with affective disorder may result from culturally conditioned or independent genetic factors producing alcoholism. For this reason, the presence of alcoholism in relatives of specific types of affective disorders in some studies does not necessarily suggest that these types of affective disorders are genetically distinct.

Schizoaffective disorder has numerous synonyms, including cycloid psychosis and atypical psychosis (Perris, 1974a). In a chart-review twin study, Cohen et al. (1972) found no cases of primary affective disorder, schizoaffective illness, and process schizophrenia in which one twin (monozygotic or dizygotic) had one of the three illnesses and the co-twin had another. However, increases of schizoaffective disorder (Angst, 1966) or acute psychosis (Gershon et al., 1975b) have been found in relatives of affective disorder patients. Perris (1974b), in a family study of schizoaffective illness, also found a specific increase in schizoaffective and not other disorders in the relatives. McCabe and Cadoret (1976) reviewed seven family studies of schizoaffective patients which showed, in aggregate, prevalence in relatives of 3.6 percent affective disorder, 2.9 percent atypical psychosis, and 2.5 percent schizophrenia. Genetic heterogeneity of schizoaffective disorders may be implied by these figures, because there are slight elevations of morbid risk of all three disorders but not to the degree found in relatives of affective disorder or process schizophrenia probands. Tsuang et al. (1976) in a chart-review study reports that atypical psychotics with affective features and/or a history of remitting illness have elevated affective illness in their relatives (7.6 percent) as compared with relatives of schizophrenics (3.1 percent).

We would conclude that some cases of schizoaffective illness are manifestations of the familial tendency to affective disorder, but that this disorder is not found exclusively or even predominantly in the spectrum of affective illness.

Minor depressive episodes which are symptomatic but do not meet criteria for unipolar illness are more frequent in families of persons with affective disorder than in controls (Gershon et al., 1975b), although mild depressive personality disturbances do not appear to be genetically transmitted (Price, 1968; Gershon et al., 1975b).

The cyclothymic personality, consisting of mild but recurrent elevations and depressions in mood state, has long been noted in the relatives of patients with affective disorder (Kallmann, 1950, 1954). In a recent study this entity was found almost exclusively in relatives of affective disorder patients, but not in relatives of controls (Gershon et al., 1975b).

These two entities, minor depression and cyclothymic personality, appear to be part of the spectrum of affective illness, and the hypothesis of a shared genetic diathesis with affective disorder has been supported by genetic models (Gershon et al., 1975a) (see below). These entities should have biologic and pharmacologic similarities with major affective disorder if they indeed share the same genetic diathesis.

Other syndromes with clinical manifestations of hyperactivity or labile mood are hyperkinetic syndrome of childhood (HSC) and the emotionally unstable character disorder (EUCD), an adolescent syndrome described by Rifkin et al. (1972, a, b). In adopted children with HSC, affective disorder was not more frequent in biologic than in adoptive families (Stewart and Morrison, 1973; Cantwell, 1975). To our knowledge, data on frequency of HSC in children of patients with affective disorder have not been published. In a case report, two unrelated hyperkinetic children of lithium-responsive bipolar parents were themselves responders to lithium for hyperkinesis in an uncontrolled open drug evaluation (Dyson and Barcai, 1970). The pharmacogenetic strategy of unmasking a spectrum illness is a valid innovation (Liebowitz et al., 1976), but systematic pharmacologic design with double-blind crossover methodology is required to accept the demonstration of a biologically related disorder.

EUCD, one of three personality disorders recognized by Rifkin et al. (1972a) has been characterized as showing a "prominence of persistent, transient, fluctuating symptoms of depression and hypomania." It has been hypothesized by these authors that there is a relationship between this personality disorder and affective illness because of the observed clinical similarity of the two conditions and because of the favorable therapeutic response to lithium carbonate by patients diagnosed as emotionally unstable character disorder (Rifkin et al., 1972c). There has not yet been a family study of EUCD to determine if affective illness is frequently seen in the families of EUCD probands.

Suicide as an entity associated with affective illness was examined by Perris (1966). It was his finding that the mortality rate for bipolar plus unipolar patients was higher than the population and that suicide as a cause of death was higher than the suicide rate in the general population. Suicide in the first degree relatives of bipolar, unipolar, and manic probands occurred more frequently than in the general population.

Examination of suicide rates in the relatives of manic-depressives by Zvolsky (1973) showed the rate as 7.3 percent, as compared to a general population figure in Sweden of 1.5 percent. Dunner et al. (1976) found that relatives of bipolar II patients showed a higher morbid risk for suicide than unipolar or bipolar I patients, although the difference was not statistically significant. Gershon et al. (1975b) reported that the relatives who committed suicide themselves had major affective illness diagnoses.

Winokur et al. (1971) investigated morbid risk for sociopathy in the primary relatives of 100 depressive probands. Here, probands were divided into categories by sex and by age at onset of depression. In early onset females, there was more depression in female relatives than in male relatives. The discrepancy is "compensated for," as those authors state, by the appearance of alcoholism *or* sociopathy in the male relatives.

Sociopathy appeared in the relatives of early onset probands. Specifically, the morbid risk was 9 percent in the male relatives and 4 percent in the female relatives of early onset female probands (Winokur et al., 1971). These data implicate sociopathy as a possible spectrum entity, but other studies do not find this (Gershon et al., 1975a).

Guze et al. (1967) looked at the occurrence of manic-depressive disease in 519 first degree relatives of male criminals. The prevalence of manic-depression was given as 4 percent, with women being affected more often than men. The authors suggest that because these subjects were not asked to report disability or medical attention resulting from these depressions, it is difficult to ascertain if the reported cases of depression differ from rates in the general population. Hutchings and Mednick (1975) also examined incidence of manic-depressive psychoses in the biologic parents of criminal and noncriminal male probands. Again, the results showed no association between manic-depression and criminality.

Although alcoholism and sociopathy may be related to certain types of primary affective disorders, these disorders do not appear to be consistently found in relatives of early onset UP probands only. The early onset criterion, as defined by Winokur et al. (1971), does not appear to be consistently transmitted as an entity in family members, as discussed earlier. Considering this, it would seem that Winokur's spectrum may not be identifying a genetically homogeneous group; it may be that only a subgroup of primary affective disorders is related to alcoholism or sociopathy, but the definition of this subgroup remains to be established.

To summarize, a spectrum of pathology has been hypothesized in the transmission of major affective illness. The disorders that have been observed in association with affective disease include alcoholism, minor depression, and cyclothymic personality. The occurrence of suicide also has been linked to affective illness more often than it appears to occur in the general population. Some cases of schizoaffective disorder also appear to be transmitted with affective illness but appear independently as well.

For a related disorder to fit genetic hypotheses, it must fit a model of transmission for affective disorder, share biologic or pharmacologic characteristics, and be linked to the same chromosomal markers as major affective illness.

It is possible that we look at the tip of an iceberg in studying major affective illnesses in relatives of patients. The development of a well-defined spectrum should enable us to better test genetic hypotheses for transmission of illness, by reducing the nonpenetrance or nonheritable variance in genetic models. Also a rational and testable basis of pharmacotherapy of certain disorders in the relatives of patients with affective illness is offered by the clinical spectrum of disorders in relatives.

MATHEMATICAL MODELS OF INHERITANCE OF UNIPOLAR AND BIPOLAR ILLNESS

Mathematical models of genetic transmission applied to family study data may help answer salient questions in the genetics of affective illness. These questions include the following:

1. Do the differences in morbid risk between families of UP and BP probands imply that the two entities are genetically distinct, or is the hypothesis tenable that BP and UP illness are two forms of the same disease that differ in (genetic) severity?

2. Is there a spectrum of other disorders associated with the major affective illnesses, which is transmitted by the same genetic process?

3. Is BP illness transmitted at a single X-chromosome locus?

4. Can an autosomal transmission sex-effect model account for the sex differences in rates of illness in the population and in relatives of patients?

By a genetic model we mean a set of hypotheses which specify the mode of genetic transmission of a characteristic, and the expected genotype (or genetic loading in MF inheritance) in randomly sampled patients, controls, and each type of relative, and based on these hypotheses specify the expected prevalences of illness in the population and in the various classes of relatives. As we have noted elsewhere (Gershon et al., 1975a), "In all-or-none disease states in which the proportion of affected relatives is lower than predicted by classical mendelian ratios, a penetrance variable must be introduced into genetic analyses [based on a single major locus (SML)]. Analysis of prevalences in relatives in such data does not permit a unique solution (SML) inheritance, since the number of parameters that can be derived from the observations is less than the number of genetic parameters (James, 1971). For multifactorial (MF) inheritance, such data would constitute an untestable genetic model (Reich et al., 1972).

"A solution to this dilemma is enabled by the substitution of a hypothetical quantitative variable for the qualitative diagnosis, as in recent developments of models of continuously variable liability to disease states (Falconer, 1965). In these models, a liability to the disease state exists for every person. This liability consists of a linear combination of genetic and random (presumably environmental) components. In every case in which the value of this liability passes a threshold, the disease state is manifest. Liability is defined to be normally distributed in MF inheritance, and normally distributed around a mean liability for each genotype in SML inheritance. The assumption of a threshold of liability does not, in itself, produce a testable genetic model (James, 1971; Reich et al., 1972; Kidd and Cavalli-Sforza, 1972), but with the introduction of additional threshold(s) to the liability continuum, testable models are produced (Reich et al., 1972). In the psychiatric disorders, such additional thresholds may be provided by intermediate states between illness and health, or by demarcation of states of greater and lesser severity of liability. The definition of states of different severity of liability within the major affective disorders may be possible by use of the UP-BP distinction among patients with affective illness, as discussed below (Gershon et al., 1975a).

If UP and BP affective disorders were fitted to such a model, one implication would be that the UP relatives of BP patients are indistinguishable from other UP patients, both clinically and biologically. This implication is testable and may allow distinction of single and multiple genetic diatheses even when a multiple threshold model fits the observed prevalences.

To test this type of model, the multidimensional parameter space is searched for the set of parameter values which predict prevalences in relatives of patients and in the population that best fit those prevalences actually observed. The goodness-of-fit of the observed and predicted values is the test of whether the model can be rejected or not.

The models tested to this time explicitly assume that the disorder evaluated is not a mixture of genetically distinct entities. Models of two independent genetic entities causing clinically indistinguishable disorders are apparently indeterminate in the absence of some marker to distinguish the two forms.

The question whether UP and BP are related entities with a shared genetic diathesis was tested as the hypothesis that BP and UP illness represent different thresholds on the same genetic-environmental liability scale (Fig. 1). This hypothesis could be tested in the data of only three investigations (Perris, 1966; Angst, 1966; Gershon et al., 1975b), because other family studies did not have random

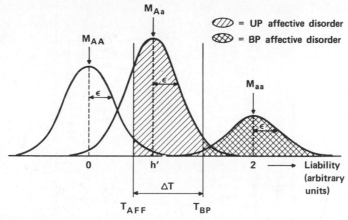

Figure 1. Parameters of single major locus model with two alleles (adapted from Kidd et al., unpublished data). Horizontal axis is a scale of liability to a disorder, which is a function of genetic and independent (random or environmental) components. Thresholds shown are for affective disorders, in which T_{AFF} = threshold for all affective illness, and T_{BP} = threshold for bipolar illness. M_{AA}, M_{Aa} and M_{aa} are the mean liability values for each genotype. ϵ is the square root of the independent (random or environmental) variance of liability, which in the model shown has the same value for each genotype. h' is the liability value for the heterozygote Aa; the liability values for the homozygotes are set at arbitrary values of 0 and 2. For each genotype, the hatched and crosshatched areas represent the proportion of persons with that genotype who will have unipolar (UP) or bipolar (BP) affective disorder.

sampling of patients for both BP and UP illness. An acceptable fit of two-threshold models of autosomal SML and MF inheritance could be found with the data of Angst and of Gershon et al., but not with the data of Perris (Gershon et al., 1975a) (Table 4).

Spectrum disorders, if they are manifestations of the same diathesis as UP and BP illness, should fit the same genetic model. This could be tested in the data of Gershon et al. (1975b), in which moderate depression, cyclothymic personality, and undiagnosed single episodes of acute psychosis were more prevalent in the families of UP and BP patients than in families of controls. A third threshold for these disorders was introduced into the SML and MF genetic models, which remained compatible with the additional data, lending this model further plausibility (Gershon et al., 1975a).

Hypotheses of a single genetic diathesis to affective illness, which produces either BP or UP disorder according to the net genetic and random liability of an individual, are thus compatible with some but not all of the family study data in these disorders. The data of Perris, with which these hypotheses are incompatible, are problematic in that the classification system excludes many secondary cases of depression. Successful application of a threshold model

Table 4. Threshold Models of Affective Disorder[*]

Patients Studied:	UP and BP Probands and Their Relatives		BP Probands and Their Relatives		
Mode of Transmission:	Single Major Locus (Autosomal)	Multifactorial	X-Chromosome Single Locus		
Model:	Multiple Thresholds	Multiple Thresholds	I. One Threshold for BP Only	II. One Threshold for Both BP and UP	III. Two Thresholds; BP and UP Have Separate Thresholds
Data:					
Gershon et al., 1975b	Fits	Fits	Fits	No fit	No fit
Winokur et al., 1969	Insufficient data	Insufficient data	Fits	Fits	Fits
Mendlewicz and Rainer, 1974	Insufficient data	Insufficient data	Insufficient data	No fit	Insufficient data
Angst, 1966	Fits	Fits	Insufficient data	Insufficient data	Insufficient data
Perris, 1966	No fit	No fit	Insufficient data	Insufficient data	Insufficient data

[*]Adapted from Gershon et al. (1975a) and van Eerdewegh et al. (1976).

demonstrates only that the genetic hypotheses tested cannot be ruled out, but does not imply that only the applied model is true.

It is of interest to apply alternate models, of X-chromosome transmission and of sex-effects, to family study data on affective illness. These models can predict different prevalences according to sex, as is found in population studies, but which is not predicted by the models tested so far. By sex-effect, we mean a tendency of one sex to be more likely to manifest an illness with a given amount of genetic and environmental predisposition. In threshold models this is represented by different thresholds for males and females, and can be applied in X-chromosome and autosomal (SML or MF) transmission models.

The hypothesis that in families of BP patients both BP and UP illness are transmitted at a single locus on the X-chromosome is of much current interest, as discussed above. Three forms of the hypothesis have been tested (van Eerdewegh et al., 1976):

Model I — one threshold for BP illness: Only two psychiatric states are defined: BP and not-BP. Unipolar illness is not explicitly considered in this model; it need not be related to liability to BP illness. One advantage of this model is that it would not be falsified by the presence of multiple sources of UP illness in relatives of BP patients (i.e., if UP illness from purely environmental causes, and as a separate genetic illness, and as a manifestation of the same genetic diathesis that causes BP were all found in BP families).

Model II — one threshold for UP and BP illness: UP and BP forms are genetically and environmentally identical (within families of BP probands) meaning they have the same genetic loading and express themselves at the same liability scale values. This model is an underlying assumption for all reported linkage studies (Winokur et al., 1969; Mendlewicz et al., 1972, 1975; Mendlewicz and Fleiss, 1974). Model II and Model I are exactly opposite hypotheses (from a logical point of view) concerning the UP form of the illness.

Model III — two thresholds for UP and BP illness: This model assumes that UP and BP illness share the same genetic diathesis, but express themselves at 2 different liability scale values, similar to the autosomal SML model in Figure 1.

Three sets of published family study data on BP illness contained sufficient information on probands and relatives according to sex, and used acceptable diagnostic criteria (Winokur et al., 1969; Mendlewicz and Rainer, 1974; Gershon et al., 1975b). Because of heterogeneity of data, each set of data was tested separately.

Considering bipolar illness only (Model I), the X-chromosome hypothesis was compatible with the two studies in which it could be tested (Table 4). However, the X-chromosome hypotheses of BP illness which included UP illness in relatives fit the data of Winokur but not Gershon (Models II and III) or Mendlewicz (Model II). The incompatibility of Mendlewicz data with X-chromosome transmission was largely due to a high proportion of father-son transmission of illness. This implies that if there were an X-chromosome transmission subgroup in the population studied by Mendlewicz et al. (1972), Mendlewicz and Fleiss (1974), and Mendlewicz et al. (unpublished data), it could represent only a fraction of all bipolar illness. In view of this, it is puzzling that the informative pedigrees from this sample are remarkably uniform in their apparent close linkage to the X-chromosome markers studied.

Bipolar affective illness afflicts more women than men in most studies, as reviewed elsewhere (Gershon et al., 1976). In autosomal transmission models, it is necessary to invoke a sex-effect on liability threshold or some other protective mechanism that makes men less likely than women to manifest illness, given a certain genetic predisposition (Reich et al., 1975). X-chromosome transmission, on the other hand, can account for male-female differences on the basis of differences between the number of men and women in the population with the allele for illness, but a sex-effect on liability threshold may still be considered.

Using the X-chromosome transmission models described above, introduction of a sex-effect did not result in a better fit of the model to any of the data sets studied. However, there were differences from the no-sex-effect models in the penetrances of specific genotypes.

A one-threshold model of autosomal transmission, whether SML or MF, is indeterminate as noted above. Introducing two thresholds through a sex-effect allows best-fit parameters to be determined (Kidd et al., unpublished data; Kidd and Spence, 1976), but makes it difficult to interpret whether the sex-effect has improved the fit of the model to the data. We therefore considered that if there was overlap within the limits of error of the male and female thresholds, a sex-effect was not necessary in the data. Leckman and Gershon (1976) found such overlap for the data of Gershon, Mendlewicz, and Winokur, and also for data published by Goetzl et al. (1974). There was one published data set (James and Chapman, 1975) with large sex-discrepancies between the morbid risks in relatives of male vs. female probands, in which introduction of sex-effect autosomal SML and MF models gave very close fit to the data. With this exception, autosomal sex-effect models do not account for the sex-differences in affective illness in bipolar families.

For each of the models discussed here, at least one study was found in which the model could be *excluded*. It is possible that none of the models so far tested is correct, perhaps because of genetic heterogeneity of illnesses included in "affective illness," or penetrance factors not appreciated in our models. On the other hand, there may be genetic and environmental differences between populations studied, which result in a particular model being generally valued in one population but not another. In this case, we could still require that interpretation of biologic data from a particular population not rest on assumptions that can be ruled out in that population using genetic models, as in the case of the X-linkage data discussed above. This constraint on the interpretation of biologic and chromosomal linkage data may be the major current application of threshold models in the mood disorders.

STUDIES OF LINKAGE TO CHROMOSOMAL MARKERS

The demonstration of linkage of affective illness with a known genetic marker would be more compelling evidence for a genetic factor in these disorders, as well as demonstrate the mode of transmission. Studies of linkage to autosomal and X-linked marker genes have been reported.

Autosomal Linkage Studies

Studies of the ABO blood group system have yielded conflicting reports of associations with affective illness. Parker et al. (1961) reported an association of manic-depressive illness with blood group O, which was replicated by one study (Masters, 1967). Irvine and Miyashita (1965) could not find a blood group association in manic-depressive illness, but reported an association of blood group O in involutional melancholia. Tanna and Winokur (1968), however, found type B associated with affectively ill probands who had positive family histories of affective illness, but no group O association. Other studies (Thomas and Hewitt, 1939; Van Eerdewegh et al., unpublished data) fail to show any association of blood type with affective illness. Blood group studies may be complicated by racial and geographic stratification, which can account for differences of 5 to 20 percent within the population of the same locale (Manuila and Lexander, 1958), as well as sampling and technical errors. ABO blood type associations with affective illness appear unlikely at this time.

Interest in the HLA tissue antigen system has been stimulated by reports of association of certain HLA alleles with neurologic and rheumatoid diseases (Svejgaard et al., 1975). A finding of HLA association with affective illness would implicate changes on the cell membrane surface, as well as suggest a role of immunity in the development of affective illness (Svejgaard and Ryder, 1976). Associations of HLA antigens with schizophrenia (Eberhard et al., 1975; Cazzullo et al., 1974) and affective disorders have been reported, but there is no agreement about which alleles are involved.

In a study of 47 affectively ill patients, Shapiro et al. (1976) reported increased BW16, B7, A3, and decreased B8. Eight out of 20 BP patients had BW16, a highly significant association. Bennahum et al. (1975) initially reported no statistically significant associations of HLA with affective illness in 12 BP patients against 67 controls. When they added 4 more BP patients, they reported (Bennahum et al., unpublished data) an increased BW17. Interestingly, none of the 16 patients had BW16. This group was not divided by polarity. Stember and Fieve (1976) report a significant increase of HLA-B5 and B13 in a group of 50 affectively ill patients, and HLA-B12 in a group of 31 bipolar patients, compared to 250 normal controls (Table 5).

Table 5. Reported HLA Associations with Affective Illness

Author	N	Locus	Antigen	Patient Diagnosis	
Stember and Fieve, 1976					250 normal controls
	50	B	5	UP + BP	P = n.s.
	31	B	12	BP only	n.s.
	50	B	13	UP + BP	n.s.
Bennahum et al., 1975					67 normal controls
	12	B	W15	BP	P = n.s.
	12	B	W17	BP	n.s.
	12	A	W10	BP	n.s.
Bennahum et al., 1976					67 normal controls
	16	B	W17	BP	P = n.s.
Shapiro et al., 1976					1967 normal controls
	47	B	W16	UP + BP	P = n.s.
	20	B	W16	BP only	P < .01
	47	A	3	UP + BP	n.s.
	47	B	7	UP + BP	n.s.
	47	B	8*	UP + BP	n.s.
van Eerdewegh et al. (unpublished)					300 normal controls
	57	B	W16	BP	P = n.s.
	57	B	W17	BP	n.s.

*Reported decreased antigen in diagnostic group.

A study at NIMH has thus far been unable to demonstrate any HLA association with affective illness in 57 probands, although a nonsignificant increase in HLA BW17 was noted (van Eerdewegh et al., unpublished data).

In comparing the frequencies of multiple antigens, the possibility of type 1 errors (rejecting the null hypothesis because of deviation owing to chance) is increased. To correct for these errors, the appropriate statistical corrections should be introduced (Svejgaard et al., 1974). No correction was made in the aforementioned studies. When a correction is applied, multiplying the observed probability value by the number of antigens tested, only the finding of BW16 in bipolar patients vs. controls ($p < 0.01$) in the study of Shapiro et al. remains statistically significant. The absence of HL-A BW16 in any of the 16 cases of Bennahum et al. raises questions about the replicability and about the racial and geographic distribution of this finding.

Recently, Tanna et al. (1976) reported on the possibility of linkage of depression spectrum disease with α-haptoglobin and complement component C3. These two loci are apparently on different chromosomes. Tanna et al. (1976) employed a sib-pair paradigm which they analyzed by a single 2×2 contingency table of all families studied pooled together, which is not a valid analytic method for sib-pair data. Complement components Bf, C2, and C4 have been reported to be associated with the HLA complex; however, linkage studies have not supported this association for C3 variants (C3^F and C3^S) (Svejgaard et al., 1975).

With the exception of an abnormality in taurine metabolism presenting as depression (Perry et al., 1975), there has not been demonstrated a consistent association of a known autosomal genetic marker with affective illness. Pedigree studies would reveal if the reported associations are actually transmitted with affective illness in families.

Linkage to X-Chromosome Markers

Based on their earlier family studies which were compatible with X-chromosome transmission in bipolar illness, Winokur and his colleagues were the first to present evidence using genetic linkage markers to support this hypothesis (Winokur and Tanna, 1969; Reich et al., 1969). A larger series of informative families was recently reported by Mendlewicz and his coworkers (Mendlewicz et al., 1972; Mendlewicz and Fleiss, 1974; Mendlewicz et al., unpublished data).

Combining theirs and Winokur's data, they concluded that in families of BP patients, affective illness is closely linked to protan and deutan color blindness, and that linkage to the Xg blood group is also present. Since families were excluded from analysis if there was apparent father-son transmission, these authors qualified their conclusion as being applicable to a subgroup of patients with BP illness.

These reported data are problematic, and the presence of linkage may be seriously questioned, as we have reviewed elsewhere (Gershon and Bunney, in press) for these reasons:

1. The reported close linkage of bipolar illness to *both* Xg and the protan-deutan region of the X-chromosome is not compatible with the known large chromosomal map distance between the Xg locus and the protan-deutan region. Recent cell culture studies of translocated chromosomes find that Xg is on the short arm of the X-chromosome and that the color-blind loci are at the distal end of the long arm (Pearson et al., 1975, Fig. 2). The enzyme HPRT (hypoxanthine guanine phosphoribosyl transferase) is on the long arm of the X-chromosome, closer to the centromere (and therefore closer to the short arm) than G6PD. Yet family studies show too much recombination to map HPRT either in relation to G6PD–color blindness (Pearson et al., 1975) or to the Xg locus (Nyhan et al., 1967), which implies that G6PD and Xg must be too distant from each other for a third locus to be observably linked to both. The same conclusion follows from direct studies of Xg and color blindness. Let θ be the maximum likelihood estimate of the recombination fraction. Renwick and Schulze (1964) reviewed 34 families informative for Xg and color blindness and found as a maximum likelihood estimate $\theta = 0.42$ with a lod score of +0.148. The statistical nature of the lod score is such that these estimates do not support the presence of observable linkage at this high recombination fraction, but they do allow much smaller values of θ to be rejected (Morton, 1955). Specifically, the implied map distance between Xg and color blindness (from the reported linkage of both to BP illness) is 26 map units, which is outside the 95 percent lower confidence limit for the same map distance derived from the Xg–color blindness recombination rate by Renwick and Schulze (1964). BP illness could be closely linked to either Xg or protan-deutan region, but not to both.

2. One assumption underlying the reported analysis is that in families of BP probands, UP and BP are equally likely manifestations of a single X-chromosome allele. This assumption can be tested as a hypothesis and rejected, using genetic models, for the population from which the bulk of reported cases are drawn as discussed above (van Eerdewegh et al., 1976). If this assumption were true only for a

subgroup of families, one would not expect the remarkable uniformity in pedigrees reported from this same population, in which virtually all the informative families appear to fit the assumption (Mendlewicz and Fleiss, 1974). Another problem lies in the use of the linkage analysis method of Edwards (1971), which requires assumption of complete penetrance and nonvariable age of onset in affective illness. This may introduce distortions in the estimated values of θ and in the lod scores.

3. A surprising finding in the families informative for color blindness and BP illness is that all 11 male probands are color-blind. If there were complete ascertainment of color blindness in the first degree relatives of probands, the expectation is that coupling (ill persons not color-blind) and repulsion (ill persons color-blind) should be equally likely in the probands and in the pedigrees. The finding that all male probands are in repulsion, and that the relatives of female probands also tend to be in repulsion (even though coupling or repulsion cannot be directly observed in the female probands), suggests an association rather than a linkage, or possibly a defective sampling process such that probands and families where color-blind persons were ill were more likely to be ascertained. If either explanation were correct, chromosomal linkage could not be concluded from these data. An association of color blindness with BP illness would be of great interest, but there is not an excess of color-blind persons among patients with affective disorder (Mendlewicz et al., 1972).

It appears that to conclude that BP affective disorder is linked to either color blindness or Xg, or to both, would be premature.

BIOLOGIC STRATEGIES IN THE GENETICS OF AFFECTIVE DISORDERS

The application of genetic models and chromosomal linkage markers to current data have not, to this time, given unequivocal answers to the questions of how the affective disorders are transmitted and whether they are genetically homogeneous. Apparently, we require delineation of an observable biologic basis of these disorders to make further progress with these genetic questions. Ideally we would seek a biologic variant (such as an altered protein) that could be assigned a specific locus on an identifiable chromosome. However, since stable biochemical differences suggest genetic differences (Stewart and Elston, 1973; Childs, 1976), virtually any biologic finding that was clearly associated with the tendency to affective illness in a subgroup of patients might be studied as a possible genetic marker. Perhaps surprisingly, the converse is also valid: genetic strategies may be used to demonstrate the validity of a particular biologic basis for affective disorders, even in the absence of an established mechanism of genetic transmission. In this section we will consider (1) biologic research strategies that may be applied in pedigree studies in a heterogeneous disorder with variable penetrance and (2) some biologic findings in the affective disorders, especially with regard to application of these research strategies.

Pedigree Methods for Biologic Studies of Psychiatric Illness

Consider a heterogeneous disorder, in which numerous independent biologic deficits can each produce apparently identical cases of a clinical disorder. Let us call each deficit a necessary factor. A person with a necessary factor has an increased likelihood of showing the disorder, but this likelihood is not 100 percent because of random factors, variable age of onset, and the like. Let us allow also for genetically transmitted contributing factors. Contributing factors are defined as those which increase the likelihood that a person has the clinical disorder *only* if a necessary factor is already present; otherwise, they do not affect this likelihood.

Following these definitions, a characteristic can be investigated as a possible genetic marker of vulnerability to an illness if it meets certain prior qualifications. (1) The characteristic must be associated with an increased likelihood of the psychiatric illness. (The converse, that persons with the illness should generally show the characteristic, need not be true, because there may be biologic heterogeneity in the illness.) (2) It must be heritable and must not be a secondary effect of the illness. (3) It must be observable (or evocable) in the well state, so that it is possible to determine its presence independently of the illness and possible to evaluate well relatives.

However, meeting these criteria still is not enough to demonstrate that a biologic characteristic is a necessary or contributing genetic factor in an illness; we must also demonstrate *nonindependent assortment with the illness within pedigrees*. That is, the transmission of the illness and the transmission of the characteristic must be related within pedigrees. The basis of pedigree study is the presumption of homogeneity of illness within pedigrees (Cavalli-Sforza and Bodmer, 1971; Rieder and Gershon, unpublished data; Haldane, 1949), which allows even rare causes of illness to be identified as genetic factors. This presumption has been considered elsewhere

Table 6. Single Sib Paradigm for the Evaluation of Hypothesis that Factor X Is Genetically Related to a Psychiatric Illness*

Sibs of ill probands with factor X	% ill
Sibs with factor X	A
Sibs without factor X	B
Tests of genetic relation to psychiatric illness	*Expected finding*
When factor X is a primary genetic factor in the illness	A > B ≤ population incidence
When factor X is a contributing genetic factor	A > B > population incidence
When factor X is of no importance in the genetics of the illness	A = B ≥ population incidence

*Adapted from Rieder and Gershon, unpublished data.

(Rieder and Gershon, unpublished data), where it is demonstrated that falsely positive conclusions will not follow from its use in this model.

An example of a general investigative strategy (Rieder and Gershon, unpublished data) for pedigree studies of this kind is to sample a large number of unrelated ill probands who have "factor X." We hypothesize that factor X is a genetic factor in the illness, and have prior knowledge that it meets the three criteria outlined above. We then examine one randomly sampled sibling of each proband, and look at the rate of psychiatric illness in those relatives who have factor X vs. those who do not (Table 6). If factor X is a necessary factor, the relatives who do *not* show factor X should *not* show the illness, except for sporadic cases resulting from the heterogeneity of the illness. Similar reasoning allows us to identify contributing and irrelevant factors, as indicated in Table 6.

As discussed elsewhere (Rieder and Gershon, unpublished data), "the advantages of this strategy lie in its robustness — it can be extended to quantitative variables and to more complex pedigree analyses. It is valid for virtually any mode of genetic transmission. If the illness has reduced penetrance, or unknown pleiomorphic forms, the predictions on rates of illness remain valid as long as the biologic hypothesis is true. Lastly, this strategy is designed to separate out biologically defined genetic subgroups in a heterogeneous disorder, as has proved so successful in mental retardation."

Much of the clinical investigation of affective disorder has centered on state-dependent phenomena: changes that occur within an individual while he is ill as compared to when he is well, or in pharmacologic manipulations that result in improvement or worsening in the disorder. Phenomena that are demonstrable only in the presence of active illness have limited usefulness in the genetic investigation of an illness with incomplete penetrance. For example, if a urinary metabolite is decreased only during episodes of illness, it is impossible to determine whether well relatives or controls would have the same finding, so there is no opportunity for positive evidence that a metabolic defect is present in ill but not well persons in a pedigree. However, the urinary metabolite decrease could be used to rule out the metabolic deficit as a transmitted factor in the illness. If there is more than one ill person in the pedigree, and one patient consistently shows the deficit whereas the other(s) consistently does not, the deficit is not transmitted along with the illness.

For genetic progress to be made based on the same comparisons of ill with well relatives, the same intensive study of pharmacologic responses and biochemical findings that has been devoted to patients during periods if illness should be undertaken in the well state of manic-depressive illness, and in the pre-onset state in persons at high risk for illness. Studies of possible interest are presented in Table 7 (p. 137).

Biologic Findings in Affective Illness

Are there biologically coherent groups of patients with affective illness, to whom these strategies are applicable? To answer this question, we shall briefly present the current status of biologic and genetic clinical research in affective illness in two areas which seem especially promising to us: biogenic monoamines and ion transport.

Biogenic Amines and the Clinical Pharmacology of Affective Illness. In this discussion, we offer a review of selected findings in the biochemistry and pharmacology of monoamines in patients with affective illness, with the emphasis on findings which have been applied in or may lead to executable genetic-biologic research strategies.

The hypotheses that central nervous system (CNS) functional activity of the catecholamines norepinephrine (NE) and dopamine (DA) and/or the indoleamine 5HT may be altered in depression or mania were initially presented on the basis of the biochemical pharmacology of drugs which are used in treating these disorders or which may provoke them (Schildkraut, 1965; Bunney and Davis, 1965; Lapin and Oxenkrug, 1969). The current status of catecholamine and indoleamine hypotheses of affective disorders has been the subject of recent reviews (Bunney et al., unpublished data; Mandell and Knapp, 1975; Mendels and Frazer, 1975; Baldessarini, 1975; Maas, 1975; Lapin and Oxenkrug, 1969). Recently, alternative hypotheses have been advanced that disturbance of an adrenergic-cholinergic balance (Janowsky, 1972) or formation of phenylethylamine (Fischer, 1975) underlies affective illness.

Each of the amine hypotheses has generated numerous observations of biochemical changes in monoamines and their metabolites in patients associated with worsening or improvement in affective state, which have been recently reviewed (Bunney et al., unpublished data; Mandell and Knapp, 1975; Mendels and Frazer, 1975; Baldessarini, 1975; Maas, 1975; Lapin and Oxenkrug, 1969; Goodwin and Post, 1975; Murphy and Wyatt, 1975; Wyatt and Murphy, 1975; Davis, 1975; Weil-Malherbe, 1976; Murphy, 1973). However, relatively few investigators have done longitudinal studies of patients for the purpose of identifying markers of vulnerability that persist into the well state, and which may be studied as possible genetic markers for the illness.

The "pharmacologic bridge" (Schildkraut and Kety, 1967; Schildkraut, 1965) between the biochemical pharmacology of drugs which perturb mood states and the pathophysiology of the disorders treated by these drugs, has been and remains an important heuristic device in clinical research (Mendels et al., 1975; Maas, 1975; Bunney and Murphy, 1975). Interest in biogenic monoamines as factors in mood disorders originally developed out of the finding that reserpine was provoking depressions in patients given this medication for hypertension (Achor et al., 1955; Harris, 1957). Reserpine was later found to deplete virtually all the aromatic biogenic amines in brain, including norepinephrine, dopamine, and 5HT, whereas certain drugs used to treat depressions, the monoamine oxidase inhibitors, caused an increase in brain serotonin and catecholamines, as reviewed elsewhere (Schildkraut, 1965; Bunney and Davis, 1965; Lapin and Oxenkrug, 1969; Shore, 1962). Since that time understanding of regulation of activity of monoaminergic neurons has been greatly enhanced, and correspondingly more sophisticated biologic observations and pharmacologic manipulations have been applied to these systems (Mandell, 1973; Usdin, 1974; Usdin and Bunney, 1975).

In clinical studies, two strategies to study these processes may be followed: (1) Pharmacologic agents with a specific effect on one segment of the processes of neural transmission are applied. Synthesis, release, degradation, and receptor sensitivity of catecholamine neurons can each be manipulated separately, and the effect on relief or activation of clinical mania or depression is studied. With the definition of neuroanatomically distinct functional systems, differential effects of drugs on each system can be studied. For example, the role of dopamine as a transmitter can be studied separately in neuroendocrine systems (as in release of growth hormone or prolactin), the nigrostriatal system (related to Parkinson symptoms), and mesolimbic system (possibly related to schizophrenic psychosis and to mania). (2) Monoamines, their metabolites, and their synthetic and degradative enzymes are studied in patients with psychiatric illness, and the biochemical effects of pharmacologic agents on these variables are also studied.

The catecholamine hypothesis of affective disorders states that functional activity of catecholamines is increased in mania and decreased in depression (Schildkraut, 1965; Bunney and Davis, 1965). The assumption that mania is the opposite of depression may not be warranted (Mendels and Frazer, 1975; Bunney et al., 1972; Court, 1968) and the catecholamine hypotheses of affective disorders can be considered separately for mania and for depression, and also separately for dopamine and norepinephrine.

In depression, the relation between the clinical and biochemical effects of the pharmacologic agents with specific biochemical actions is largely but not entirely consistent with the catecholamine hypotheses. αMT, which inhibits catecholamine synthesis, was found to exacerbate depression in 4 of 6 patients, as expected (Bunney et al., 1971). d-Amphetamine, which stimulates catecholamine receptors through release of newly synthesized DA, causes transient improvement in some but not all depressed patients (Maas, 1975; Fawcett et al., 1972). L-Dopa is a precursor of DA and NE which bypasses the rate limiting step of Tyrosine → dopa and thus increases synthesis of DA and NE. It is an effective agent in parkinsonism, in which there is a deficiency of DA in the nigrostriatal pathway, but L-dopa did not improve depression except in a subgroup of bipolar patients (Gershon et al., 1971a). Lithium carbonate, which increases reuptake of norepinephrine released at the nerve ending, and phenothiazines, which block dopamine receptors, are each effective antidepressants in certain types of depressed patients (Baron et al., 1975; Goodwin et al., 1972; Overall et al., 1966). These last findings are difficult to reconcile to the catecholamine hypothesis of depression.

In mania αMT decreases manic symptoms (Bunney et al., 1971) and L-dopa exacerbates them (Murphy et al., 1971; Gershon et al., 1971a), as predicted from the decrease or increase in functional CA. Lithium carbonate, butyrophenones, and phenothiazines are effective antimanic agents (Klein and Davis, 1969), again as predicted. However, DBH inhibition increases psychosis in manics (Sack and

Goodwin, 1974). Since DBH is the enzyme responsible for the last step in NE synthesis, this suggests that increased NE activity is not a generally present etiologic factor in mania. DBH inhibition would not be expected to have an effect on DA neurons, because they lack the enzyme (see below).

We would view the catecholamine hypothesis as consistent with clinical pharmacologic studies of mania, but in depression there are inconsistencies suggesting that the hypothesis is not generally applicable (although for each agent studied there are subgroups of patients who respond as predicted). This suggests that pharmacologic challenge and pharmacogenetic studies of agents affecting catecholamines may be better applied to bipolar patients than to unipolar, using strategies in which the predicted response is in the direction of mania.

Evidence that serotonin depletion is associated with both depression and mania has recently been reviewed (Mendels and Frazer, 1975; Kety, 1971; van Praag, unpublished data). MAO inhibitors and tricyclic antidepressants (TCA) appear to increase 5HT activity in CNS, although the TCA vary in their relative specificities for 5HT or NE/DA reuptake blockade, the mechanism by which monoamine activity may be enhanced (Maas, 1975). Serotonin synthesis is not subject to end-product inhibition, unlike catecholamines, so that administration of the amino acid serotonin precursor tryptophan produces proportionate increases in brain tryptophan and 5HT (Wurtman and Fernstrom, 1976). The therapeutic effects of tryptophan in depression are controversial, with some but not all studies reporting improvement (Mendels et al., 1975). In patients receiving imipramine or MAOI and improving from depression, pCPA produced transient worsening, suggesting a possible role for serotonin in the antidepressant response (Shopsin et al., 1975, 1976). In mania, tryptophan was recently noted to be effective as an anti-manic agent in a small series of patients (Wilson and Prange, 1972). Blockade of 5HT receptors with methysergide does not appear to ameliorate mania, although there were early reports to the contrary as reviewed elsewhere (Maas, 1975). Lithium carbonate initially causes an increase in cellular tryptophan uptake, and after chronic administration there is a decrease in tryptophan hydroxylase activity. The net effect is to stabilize serotonin turnover within a normal range, which may correct a hypothesized pre-existing deficit in serotonin production in affective illness (Mandell and Knapp, 1975).

Pharmacologic Response and Pharmacologic Challenge Strategies. To study the segregation of pharmacologic response and psychiatric illness within pedigrees, we require drugs whose behavioral or biochemical/physiologic effects *in the well state* vary between individuals. Extending the therapeutic pharmacology of affective disorders into pedigree studies would be generally unrewarding, because lithium, the tricyclic antidepressants, and the monoamine oxidase inhibitors all have nonspecific sedative effects in controls and in stable recovered patients with affective illness. One exception is that tricyclic antidepressants may provoke mania (more frequently in bipolar patients) after varying lengths of time administered (Bunney et al., 1970b; Prien et al., 1973; Coppen et al., 1976b). Similarly, reserpine and alphamethyldopa eventually provoke depression in a small proportion of patients receiving these drugs for hypertension (Goodwin and Bunney, 1971). Presumably this reflects an underlying vulnerability to depression, and could be studied within pedigrees. These clinical disorders would not be experimentally produced because of ethical considerations, but they imply that there may be executable pharmacologic challenge strategies in which the drug response produced is subclinical and transient.

The variable time period required for clinical disorders to be produced by reserpine or tricyclics has implications for well-state studies. These time periods may represent cumulative effects of drug administration, *or* they may reflect an *underlying vulnerability in the patient that is present only intermittently.* That is, the time interval may be characteristic of the patient and not of the drug, and the patient may not be demonstrably vulnerable during long periods of time, corresponding to the free intervals in these cyclic disorders. One implication is that longitudinal studies are needed to detect possible intermittent or rhythmic phenomena in hypothesized biologic vulnerability to illness. For pharmacologic challenge studies numerous transient challenges may be required to demonstrate whether or not a vulnerability is present.

What sort of vulnerability might be unmasked by pharmacologic challenge in the well state? Based on the clinical pharmacology of the illness, and the monoaminergic hypotheses of affective illness, we can consider several hypotheses (Table 7). In each case, we are testing the hypothesis that there is a failure of normal adaptive responses to an alteration in activity of the transmitter system studied, so that the person vulnerable to the illness will show a different response from the person who is not.

Four possible hypotheses of the vulnerable state are as follows: (1) Decreased activity of (one or more) monoaminergic neuron systems. (2) Supersensitivity of a monoamine receptor. An alternate hypothesis would be that supersensitivity is more easily induced in these persons. (3) Increased activity of monoaminergic neuron systems. (4) Increased sensitivity to antagonist neurotransmitter system.

Table 7. Some Clinical Pharmacologic Strategies for Unmasking Vulnerability to Affective Disorder

Hypothesized Vulnerable State	Strategy	Examples of Clinically Usable Pharmacologic Agents		
		Dopamine	*Norepinephrine*	*Serotonin*
A. *Decreased* functional activity of monoaminergic neurons	1. Receptor blockade	Haloperidol Pimozide	Phenoxybenzamine Propranolol	Methysergide
	2. Synthesis inhibition	α-MT	α-MT Fusaric acid	pCPA
	3. Inhibition of neuronal transmitter release	GBL		
B. *Supersensitivity* (may be more easily produced)	1. Same as A, *followed* by agonist	d-Amphetamine Piribedil Methylphenidate	d-Amphetamine Clonidine Methylphenidate	Carbohydrate loading, then Try 5-HTP Fenfluramine
C. *Increased* functional activity of monoaminergic neurons	1. Agonist administration	d-Amphetamine Piribedil Methylphenidate	d-Amphetamine Clonidine Methylphenidate	Carbohydrate loading, then Try 5-HTP Fenfluramine
		Acetylcholine	*GABA*	
D. *Altered* sensitivity to antagonist neurotransmitter system				
a. Cholinergic-adrenergic balance	1. Agonist of monoamine system, *followed* by agonist of other transmitter systems	Agonist: Physostigmine	Muscimol	
b. GABA-dopaminergic balance	1. Antagonist of other transmitter system	Antagonist: Atropine Scopolamine		

α-MT = Alphamethyl tyrosine; pCPA = Para-chlorophenylalanine; GBL = Gamma-butyrolactone; Try = Tryptophan; 5-HTP = 5-hydroxytryptophan; GABA = Gamma amino butyric acid.

Numerous other hypotheses might be considered; the four general hypotheses we consider here are chosen because they are plausible in light of current evidence as reviewed above, and because they are testable using the genetic clinical research strategy discussed earlier in this chapter. Clinical strategies and appropriate pharmacologic agents for these hypotheses are described in Table 7.

As an example of a pharmacologic challenge strategy, let us consider d-amphetamine, which has been used in research protocols to predict antidepressant response (Roberts, 1959; Fawcett et al., 1972; Kiloh et al., 1974), and recently to distinguish between schizophrenia and manic-depressive illness (Janowsky et al., 1973a, b). This substance is an example of a drug with specific biochemical and behavioral effects, which can be suitably studied in a brief clinical trial, and whose clinical psychiatric effects are transient and not a danger to the patient.

In animals, this substance produces increased motor activity and stereotypy; in man, elevated mood and improved motor performance are seen, although not in all individuals (Tecce and Cole, 1974). Amphetamine stimulates release and blocks amine reuptake at NE and DA but not 5HT neurons (Maas, 1975). Amphetamine motor effects in animals are abolished by αMT but not reserpine, implying that these effects are mediated by newly synthesized catecholamines and that amphetamine itself is an indirect agonist (Cooper et al., 1974). 5HT plays an inhibitory role in the behavioral effects of amphetamine; when brain 5HT is reduced by decreased dietary tryptophan or pCPA, the motor response to amphetamine is potentiated (Hollister et al., 1976). In single unit studies amphetamine selectively stimulates the postsynaptic but not the presynaptic dopamine receptor (Bunney and Aghajanian, 1975).

In depressed patients, a mood-brightening response to d-amphetamine is predictive of a favorable response to treatment with imipramine or desipramine (Maas, 1975), as discussed above. In manic patients methylphenidate (which has effects similar to amphetamine) infusion produced increase in manic symptoms of 5 of 10 patients (Janowsky et al., 1973a, b), and similar findings were reported after recovery. Pharmacogenetic studies have not been reported. To apply a pharmacologic challenge strategy we would hypothesize that increased sensitivity to amphetamine stimulation may be present in the well state in some bipolar patients, and that this sensitivity may be heritable and may serve as a genetic marker of vulnerability to the illness. A similar vulnerability in schizophrenia is suggested by a recent report that recovered schizophrenics show a transient (1 hour) return of florid psychotic symptoms during amphetamine infusions (van Kammen et al., unpublished data), although another study did not find this (Janowsky et al., 1973b).

Numerous CNS responses can be studied in these pharmacologic challenge strategies. Based on known involvement of monoamines in different functional systems in the CNS, one can study mood, perceptual vigilance and arousal, cortical visual evoked response, stereotypic and other extrapyramidal movements, release of monoamines and cyclic nucleotides into CSF or blood, and neuroendocrine responses. Bunney and Murphy have described in vitro test systems suitable for study of neurotransmitter receptor function in man; these include subcutaneous adipose tissue for study of catecholamine–adenyl cyclase interaction, the platelet prostaglandin E1 receptor that is inhibited by norepinephrine, and the leukocyte β-adrenergic receptor (Bunney and Murphy, 1975). Each of these could be studied in a genetic paradigm if stable interindividual differences were present.

Enzymes of Monoamine Synthesis and Metabolism.   Studies of protein or enzyme polymorphism are particularly suitable to genetic investigations of affective disorder, because an enzyme structure is determined by a single genetic code sequence. Genetically produced aberrations in enzyme activity are caused by unusual genetic coding, resulting in either an abnormal amino acid sequence for that enzyme or a change in regulation of metabolism of the enzyme as has been evidenced for tyrosine hydroxylase, dopamine-β-hydroxylase, and phenylethanolamine N-methyltransferase in mice (Barchas et al., 1975). Studies of the enzyme would reveal either or both of the following: (1) an abnormal quantity of the usual enzyme, or (2) aberrant physiochemical properties of the enzyme. In recent years, much interest has focused on the CNS amine–related enzymes which can be measured in peripheral blood: MAO, COMT, and DBH (Table 8). The precise relationship of these peripheral enzymes to their corresponding counterparts in the CNS is not known. However, an abnormality in the peripheral enzymes might reflect a parallel abnormality in CNS. There have been two recent studies on these enzymes in the CNS. Grote et al. (1974) found no difference in MAO, COMT, or DBH activity in brains of depressive suicides when compared to controls. In contrast, Gottfries et al. (1974) found that MAO activity was decreased in suicide brains. The biologic role of these enzymes is described in more detail below. Many other CNS amine–related enzymes would be of interest, such as tyrosine hydroxylase, the rate-limiting enzyme in the formation of dopamine and NE (Cooper et al., 1974), but they are not clinically measurable in blood or CSF.

MAO is a major degradative enzyme of many biogenic amines as

Table 8. Biogenic Amine Related Enzyme Activity in Affective Illness

Enzyme	Affectively Ill Subjects	Subjects vs. Controls	Reference	Segregates with Illness
Platelet MAO	Depressed inpatients and outpatients	↑	Nies et al., 1971, 1974 (personal communication)	No
	BP and UP depressed patients	BP →	Murphy and Weiss, 1972	
	BP patients	BP →	Leckman et al., unpublished data b	
	BP and UP depressed patients	BP → UP ←	Landowski et al., 1975	
	BP patients	BP ←	Belmaker et al., 1976	
Plasma MAO	Depressed women	↑	Klaiber et al., 1972	No
	BP and UP patients	No difference	Mattson et al., 1974	
	BP and UP patients	No difference	Gershon et al., 1977	
Rbc COMT	BP and UP patients	Women ↓	Cohn et al., 1970	
	BP and UP patients	For women UP < BP < controls →	Dunner et al., 1971	
	Depressed women	No difference	Briggs and Briggs, 1973	
	BP and UP patients	BP, UP ↑	Dunner et al., 1976	
	BP and UP patients	No difference	Gershon and Jonas, 1975	Yes
	BP and UP patients	No difference	Mattson et al., 1974	
	UP women	No difference	White et al., 1976	
Plasma DBH	BP and UP patients	No difference	Shopsin et al., 1972	No
	BP and UP patients	No difference	Wetterberg et al., 1972a	
	BP and UP patients	No difference	Lamprecht et al., 1974a	
	BP and UP patients	No nonrelative controls	{ Levitt and Mendlewicz, 1975 Levitt et al., 1976 }	
	BP and UP patients	Psychotically Depressed UP patients ↓	Meltzer et al., 1976	

well as of putative neurotransmitters such as NE, DA, and serotonin (Blaschko, 1963). MAO may also play a role in the regulation of synthesis of NE (Weiner and Bjur, 1972; Trendelenburg et al., 1972) and serotonin (Green and Grahame-Smith, 1975). The biologic role of MAO in the metabolism of neurotransmitter amines has been reviewed elsewhere (Kopin, 1964; Tipton, 1973; Youdim, 1976). Studies of immunologic reactions (Hartman, 1972; Hartman et al., 1969; McCauley and Racker, 1973; Youdim and Collins, 1975), electrophoretic mobility (Youdim and Collins, 1975; Borges and D'Iorio, 1973) and substrate and inhibitor specificities (Johnston, 1968; Hall et al., 1969; Squires, 1972; Neff and Goridis, 1972; Youdim et al., 1972) favor the existence of two or more forms of mitochondrial MAO. The "type A" and "type B" forms of the enzyme were originally identified by Johnston (1968), who demonstrated two distinct sensitivities to inhibition in MAO from rat brain. As reviewed by Murphy and Donnelly (1974), the evidence suggests that most tissues, including brain, have varying proportions of both type A and B enzymes; however, human platelet MAO is homogeneous electrophoretically (Collins and Sandler, 1971) and appears to consist only of the "B" form in its substrate and inhibitor characteristics (Edwards and Chang, 1975; Donnelly and Murphy, 1976).

Both platelet MAO (Nies et al., 1973, 1974; Wyatt et al., 1973; Murphy and Donnelly, 1974) and plasma MAO (Nies et al., 1973; Gershon et al., 1977) activities are heritable. Platelet MAO activity has been reported by Murphy and Wyatt (1975) to be a relatively stable characteristic of the individual; the changes that did occur (in 15 to 20 percent of the patients) were not in relation to the clinical state of the patient. Landowski et al. (1975), however, found that platelet MAO of bipolar depressives, which was lower than controls, rose to the same level as controls when the depression remitted.

Platelet MAO has been measured in groups of patients with affective disorder. Although the studies are not all in agreement, alterations in platelet MAO activity have been described.

Murphy and Weiss (1972) found that BP depressives had *lower* platelet MAO than UP depressives and controls, a finding later confirmed by Leckman et al. (unpublished data b) in the same population. The platelet MAO of the UP patients (Murphy and Weiss, 1972) was not significantly different from that of controls. Unipolar patients were not included in Leckman's study. Landowski et al. (1975) also found that lower platelet MAO differentiated BP depressed patients from UP depressed patients and controls. In that study, the UP depressed group had a higher platelet MAO than either the bipolar depressed group or controls. In contrast, Belmaker et al. (1976) found increased platelet MAO in BP patients as compared to controls. Nies et al. (1971, 1974) measured the platelet MAO activity of a large group of depressed inpatients and outpatients with a range of depressive diagnoses and found their platelet MAO to be greater than normals matched for age. Twenty-six bipolar depressed patients who were included in this group also had significantly higher platelet MAO activity than controls (Nies et al., 1974; Nies, personal communication). These discrepancies may be due to population differences in the predominant biologic factors in mood disorders; Murphy and Leckman's studies were done in Bethesda, Maryland, Landowski's in Poland, Belmaker's in Jerusalem, Israel, and Nies' in Vermont.

Leckman et al. (unpublished data b), in a study of bipolar probands and their first degree relatives, failed to show nonindependent segregation of platelet MAO with affective illness. That is, both ill and well relatives tended to have low platelet MAO. According to this evidence, platelet MAO activity cannot by itself be used as a marker for increased individual vulnerability.

Plasma MAO and platelet MAO differ in substrate affinities, in inhibitor responses, and in cofactor requirements, and they appear to be distinct enzymes (Murphy and Donnelly, 1974). Plasma MAO activity measured with benzylamine as the substrate is not correlated with platelet MAO activity using benzylamine or tryptamine as the substrate (Murphy and Donnelly, 1974).

Plasma MAO was reported by Klaiber et al. (1972) to be increased in premenopausal women with depression. Gershon et al. (1977) and Mattson et al. (1974) found that BP and UP patients were no different from each other or from controls in plasma MAO activity.

Gershon et al. (1977) demonstrated independent assortment of plasma MAO activity with respect to affective disorders within families, which precludes the use of plasma MAO as a marker for increased individual vulnerability.

Shih and Eiduson (1971) have suggested that plasma MAO isoenzyme patterns may differ in various subgroups of depressive patients. Belmaker and Ebstein (unpublished data) and Ebstein et al. (1976), however, have been unable to identify a mutant form of plasma MAO, platelet MAO, or erythrocyte COMT in schizophrenic or manic-depressive individuals, by electrophoretic methods.

It has been suggested that COMT may be associated with the adrenergic receptor (Axelrod, 1966) as well as functioning as a major degradative enzyme of intraneuronal catecholamines (Hertting and Axelrod, 1961; Axelrod, 1966). The evidence for its receptor role is inconclusive (Cuatrecasas, 1974). COMT is found in human red blood cells in addition to other non-neural tissue (Axelrod and Cohn, 1971) and has a broad substrate specificity for catechol compounds.

Red blood cell COMT activity has been shown to be heritable (Weinshilboum et al., 1974; Gershon and Jonas, 1975; Grunhaus et al., 1976) and a stable characteristic of the individual (Cohn et al., 1970; Dunner et al., 1971).

Red blood cell COMT activity has been reported in several studies (Cohn et al., 1970; Dunner et al., 1971; Briggs and Briggs, 1973) to be decreased in women but not in men with primary affective disorders. Dunner et al. (1971) reported both bipolar and unipolar female patients had decreased erythrocyte COMT levels as compared with controls. The erythrocyte COMT levels in the unipolar group were significantly lower than in the bipolar group. Dunner et al. (1976) were unable to replicate these findings. Gershon and Jonas (1975), in their studies on the Jerusalem population, found *increased* erythrocyte COMT levels in a group of men and women with affective disorder. There was no unipolar-bipolar difference in red blood cell COMT activity, and men had higher activity than women in this study. Ebstein et al. (1976) also studied the Jerusalem population, including some of the patients previously studied by Gershon and Jonas (1975). They found an increase in the red blood cell COMT activity in 12 bipolar patients as compared to 15 controls. Although the 20 percent increased activity was almost identical to the report of Gershon and Jonas, the increase was not statistically significant. A recent report by White et al. (1976) failed to demonstrate a significantly different level of COMT in unipolar depressed women from controls. Likewise, Mattson et al. (1974) found no difference in the COMT activity among unipolar patients, bipolar patients, and controls. Population differences may play a role in these discrepancies.

Gershon and Jonas (1975) found that increased erythrocyte COMT activity distinguished healthy relatives from probands and ill relatives. The nonindependent assortment suggests that COMT may be a marker of genetically determined vulnerability to affective illness in the population studied.

The nonuniformity of alterations in platelet MAO and erythrocyte COMT activity may reflect genetic heterogeneity of affective disorders or environmental differences. For this reason, Gershon (1976) stresses the value of crossnational comparative biologic and population-genetic studies.

The nonspecific enzyme DBH catalyzes the conversion of DA to NE (Kaufman and Friedman, 1965) as well as β-hydroxylating other phenylethylamines to their corresponding phenylethanolamines (Levin and Kaufman, 1961). DBH is found in the noradrenergic neurons of the brain (Hartman, 1973; Coyle and Axelrod, 1972), in sympathetic neurons (Potter and Axelrod, 1963; Molinoff et al.,

1970), and in the chromaffin granules of the adrenal medulla (Oka et al., 1967; Viveros et al., 1968).

DBH is released by exocytosis along with catecholamines from the adrenal medulla (Viveros et al., 1968) and from sympathetic nerve terminals (Weinshilboum et al., 1971; Gewirtz and Kopin, 1960; Smith et al., 1970). The source of serum DBH is most likely from sympathetic nerves rather than from adrenal medulla or CNS. 6-Hydroxydopamine, a drug which destroys sympathetic nerve terminals (Thoenen and Tranzer, 1968), lowers serum DBH activity by 25 percent, but removal of the adrenal medulla does not reduce serum DBH activity (Weinshilboum and Axelrod, 1971c). Intraventricular 6-hydroxydopamine, which destroys central noradrenergic neurons, does not alter serum DBH activity (Lamprecht et al., 1974b).

DBH activity is measurable in human plasma or serum (Weinshilboum and Axelrod, 1971b; Goldstein et al., 1971; Nagatsu and Udenfriend, 1972; Molinoff et al., 1970) and has been shown, despite wide interindividual variation, to be a stable intraindividual characteristic, regardless of clinical state (Shopsin et al., 1972; Wetterberg et al., 1972a; Levitt and Mendlewicz, 1975; Meltzer et al., 1976; Weinshilboum and Axelrod, 1971a; Goldstein et al., 1971; Nagatsu and Udenfriend, 1972; Levitt et al., 1974; Horwitz et al., 1973; Levitt et al., 1976).

Serum DBH activity has been shown to be heritable (Weinshilboum et al., 1973; Ross et al., 1973; Levitt and Mendlewicz, 1975; Ogihara et al., 1975) and has been associated with several diseases thought to have a genetic component. Serum DBH activity is reported to be decreased in familial dysautonomia (Weinshilboum and Axelrod, 1971a) and Down's syndrome (Wetterberg et al., 1972b) and increased in autosomal dominant torsion dystonia (Wooten et al., 1973), Huntington's chorea (Lieberman et al., 1972; Shokeir, 1975) and Lesch-Nyhan syndrome (Rockson et al., 1974).

Several studies have reported that there is no significant difference in the serum or plasma DBH activity between either affectively ill and controls (Shopsin et al., 1972; Wetterberg et al., 1972a; Lamprecht et al., 1974a) or unipolar and bipolar patients (Shopsin et al., 1972; Levitt and Mendlewicz, 1975; Lamprecht et al., 1974a; Levitt et al., 1976). In a recent report by Meltzer et al. (1976), there was a significant decrease in serum DBH activity of UP psychotically depressed patients compared to controls and other depressive groups.

In a study of pairs of same-sex siblings (Levitt and Mendlewicz, 1975; Levitt et al., 1976) discordant for affective illness, plasma DBH failed to distinguish between UP and BP patients and their well siblings, which is compatible with independent assortment of plasma DBH in UP and BP illness. Also in this study, there were four MZ twin pairs discordant for affective illness (two twins with a unipolar diagnosis and two twins with a bipolar diagnosis) but concordant for plasma DBH activity.

Weinshilboum et al. (1975) reported that very low serum DBH is likely inherited by a single autosomal recessive gene. It would be of interest to study pedigrees of families with very low serum DBH and affective disorder to determine whether the two factors segregate together.

Of the three enzymes MAO, COMT, and DBH, erythrocyte COMT activity alone has been found to segregate with affective illness (Gershon and Jonas, 1975; see Table 8) and seems a possible genetic marker for affective illness in the populations studied.

   CSF + Urinary Metabolites of Monoamines. The major metabolic pathways of CNS monoamines are well known: 5HT→5-HIAA, DA→DOPAC→HVA, and NE→MHPG (principal metabolite) and VMA (Cooper et al., 1974). Significant amounts of the acid metabolites are transported into the CSF and from there into the bloodstream, where they are excreted in the urine. Clinical studies of these metabolites in urine and CSF have therefore been of much interest in view of the monoamine hypotheses of affective disorders. The advantage of urinary studies of metabolites is that the amount excreted per unit time is directly related to the rate of production of the metabolite; the disadvantage is the nonspecificity of the source of the metabolite. As reviewed elsewhere, only the NE metabolite MHPG in urine in man may provide an index of CNS turnover of a monoamine (Goodwin and Post, 1975; Ebert and Kopin, 1975).

The source of CSF monoamine metabolites has been the subject of recent reviews (Goodwin and Post, 1975; Garelis et al., 1974) which note that significant amounts of 5-HIAA and NE metabolites are produced in the cord and appear in lumbar CSF. In patients with blockage of CSF flow in the spinal space, HVA does not appear in lumbar CSF below the blockage, suggesting predominant origin in rostral areas (Post et al., 1973), but recent studies in rhesus monkeys have demonstrated a spinal cord origin for a small proportion of HVA in lumbar CSF (Kessler et al., 1976).

Furthermore, the physiologic meaning of metabolite concentrations is unclear, because they are determined by multiple feedback mechanisms governing neural firing rate and monoamine synthesis, and possibly by variations in the transport system for monoamines. Nevertheless, there has been much interest in these measurements as possible indicators of activity of CNS monoamine neurons. A more

dynamic measurement of the acid metabolites is provided by ad-
ministering probenecid, which blocks the transport of organic acids
out of CNS (Werdinius, 1967), so that the rate of accumulation of
these acids in CSF becomes an index of turnover of the corresponding monoamines (Goodwin et al., 1973). Although increases or
decreases in turnover do *not* necessarily imply corresponding
changes in the rate or magnitude of postsynaptic response (Roth et
al., 1973) since multiple feedback loops exist, nonetheless such
changes are of interest and in combination with pharmacologic and
other data may be interpretable.

5-HIAA.   In depression, decreased CSF 5-HIAA and decreased
accumulation of 5-HIAA after probenecid have been reported by several investigators but not by others, as reviewed by Post and Goodwin (in press). This apparent inconsistency may reflect heterogeneity
in the pathophysiologic basis of affective illness, with different populations having greater or smaller proportions of depressed patients
with a specific functional disorder reflected in serotonin metabolism.
The findings of a bimodal distribution in CSF 5-HIAA in depression
in two studies (van Praag and Korf, 1971; Asberg et al., 1976) with a
significant proportion of, but not all, depressed patients showing
decreased CSF 5-HIAA, is compatible with this hypothesis. Both
sets of investigators find supporting evidence that low 5-HIAA patients are distinguished in clinical characteristics (Asberg et al.,
1976; van Praag, unpublished data) by an antidepressant response to
the serotonin precursor 5HTP in depression (van Praag, unpublished
data) and by specific therapeutic response to tricyclic antidepressants, according to whether the antidepressant has a marked effect on
5HT reuptake (van Praag, unpublished data; Asberg et al., 1976).

Bipolar-unipolar differences have not been consistently noted in
CSF studies on monoamine metabolites as noted above, but there is
a tendency in several studies for low 5HIAA accumulation after
probenecid to be found in BP rather than UP patients (Goodwin and
Post, 1975; van Praag et al., 1973; Bowers, 1974).

Do these findings characterize these patients even in the well
state, as is required for demonstrating the role of a genetic factor
using our genetic paradigms? Of the five studies reporting reduced
CSF 5-HIAA in depression (Ashcroft et al., 1973; Subrahmanyam,
1975; Coppen et al., 1972a; Dencker et al., 1966; van Praag and Korf,
1974), four report data in the patients on recovery. In three studies
(Ashcroft et al., 1973; Subrahmanyam, 1975; Coppen et al., 1972a)
CSF 5-HIAA has not changed from the depressed state; in the fourth
(Dencker et al., 1966) the results were mixed.

HVA.   Only two of the nine clinical studies reviewed by Post and Goodwin (in press) reported low CSF HVA in depression, but in six of eight studies the rate of HVA accumulation (after probenecid administration) was decreased. Data on the well state have not been reported.

MHPG.   Urinary MHPG excretion, which may be an index of NE turnover in CNS (Ebert and Kopin, 1975) has been reported decreased in depression (Maas et al., 1968) and in the depressed phase in bipolar patients (Stoddard et al., 1974; Schildkraut et al., 1973; Maas et al., 1973; Maas, 1975), as reviewed elsewhere (Maas, 1975). However, this parameter tends to return to normal upon recovery (Greenspan et al., 1970), although not all studies agree (Subrahmanyam, 1975). Urinary MHPG in depressed patients is subject to variation owing to motor activity and stress (Ebert et al., 1972; Post and Goodwin, 1973; Muscettola et al., 1976; Maas, 1975), although this may not be the case in healthy subjects (Muscettola, 1976; Maas et al., 1973).

CSF MHPG has been reported decreased in two of four studies of depressed patients reviewed by Goodwin and Post, and this finding appears to persist in the well state in a small series of patients, (N =5) studied by them (Post and Goodwin, in press; Goodwin and Post, 1975). VMA in CSF is also reported reduced in depression (Jimerson et al., 1975).

TWO SUBGROUPS DEFINED BY METABOLITES AND DRUG RESPONSE.   The low CSF 5-HIAA subgroup may represent one biologically coherent subtype among depressive illness; another subgroup may be defined by low urinary MHPG excretion when depressed (Maas, 1975). The exciting hypothesis that these groups represent specific and separate deficits in monoamine activity at CNS synapses is suggested by the following evidence: (1) These groups tend not to overlap—depressed patients with decreased urinary MHPG have higher CSF 5-HIAA accumulation after probenecid than patients with normal or increased urinary MHPG (Goodwin et al., unpublished data). (2) Antidepressants with specific effects on NE or 5HT reuptake have the predicted therapeutic effects. Blockade of reuptake delays inactivation of released monoamines, presumably potentiating their activity at receptor sites. In patients with low urinary MHPG, imipramine and desipramine (the active metabolite of imipramine) are effective antidepressants, whereas amitriptyline tends not to be, and the opposite is true in patients with normal or high MHPG (Maas et al., 1972; Schildkraut, 1973; Beckmann and Goodwin, 1975). Desmethylimipramine has a relatively specific effect on blockade of reuptake at NE but not 5HT neurons, whereas the opposite is true of amitriptyline (Maas, 1975). Low CSF 5-HIAA patients, on the other hand, do not respond to nortriptyline (Asberg et al., 1976), which has weak 5HT uptake inhibition. Among depressed patients, these patients do respond to chlorimipramine, a relatively specific 5HT reuptake blocker among the clinically used tricyclic antidepressants (van Praag, unpublished data). In the chlorimipramine study, nonresponders (without reduced 5HIAA) were then given nortriptyline (which has more NE blockade activity) to which they responded (van Praag, unpublished data), which is compatible with the hypothesis that each patient tended to have only one of the two hypothesized monoamine deficits. Systematic randomized crossover studies between the two types of antidepressant (e.g., nortriptyline and quipazine or chlorimipramine), with measurement of urinary MHPG and CSF 5HIAA are still required to test this hypothesis thoroughly. (3) The d-amphetamine mood brightening response in depression seems specific to the low MHPG group (Maas, 1975).

Can genetic strategies be used to investigate the existence and transmission of the two hypothesized independent subtypes of affective illness? In the case of 5-HIAA in CSF, further study is needed to establish the stability of this finding in the well state, and to determine whether resting CSF 5-HIAA concentrations or some related parameter (such as probenecid-induced accumulation of CSF 5-HIAA) best characterize this subgroup of patients. Studies of the heritability of this parameter and its transmission in pedigrees could then proceed.

The specificity of antidepressant response, which supports the existence of separate biologic subtypes, does not appear applicable to a genetic paradigm, because in the well state we do not know of a response to antidepressants that will distinguish these persons from normals. Similarly, the low urinary MHPG subgroup does not appear susceptible to the genetic paradigm described above, as the finding seems to appear only in the ill state under strictly controlled conditions. However, if it could be demonstrated that ill relatives did *not* show the same low urinary MHPG during depression, or the same antidepressant response, the hypothesis that this was a necessary factor in the genetic transmission of depression in this group would be disproved.

Ion Transport.   Alterations in ion transport across the cell membrane is another area of interest in searching for a biologic characteristic revealing vulnerability to an affective disorder. The therapeutic response to Li carbonate in bipolar and some unipolar patients has stimulated investigations of the characteristics of Li responders and a possible ion transport disturbance in affective illness.

Mendels and Frazer (1974) have postulated that the human

erythrocyte can be used as a model for neuronal cation transport and have presented evidence (Frazer et al., 1973) from studies in rats that red blood cell lithium level is better than plasma lithium level in predicting the concentration of Li in brain. In a clinical study of acutely depressed unipolar and bipolar patients, Mendels and Frazer (1973) found that the red blood cell/plasma Li level (Li index) was significantly *higher* in the patients who had a therapeutic response to lithium. They suggest that their results may reflect differences in cell membrane properties in a subgroup of the affectively ill population. This was not replicated by Rybakowski et al. (1974b). Casper et al. (1976) found that a *higher* lithium index distinguished clinical responders from nonresponders in a group of patients with primary affective disorder or schizoaffective illness. Others have reported the value of the Li index in prophylactic response to Li carbonate in major affective illness as both predictive (Mendels et al., 1976) and nonpredictive (Cazzullo et al., 1975; Knorring et al., 1976; Rybakowski and Strzyzewski, 1976). Studies have also compared the lithium index of UP and BP patients with conflicting results as to whether the Li index distinguishes between the two groups (Ramsey et al., 1976; Elizur et al., 1972; Rybakowski et al., 1974b; Leckman et al., unpublished data a). Two studies have examined the Li index in affective illness as compared to controls. Lyttkens et al. (1973) found that bipolar females had a significantly *higher* lithium index than female controls. Elizur et al. (1972) reported that the Li index of bipolar patients who are either manic or depressed is *lower* than that of bipolar patients in remission and controls.

Dorus et al. (1974, 1975) in MZ-DZ twin studies, have demonstrated a substantial genetic component of the in vitro and in vivo uptake of the Li ion by the human erythrocyte. Further investigation is needed to determine whether the Li index is a stable characteristic of the individual and whether an alteration of the Li index segregates with affective disorder within families.

Hokin-Neaverson et al. (1974) have reported that the mean sodium pump activity of a group of bipolar patients was significantly lower than that of controls, although there was considerable overlap of individual values. The sodium pump values did not seem to be related to the manic or remission phases of the illness, or to lithium or phenothiazine therapy.

Further study of the sodium pump activity in the well and ill state may prove useful in delineating a subgroup of the affective disorder population with significant membrane transport disturbance that is genetically transmitted.

SUMMARY

Recent attempts to identify biologic factors which are inherited in the affective disorders have been stimulated by the considerable evidence for a genetic predisposition in these disorders. Twin and family studies have provided support for this hypothesis and impetus for investigators to isolate subgroups of the affective disorders which can be shown to demonstrate genetic transmission.

The unipolar (UP) and bipolar (BP) forms of affective illness appear not to be genetically and physiologically identical, although the degree of overlap in family and biologic-pharmacologic studies is considerable. It appears likely that at least a subgroup of UP illness shares its genetic diathesis with BP illness. A demonstrable physiologic vulnerability or pharmacologic response may eventually prove to be useful in defining genetic subgroups of patients with affective disorders. Among the promising biologic findings in these disorders which we have reviewed, none is clearly established as an identifying marker of an "affective genotype."

Linkage of BP illness to markers on the X-chromosome has been reported, but the evidence has internal inconsistencies which must be resolved before the phenomenon can be accepted. Association of BP illness with specific HLA types has also been reported, but efforts at replication have been unsuccessful. Similarly, mathematical models of transmission applied to family study data do not consistently support the same mode of transmission when applied to data collected at different centers.

Recent biologic-genetic studies in affective illness have concentrated on physiologic characteristics that (1) distinguish patients with these disorders from controls, (2) are stable characteristics of the individual in the well state, and (3) are heritable. Changes in activity of enzymes of monoamine metabolism observed in peripheral blood, erythrocyte catechol-O-methyltransferase (COMT) and platelet monoamine oxidase (MAO), satisfy these requirements. In the initial reported studies, increased COMT activity segregated with the illness within families, but decreased platelet MAO activity did not, suggesting that COMT may be a transmitted marker of vulnerability. Replication is required. Application of genetic strategies to other biologic pharmacologic characteristics of affective illness appears promising.

ACKNOWLEDGMENT

We acknowledge appreciation for the excellent editorial assistance of Janice N. Ohler and the excellent secretarial assistance of Diane Mueller in the preparation of this manuscript.

References

Achor, R. W. P., N. O. Hanson, and R. W. Gifford, Jr. 1955. Hypertension treated with rauwolfia serpentina and with reserpine. JAMA 159:841–845.

Angst, J. 1966. Zur Ätiologie und Nosologie endogoner depressiver Psychosen. In Monographien aus dem Gesamtgebiete der Neurologie und Psychiatrie. Berlin, Springer-Verlag, No. 112.

Asano, N. 1967. Clinico-Genetic Study of Manic-Depressive Psychoses. In Clinical Genetics in Psychiatry, Mitsuda, H. (Ed.), pp. 262–275. Kyoto, Bunko-sha Co., Ltd.

Asberg, M., P. Thoren, L. Traskman, L. Bertilsson, and V. Ringberger. 1976. Serotonin depression—a biochemical subgroup within the affective disorders? Science 191:478–480.

Ashcroft, G. W., I. M. Blackburn, D. Eccleston, A. Glen, W. Hartley, N. Kinloch, M. Lonergan, L. Murray, and A. I. Pullar. 1973. Changes on recovery in the concentration of tryptophan and the biogenic amine metabolites in the cerebrospinal fluid of patients with affective illness. Psychol. Med. 3:319–325.

Axelrod, J. 1966. Methylation reactions in the formation and metabolism of catecholamines and other biogenic amines. Pharmacol. Rev. 18:95–113.

Axelrod, J., and C. K. Cohn. 1971. Methyltransferase enzymes in red blood cells. J. Pharmacol. Exp. Ther. 176:650–654.

Baldessarini, R. J. 1975. The basis for amine hypotheses in affective disorders. Arch. Gen. Psychiat. 32:1087–1093.

Barchas, J. D., R. D. Ciaranello, S. Kessler, and D. A. Hamburg. 1975. Genetic Aspects of Catecholamine Synthesis. In Genetic Research in Psychiatry, Fieve, R. R., D. Rosenthal, and H. Brill (Eds.), pp. 27–62. Baltimore, Johns Hopkins University Press.

Baron, M., E. S. Gershon, V. Rudy, W. Z. Jonas, and M. Buchsbaum. 1975. Lithium carbonate response in depression: Prediction by unipolar/bipolar illness, averaged evoked response, catechol-O-methyltransferase, and family history. Arch. Gen. Psychiat. 32:1107–1111.

Beckmann, H., and F. K. Goodwin. 1975. Antidepressant response to tricyclics and urinary MHPG in unipolar patients. Arch. Gen. Psychiat. 32:17–21.

Belmaker, R. H., K. Ebbsen, R. Ebstein, and R. Rimon. 1976. Platelet monoamine oxidase in schizophrenia and manic-depressive illness. Brit. J. Psychiat. 129:227–232.

Belmaker, R. H., and R. Ebstein. 1977. The Search for Genetic Polymorphisms of Human Biogenic Amine-Related Enzymes. In The Impact of Biology on Modern Psychiatry, Gershon, E. S., R. H. Belmaker, S. S. Kety, and M. Rosenbaum (Eds.). New York, Plenum Press.

Bennahum, D. A., G. M. Troup, R. T. Rada, R. Kellner, and W. Kyner. 1975. Human leukocyte antigens (HLA) in psychiatric illness. Clin. Res. 23:260A.

Bennahum, D. A., G. M. Troup, R. T. Rada, R. Kellner, and W. Kyner. Unpublished data. The histocompatibility antigens of schizophrenic and manic-depressive patients.

Blaschko, H. 1963. Amine Oxidase. In The Enzymes, Boyer, P. D., H. Larely, and K. Myrback (Eds.), pp. 337–351. New York, Academic Press.

Borges, J., M. Diaz, and A. D'Iorio. 1973. Polyacrylamide gel electrophoresis of rat liver mitochondrial monoamine oxidases. Canad. J. Biochem. 51:1089–1095.

Bowers, M. B. 1970. Cerebrospinal fluid 5-hydroxyindoles and behavior after L-tryptophan and pyridoxine administration to psychiatric patients. Neuropharmacology 9:599–604.

Bowers, M. B. 1974. Lumbar CSF 5-hydroxyindoleacetic acid and homovanillic acid in affective syndromes. J. Nerv. Ment. Dis. 158:325–330.

Briggs, M. H., and M. Briggs. 1973. Hormonal influences on erythrocyte catechol-O-methyl transferase activity in humans. Experientia 29:278–280.

Broadhurst, A. D. 1970. L-Tryptophan versus E.C.T. Lancet 1:1392–1393.

Buchsbaum, M., F. K. Goodwin, D. L. Murphy, and G. Borge. 1971. Average evoked response in affective disorders. Am. J. Psychiat. 128:19–25.

Buchsbaum, M., S. Landau, D. L. Murphy, and F. K. Goodwin. 1973. Average evoked response in bipolar and unipolar affective disorders: Relationship to age, sex, age of onset, and monoamine oxidase. Biol. Psychiat. 7:199–212.

Bunney, B. S., and G. K. Aghajanian. 1975. Evidence for Drug Actions on Both Pre- and Postsynaptic Catecholamine Receptors in the CNS. In Pre- and Postsynaptic Receptors, Usdin, E., and W. E. Bunney, Jr. (Eds.), pp. 89–122. New York, Marcel Dekker, Inc.

Bunney, W. E., Jr. 1976. To be presented at Annual Meeting of Am. Col. of Neur. Psychopharmacol. Personal communication.

Bunney, W. E., Jr., H. K. H. Brodie, D. L. Murphy, and F. K. Goodwin. 1971. Studies of alpha-methyl tyrosine, L-dopa and L-tryptophan in depression and mania. Am. J. Psychiat. 127:872–881.

Bunney, W. E., Jr., and J. M. Davis. 1965. Norepinephrine in depressive reactions. A review. Arch. Gen. Psychiat. 13:483–494.

Bunney, W. E., Jr., F. K. Goodwin, and D. L. Murphy. 1972. The "switch process" in manic-depressive illness. Arch. Gen. Psychiat. 27:312–317.

Bunney, W. E., Jr., and B. L. Gulley. 1977. In Biochemistry of Mental Disorders: New Vistas, Isdin, E., and A. Mandell (Eds.). In press.

Bunney, W. E., Jr., and D. L. Murphy. 1975. Strategies for the Systematic Study of Neurotransmitter Receptor Function in Man. In Pre- and Postsynaptic Receptors, Usdin, E., and W. E. Bunney, Jr. (Eds.). New York, Marcel Dekker, Inc.

Bunney, W. E., Jr., D. L. Murphy, H. Brodie, and F. K. Goodwin. 1970a. L-Dopa in depressed patients. Lancet 1:352.

Bunney, W. E., Jr., D. L. Murphy, and F. K. Goodwin. 1970b. The switch process from depression to mania: Relationship to drugs which alter brain amines. Lancet 1:1022–1027.

Cadoret, R. 1976. Genetics of Affective Disorders. In Biological Foundations of Psychiatry, Grenell, R. G., and S. Gabay (Eds.), pp. 645–652. New York, Raven Press.

Cantwell, D. P. 1975. Genetic Studies of Hyperactive Children: Psychiatric Illness in Biologic and Adopting Parents. In Genetic Research in Psychiatry, Fieve, R. R., D. Rosenthal, and A. A. Brill (Eds.), pp. 273–280. Baltimore, Johns Hopkins University Press.

Carpenter, W. T., J. S. Strauss, and S. Muleh. 1973. Are there pathognomonic symptoms in schizophrenia? An empiric investigation of Schneider's first-rank symptoms. Arch. Gen. Psychiat. 28:847–852.

Carroll, B. J., G. C. Curtis, and J. Mendels. 1976. Neuroendocrine regulation in depression. Arch. Gen. Psychiat. 33:1039–1044.

Carroll, B. J., R. M. Mowbray, and B. Davies. 1970. Sequential comparison of L-tryptophan with ECT in severe depression. Lancet 1:967–969.

Casper, R. C., G. Pandey, L. Gosenfeld, and J. M. Davis. 1976. Intracellular lithium and clinical response. Lancet 2:418–419.

Cavalli-Sforza, L. L., and W. F. Bodmer. 1971. The Genetics of Human Populations, pp. 860–866. San Francisco, W. H. Freeman.

Cazzullo, C. L., E. Smeraldi, and G. Penati. 1974. The leucocyte angigenic system HLA as a possible genetic marker of schizophrenia. Brit. J. Psychiat. 125:25–27.

Cazzullo, C. L., E. Smeraldi, E. Sachetti, and S. Bottinelli. 1975. Intracellular lithium concentration and clinical response. Brit. J. Psychiat. 126:298–300.

Childs, B. 1976. Medical genetics. In Worden, F. G., S. Matthysse, B. Childs, and E. S. Gershon (Eds.). Neurosciences Res. Prog. Bull. 14:13–18.

Cohen, S. M., M. G. Allen, and W. M. Pollin. 1972. Relationship of schizoaffective psychosis to manic depressive psychosis and schizophrenia. Arch. Gen. Psychiat. 26:539–546.

Cohn, C. K., D. L. Dunner, and J. Axelrod. 1970. Reduced catechol-O-methyltransferase activity in red blood cells of women with primary affective disorder. Science 170:1323–1324.

Collins, G. G. S., and M. Sandler. 1971. Human blood platelet monoamine oxidase. Biochem. Pharmacol. 20:289–296.

Cooper, J. R., F. E. Bloom, and R. H. Roth. 1974. The Biochemical Basis of Neuropharmacology. New York, Oxford University Press.

Coppen, A., R. Gupta, S. Montgomery, and J. Bailey. 1976a. A double-blind comparison of lithium carbonate and Ludiomil in the prophylaxis of unipolar affective illness. Pharmakopsychiatr. Neuropsychopharmakol. 9:94–99.

Coppen, A., S. A. Montgomery, R. K. Gupta, and J. E. Bailey. 1976b. A double-blind comparison of lithium carbonate and maprotiline in the prophylaxis of the affective disorders. Brit. J. Psychiat. 128:479–485.

Coppen, A., A. J. Prange, P. C. Whybrow, and R. Noguera. 1972a. Abnormalities of indoleamines in affective disorders. Arch. Gen. Psychiat. 26:474–478.

Coppen, A., P. Whybrow, R. Noguera, R. Maggs, and A. Prange. 1972b. The comparative antidepressant value of L-tryptophan and imipramine with and without attempted potentiation by liothyronine. Arch. Gen. Psychiat. 26:234–241.

Court, J. H. 1968. Manic depressive psychosis: An alternative conceptual model. Brit. J. Psychiat. 114:1523–1530.

Coyle, J. T., and J. Axelrod. 1972. Dopamine-β-hydroxylase in the rat brain: Developmental characteristics. J. Neurochem. 19:449–459.

Crowe, R. R. 1975. Adoption studies in psychiatry. Biol. Psychiat. 10:353–371.

Cuatrecasas, P., G. P. Tell, V. Sica, I. Parikh, and K. J. Chang. 1974. Noradrenaline binding and the search for catecholamine receptors. Nature 247:92–97.

Davis, J. M. 1975. Critique of single amine theories: Evidence of a cholinergic influence in the major mental illnesses. In Biology of the Major Psychoses, Freedman, D. X. (Ed.). Res. Publ. Assoc. Res. Nerv. Ment. Dis. 54:333–346. New York, Raven Press.

Davis, J. M., and J. O. Cole. 1976. Antipsychotic Drugs, Antidepressant Drugs. In Comprehensive Textbook of Psychiatry, Freedman, A. M., H. I. Kaplan and B. J. Sadock (Eds.), Chapter 31:2. Baltimore, Williams and Wilkins.

Dencker, S. J., V. Malm, B. E. Roos, and B. Werdinius. 1966. Acid monoamine metabolites of cerebrospinal fluid in mental depression and mania. J. Neurochem. 13:1545–1548.

Detre, T., J. Himmelhoch, M. Swartzburg, C. M. Anderson, R. Byck, and D. J. Kupfer. 1972. Hypersomnia and manic-depressive disease. Am. J. Psychiat. 128:1303.

Donnelly, C. H., and D. L. Murphy. Substrate and inhibitor-related characteristics of human platelet monoamine oxidase. Biochem. Pharmacol. In press.

Dorus, E., G. N. Pandey, and J. M. Davis. 1975. Genetic determinant of lithium ion distribution: An in vitro and in vivo monozygotic-dizygotic twin study. Arch. Gen. Psychiat. 32:1097–1102.

Dorus, E., G. N. Pandey, A. Frazer, and J. Mendels. 1974. Genetic determinant of lithium ion distribution: I. An in vitro monozygotic-dizygotic twin study. Arch. Gen. Psychiat. 31:463–465.

Dunner, D. L., C. K. Cohn, E. S. Gershon, and F. K. Goodwin. 1971. Differential catechol-O-methyltransferase activity in unipolar and bipolar affective illness. Arch. Gen. Psychiat. 25:348–353.

Dunner, D. L., and R. R. Fieve. 1975. Affective disorder: Studies with amine precursors. Am. J. Psychiat. 132:180–183.

Dunner, D. L., E. S. Gershon, and F. K. Goodwin. 1976. Heritable factors in the severity of affective illness. Biol. Psychiat. 11:31–42.

Dunner, D. L., F. K. Goodwin, E. S. Gershon, D. L. Murphy, and W. E. Bunney, Jr. 1972. Excretion of 17-OHCS in unipolar and bipolar depressed patients. Arch. Gen. Psychiat. 26:360–363.

Dunner, D. L., M. Levitt, J. Cumbaraci, and R. R. Fieve. In press. Erythrocyte catechol-O-methyltransferase in primary affective disorder. Biol. Psychiat.

Dyson, W. L., and A. Barcai. 1970. Treatment of children of lithium-responding parents. Current Ther. Res. 12:286–290.

Eberhard, G., G. Franzen, and B. Low. 1975. Schizophrenia susceptibility and HL-A antigen. Neuropsychobiology 1:211–217.

Ebert, M. H., and I. J. Kopin. 1975. Differential labelling of origins of urinary catecholamine metabolites by dopamine-C14. Trans. Assoc. Am. Physicans 88:256–264.

Ebert, M. H., R. M. Post, and F. K. Goodwin. 1972. Effect of physical activity on urinary excretion of MHPG. Lancet 2:766.

Ebstein, R., R. H. Belmaker, D. Benbenisty, and R. Rimon. 1976. Electrophoretic pattern of red blood cell catechol-O-methyltransferase in schizophrenia and manic-depressive illness. Biol. Psychiat. 11:613–623.

Edwards, D. J., and S. Chang. 1975. Multiple forms of monoamine oxidase in rabbit platelets. Life Sci. 17:1127–1134.

Edwards, J. H. 1971. The analysis of X-linkage. Ann. Hum. Genet. 34:229.

Elizur, A., B. Shopsin, S. Gershon, and A. Ehlenberger. 1972. Intra : extracellular lithium ratios and clinical course in affective states. Clin. Pharmacol. Ther. 13:947–952.

Elston, R. C., and J. Stewart. 1971. A general model for the genetic analysis of pedigree data. Hum. Hered. 21:523–542.

Falconer, D. S. 1965. The inheritance of liability to certain diseases estimated from the incidence among relatives. Ann. Hum. Genet. 29:51.

Fawcett, J., J. W. Maas, and H. Dekirmenjian. 1972. Depression and MHPG excretion. Arch. Gen. Psychiat. 26:246–251.

Feighner, J. P., E. Robins, and S. B. Guze. 1972. Diagnostic criteria for use in psychiatric research. Arch. Gen. Psychiat. 26:57–63.

Fieve, R. R. 1973. Overview of Therapeutic and Prophylactic Trials with Lithium in Psychiatric Patients. In Lithium: Its Role in Psychiatric Research and Treatment, Gershon, S., and B. Shopsin (Eds.), pp. 317–350. New York, Plenum Press.

Fieve, R. R. 1976. Lithium therapy. In Comprehensive Textbook of Psychiatry, Friedman, A. M., H. I. Kaplan, and B. J. Sadock (Eds.), Vol. 2, Chapter 31.8. Baltimore, Williams and Wilkins.

Fieve, R. R., T. Kumbaraci, and D. Dunner. 1976. Lithium prophylaxis of depression in bipolar I, bipolar II, and unipolar patients. Am. J. Psychiat. 133:925–929.

Fischer, E. 1975. The phenylethylamine hypothesis of thymic homeostasis. Biol. Psychiat. 10:667–674.

Frazer, A., J. Mendels, S. K. Secunda, C. M. Cochrane, and C. P. Bianchi. 1973. The prediction of brain lithium concentrations from plasma or erythrocyte measures. J. Psychiat. Res. 10:1–7.

Fremming, K. 1951. The expectation of mental infirmity in a sample of the Danish population. Occ. Papers on Eugenics, 7. London, Cassell and Co., Ltd.

Garelis, E., S. N. Young, S. Lal, and T. L. Sourkes. 1974. Monoamine metabolites in lumbar CSF: The question of their origin in relation to clinical studies. Brain Res. 79:1–8.

Gayford, J. J., A. L. Parker, E. M. Phillips, and A. R. Rowsell. 1973. Whole blood 5-hydroxy-tryptamine during treatment of endogenous depressive illness. Brit. J. Psychiat. 122:597–598.

Gershon, E. 1977. Genetic and Biologic Studies of Affective Illness. In Impact of Biology on Modern Psychiatry, Gershon, E. S., R. H. Belmaker, S. S. Kety, and M. Rosenbaum (Eds.). New York, Plenum Publishing Co.

Gershon, E., M. Baron, and J. Leckman. 1975a. Genetic models of the transmission of affective disorders. J. Psychiat. Res. 12:301–317.

Gershon, E., R. H. Belmaker, R. Ebstein, and W. Z. Jonas. 1977. Plasma monoamine oxidase activity unrelated to genetic vulnerability to primary affective illness. Arch. Gen. Psychiat. In press.

Gershon, E., and M. Buchsbaum. 1976. A Genetic Study of Average Evoked Response Augmenting/Reducing in Affective Disorders. In Psychopathology and Brain Dysfunction, Shagass, C., and S. Gershon (Eds.), (American Psychopathological Association, 66th Annual Meeting). New York, Raven Press.

Gershon, E., and W. E. Bunney, Jr. In press. The question of X-linkage in bipolar manic-depressive illness. J. Psychiat. Res.

Gershon, E., W. E. Bunney, Jr., F. K. Goodwin, D. L. Murphy, D. L. Dunner, and G. M. Henry. 1971a. Catecholamines in Affective Illness: Studies with L-Dopa and Alpha-methyl-para-tyrosine. In Brain Chemistry and Mental Disease, Ho, B. T., and W. M. McIsaac (Eds.), pp. 135–163. New York, Plenum Publishing Co.

Gershon, E., W. E. Bunney, Jr., J. Leckman, M. van Eerdewegh, and B. DeBauche. 1976. The inheritance of affective disorders: A review of data and of hypotheses. Behav. Genet. 6:227–261.

Gershon, E., D. L. Dunner, and F. K. Goodwin. 1971b. Toward a biology of affective disorders. Arch. Gen. Psychiat. 25:1–15.

Gershon, E., and W. Jonas. 1975. A clinical and genetic study of erythrocyte soluble catechol-O-methyl transferase activity in primary affective disorder. Arch. Gen. Psychiat. 32:1351–1356.

Gershon, E., and J. L. Liebowitz. 1975. Sociocultural and demographic correlates of affective disorders in Jerusalem. J. Psychiat. Res. 12:37–50.

Gershon, E., A. Mark, N. Cohen, N. Belizon, M. Baron, and K. E. Knobe. 1975b. Transmitted factors in the morbid risk of affective disorders: A controlled study. J. Psychiat. Res. 12:283–299.

Gewirtz, G. P., and I. J. Kopin. 1970. Release of dopamine-β-hydroxylase with norepinephrine during cat splenic nerve stimulation. Nature 227:406–407.

Goetzl, U., R. Green, P. Whybrow, and R. Jackson. 1974. X-linkage revisited. A further family study of manic-depressive illness. Arch. Gen. Psychiat. 31:665–672.

Gold, P., F. K. Goodwin, T. Wehr, R. Rebar, and R. Sack. Unpublished data a. Growth hormone and prolactin response to L-dopa in affective illness.

Gold, P., R. Rebar, T. Wehr, and F. K. Goodwin. Unpublished data b. TRH responses: UP-BP differences and CSF correlates. New Research Abstract NR19, A.P.A. 1976.

Goldstein, M., L. S. Friedman, and M. Bonnay. 1971. An assay for dopamine-β-hydroxylase activity in tissues and serum. Experientia 27:632–633.

Goodwin, F. K., and H. Beckmann. 1975. Urinary MHPG in unipolar and bipolar affective disorders. Sci. Proc. A.P.A. 128:96–97.

Goodwin, F. K., and W. E. Bunney, Jr. 1971. Depressions following reserpine: A reevaluation. Semin. Psychiat. 3:435–448.

Goodwin, F. K., D. L. Murphy, H. K. H. Brodie, and W. E. Bunney, Jr. 1970. L-Dopa-catecholamines, and behavior: A clinical and biochemical study in depressed patients. Biol. Psychiat. 2:341–366.

Goodwin, F. K., D. L. Murphy, D. L. Dunner, and W. E. Bunney, Jr. 1972. Lithium response in unipolar versus bipolar depression. Am. J. Psychiat. 129:44–47.

Goodwin, F. K., and R. M. Post. 1975. Studies of Amine Metabolites in Affective Illness and in Schizophrenia: A Comparative Analysis. In Biology of the Major Psychoses, Freedman, D. X. (Ed.). Research Publication Assoc. Res. Nerv. and Mental Dis. Vol. 54 pp. 299–332. New York, Raven Press.

Goodwin, F. K., R. M. Post, D. L. Dunner, and E. K. Gordon. 1973. Cerebrospinal fluid amine metabolites in affective illness: The probenecid technique. Am. J. Psychiat. 130:73–78.

Goodwin, F. K., R. M. Post, and T. Wehr. Unpublished data. Clinical Approaches to the Evaluation of Brain Amine Function in Mental Illness: Some Conceptual Issues. In Essays in Neurochemistry and Neuropharmacology, Lovenberg, W., and M. Youdim (Eds.). London, John Wiley and Sons, Ltd.

Gottfries, C. G., L. Oreland, A. Wiberg, and B. Winblad. 1974. Brain-levels of monoamine oxidase in depression. Lancet 2:360–361.

Green, A. R., and D. G. Grahame-Smith. 1975. In Handbook of Psychopharmacology, Iversen, L. L., G. Iversen, and S. Snyder (Eds.), pp. 169–245. New York, Plenum Press.

Greenspan, K., J. J. Schildkraut, E. K. Gordon, L. Baer, M. Aronoff, and J. Durell. 1970. Catecholamine metabolism in affective disorders. J. Psychiat. Res. 7:171–183.

Grote, S. S., S. G. Moses, E. Robins, R. W. Hudgens, and A. B. Croninger. 1974. A study of selected catecholamine metabolizing enzymes: A comparison of depressive suicides and alcoholic suicides with controls. J. Neurochem. 23:791–802.

Grunhaus, L., R. Ebstein, R. Belmaker, S. G. Sandler, and W. Jonas. 1976. A twin study of human red blood cell catechol-O-methyl transferase. Brit. J. Psychiat. 128:494–498.

Guze, S. B., E. D. Wolfgram, J. K. McKinney, and D. P. Cantwell. 1967. Psychiatric illness in the families of convicted male criminals: A study of 519 first-degree relatives. Dis. Nerv. Syst. 28:651–659.

Haldane, J. B. S. 1949. A test for homogeneity of records of familial abnormalities. Ann. Eugen. 14:339–341.

Hall, D. W. R., B. W. Logan, and G. H. Parsons. 1969. Further studies on the inhibition of monoamine oxidase by M S B 9302 (Clorgyline). Biochem. Pharmacol. 18:1447–1454.

Harris, T. H. 1957. Depression induced by the rauwolfia compounds. Am. J. Psychiat. 113:950.

Hartman, B. K. 1972. The discovery and isolation of a new monoamine oxidase from brain. Biol. Psychiat. 4:147–155.

Hartman, B. K. 1973. Immunofluorescence of dopamine-β-hydroxylase: Application of improved methodology to the localization of the peripheral and central noradrenergic nervous system. J. Histochem. Cytochem. 21:312–332.

Hartman, B. K., K. J. Yasunobu, and S. Udenfriend. 1969. Immunological identity of the multiple forms of beef liver mitochondrial monoamine oxidase. Arch. Biochem. Biophys. 147:797–804.

Helgassen, T. 1964. Epidemiology of mental disorders in Iceland. Acta Psychiat. Scand. 40: Suppl. 173.

Helzer, J. E., and G. Winokur. 1974. A family interview study of male manic depressives. Arch. Gen. Psychiat. 31:73–77.

Hertting, G., and J. Axelrod. 1961. Fate of tritiated noradrenaline at the sympathetic nerve endings. Nature 192:172–173.

Hokin-Neaverson, M., D. A. Spiegel, and W. C. Lewis. 1974. Deficiency of erythrocyte sodium pump activity in bipolar manic-depressive psychosis. Life Sci. 15:1739–1748.

Hollister, A. S., G. R. Breese, C. M. Kuhn, B. R. Cooper, and S. M. Schanberg. 1976. An inhibitory role for brain serotonin-containing systems in the locomotor effects of d-amphetamine. J. Pharm. Exp. Ther. 198:12–22.

Horwitz, D. R., R. W. Alexander, W. Lovenberg, and H. R. Keiser. 1973. Human serum dopamine-β-hydroxylase. Circ. Res. 32:594–599.

Hutchings, B., and S. A. Mednick. 1975. Registered Criminality in the Adoptive and Biological Parents of Registered Male Criminal Adoptees. In Genetic Research in Psychiatry, Fieve, R. R., D. Rosenthal, and A. A. Brill (Eds.), pp. 105–116. Baltimore, Johns Hopkins University Press.

Irvine, D. G., and H. Miyashita. 1965. Blood types in relation to depressions and schizophrenia: A preliminary report. Canad. Med. Assoc. J. 92:551–554.

James, J. W. 1971. Frequency in relatives for an all-or-none trait. Ann. Hum. Genet. 35:47–49.

James, N. M., and C. J. Chapman. 1975. A genetic study of bipolar affective disorder. Brit. J. Psychiat. 126:449–456.

Janowsky, D. S., J. M. Davis, M. K. El-Yousef, and H. J. Sekerke. 1972. A cholinergic-adrenergic hypothesis of mania and depression. Lancet 2:632–635.

Janowsky, D. S., M. K. El-Yousef, J. M. Davis, and H. J. Sekerke. 1973a. Antagonistic effects of physostigmine and methylphenidate in man. Am. J. Psychiat. 130:1370–1376.

Janowsky, D. S., M. K. El-Yousef, J. M. Davis, and H. J. Sekerke. 1973b. Provocation of schizophrenic symptoms by intravenous administration of methylphenidate. Arch. Gen. Psychiat. 28:185–191.

Jimerson, D. C., E. K. Gordon, R. M. Post, and F. K. Goodwin. 1975. Central noradrenergic function in man: Vanillylmandelic acid in CSF. Brain Res. 99:434–439.

Johnston, J. P. 1968. Some observations upon a new inhibitor of monoamine oxidase in brain tissue. Biochem. Pharmacol. 17:1285–1297.

Kallman, F. 1950. The Genetics of Psychoses: An Analysis of 1,232 Twin Index Families. In Congres Internationale de Psychiatrie (Paris, 1950). Paris, Hermann and Cie. Also: Genetic Aspects of Psychosis. In The Biology of Mental Health and Disease. The 27th Annual Conference of the Milband Memorial Fund. New York, Paul B. Hoeber, Inc. Medical Book Department of Harper & Row.

Kallman, F. 1954. Genetic Principles in Manic-Depressive Psychoses. In Depression, Hoch, P. H., and J. Zubin (Eds.). New York, Grune & Stratton, Inc.

Kaufman, S., and S. Friedman. 1965. Dopamine-β-hydroxylase. Pharmacol. Rev. 17:71–100.

Kendell, R. E. 1976. The classification of depressions: A review of contemporary confusion. Brit. J. Psychiat. 129:15–28.

Kessler, J. A., E. K. Gordon, J. L. Reid, and I. J. Kopin. 1976. Homovanillic acid and 3-methoxy-4-hydroxyphenylethyleneglycol production by the monkey spinal cord. J. Neurochem. 26:1057–1061.

Kety, S. S. 1971. Brain Amines and Affective Disorders. In Brain Chemistry and Mental Disease, Ho, B. T., and W. M. McIsaac (Eds.). Advances in Behavioral Biology, Vol. 1, pp. 237–244. New York, Plenum Press.

Kidd, K. K., and L. L. Cavalli-Sforza. 1972. Genetic models for schizophrenia. Neurosci. Res. Program Bull. 10:405.

Kidd, K. K., T. Reich, and S. Kessler. Unpublished data. Sex effect and the single gene.

Kidd, K. K., and M. A. Spence. 1976. Genetic analyses of pyloric stenosis suggesting a specific maternal effect J. Med. Genet. 13:290–294.

Kiloh, L. G., M. Neilson, and G. Andrews. 1974. Response of depressed patients to methylamphetamine. Brit. J. Psychiat. 125:496–499.

Klaiber, E. L., D. M. Broverman, W. Vogel, Y. Kabayashi, and D. Moriarty. 1972. Effects of estrogen therapy on plasma MAO activity and EEG driving responses of depressed women. Am. J. Psychiat. 128:1492–1498.

Klein, D. F., and J. M. Davis. 1969. Diagnosis and Drug Treatment of Psychiatric Disorders. Williams & Wilkins.

Knorring, L., L. Oreland, C. Perris, and A. Wiberg. 1976. Evaluation of the lithium RBC/plasma ratio as a predictor of the prophylactic effect of lithium treatment in affective disorders. Pharmacopsychiatry 9:81–84.

Kopin, I. J. 1964. Storage and metabolism of catecholamines: The role of monoamine oxidase. Pharmacol. Rev. 16:179–191.

Kupfer, D. 1976. REM latency: A psychobiologic marker for primary depressive disease. Biol. Psychiat. 11:2:159–174.

Kupfer, D., D. Pickar, J. Himmelhoch, and T. P. Detre. 1975. Are there two types of unipolar depression? Arch. Gen. Psychiat. 32:866–871.

Lamprecht, F., M. H. Ebert, I. Turek, and I. J. Kopin. 1974a. Serum dopamine-β-hydroxylase in depressed patients and the effect of electroconvulsive shock treatment. Psychopharmacologia 40:241–248.

Lamprecht, F., R. J. Matta, B. Little, and T. P. Zahn. 1974b. Plasma dopamine-beta-hydroxylase (DBH) activity during the menstrual cycle. Psychosom. Med. 36:304–310.

Landowski, J., W. Lysiak, and S. Angielski. 1975. Monoamine oxidase activity in blood platelets from patients with cyclophrenic depressive syndromes. Biochem. Med. 14:347–354.

Lapin, I. P., and G. F. Oxenkrug. 1969. Intensification of the central serotonergic processes as a possible determinant of the thymoleptic effect. Lancet 1:132–136.

Leckman, J. F., and E. S. Gershon. 1976. Autosomal models of sex effect in bipolar-related major affective illness. Abstract in Sci. Proc. Am. Psychiat. Assoc. 129:127–128.

Leckman, J. F., E. S. Gershon, A. Frazer, and J. Mendels. Unpublished data a. Failure of the rbc/plasma ratio to predict clinical polarity among patients with primary affective disorder: A prospective study.

Leckman, J. F., E. S. Gershon, D. S. Murphy, and A. S. Nichols. Unpublished data b. Reduced platelet monoamine oxidase activity in first degree relatives of individuals with bipolar affective disorders: A preliminary report. Abstract in Sci. Proc. Am. Psychiat. Assoc. 129:128–129.

Lee, C. R., S. E. Hill, M. Dimitraakoudi, F. A. Jenner, and R. J. Pollitt. 1975. The relationship of plasma to erythrocyte lithium levels in patients taking lithium carbonate. Brit. J. Psychiat. 127:596–598.

Leonhard, K. 1957. Aufreilung der Endogenen. Psychosen. 1st Ed. Berlin.

Leonhard, K., I. Korff, and H. Schulz. 1962. Die Temperamente in den Familien der monopolaren and bipolaren phasischen Psychosen. Psychiatria et Neurologia 143:416–434.

Levin, E. Y., and S. Kaufman. 1961. Studies on the enzyme catalyzing the conversion of dopamine to norepinephrine. J. Biol. Chem. 236:2043–2049.

Levitt, M., D. L. Dunner, J. Mendlewicz, D. B. Frewin, W. Lauelor, J. L. Fleiss, F. Stallone, and R. R. Fieve. 1976. Plasma dopamine β-hydroxylase activity in affective disorders. Psychopharmacologia 46:205–210.

Levitt, M., D. B. Frewin, C. C. Co, W. K. Luke, and J. A. Downey. 1974. Plasma dopamine-β-hydroxylase activity in paraplegic and quadriplegic subjects. Aust. N.Z. J. Med. 4:48–52.

Levitt, M., and J. Mendlewicz. 1975. A genetic study of plasma dopamine-β-hydroxylase in affective disorder. Mod. Probl. Pharmacopsychiat. 10:89–98.

Lieberman, A. N., L. S. Freedman, and M. Goldstein. 1972. Serum dopamine-β-hydroxylase activity in patients with Huntington's chorea and Parkinson's disease. Lancet 1:153–154.

Liebowitz, J., V. Randy, E. Gershon, and A. Gillis. 1976. A pharmacogenetic case report: Lithium responsive post-psychotic antisocial behavior. Comp. Psychiat. 17:655–660.

Lyttkens, S., U. Soderberg, and S. Wetterberg. 1973. Increased lithium erythrocyte/plasma ratio in manic-depressive psychosis. Lancet 1:40.

Maas, J. W. 1975. Biogenic amines and depression. Arch. Gen. Psychiat. 32:1357–1361.

Maas, J. W., H. Dekirmenjian, and J. A. Fawcett. 1973. Relation of exercise to MHPG excretion in normal subjects. Arch. Gen. Psychiat. 29:391–396.

Maas, J. W., H. Dekirmengian, and F. Jones. 1973. The Identification of Depressed Patients Who Have a Disorder of NE Metabolism and/or Disposition. In Frontiers of Catecholamine Research, Usdin, E., and S. Snyder (Eds.), pp. 1091–1096. New York, Pergamon Press.

Maas, J. W., J. A. Fawcett, and H. Dekirmenjian. 1968. 3-Methoxy-4-hydroxyphenyl-glycol (MHPG) excretion in depressive patients: A pilot study. Arch. Gen. Psychiat. 19:129–134.

Maas, J. W., J. A. Fawcett, and H. Dekirmenjian. 1972. Catecholamine metabolism, depressive illness and drug response. Arch. Gen. Psychiat. 26:252–262.

Mandell, A. J. 1973. New Concepts in Neurotransmitter Regulation. New York, Plenum Press.

Mandell, A. J., and S. Knapp. 1975. Current research in the indoleamine hypothesis of affective disorders. Psychopharmacol. Comm. 1:587–597.

Manuila A., and M. D. Lexander. 1958. Blood groups and disease — hard facts and delusions. JAMA 167:2047–2053.

Masters, A. B. 1967. The distribution of blood groups in psychiatric illness. Brit. J. Psychiat. 113:1309–1315.

Mattson, B., T. Mjorndal, L. Oreland, and C. Perris. 1974. Catechol-O-methyltransferase and plasma monoamine oxidase in patients with affective disorders. Acta Psychiat. Scand. 255:187–192.

Matussek, N. 1971. L-Dopa in the treatment of depression. In Advances in Neuropharmacology, Vinar, O., Z. Votova, and P. B. Bradley (Eds.). Amsterdam, North-Holland Publ., 111–119.

McCabe, M. S., and R. J. Cadoret. 1976. Genetic investigations of atypical psychoses. I. Morbidity in parents and siblings. Comp. Psychiat. 17:347–352.

McCauley, R., and E. Racker. 1973. Separation of two monoamine oxidases from bovine brain. Molec. Cell. Biochem. 1:73–81.

Meltzer, H. Y., H. W. Cho, B. J. Carroll, and P. Russo. 1976. Serum dopamine-β-hydroxylase activity in the affective psychoses and schizophrenia. Arch. Gen. Psychiat. 33:585–591.

Mendels, J. 1974. Lithium in the Treatment of Depressive States. In Lithium Research and Therapy, Johnson, N. (Ed.). New York, Academic Press.

Mendels, J. 1976. Lithium in the treatment of depression. Am. J. Psychiat. 133:373–378.

Mendels, J., and A. Frazer. 1973. Intracellular lithium concentration and clinical response: Towards a membrane theory of depression. J. Psychiat. Res. 10:9–18.

Mendels, J., and Frazer. 1974. Alterations in cell membrane activity in depression. Am. J. Psychiat. 131:1240–1246.

Mendels, J., and A. Frazer. 1975. Reduced central serotonergic activity in mania. Brit. J. Psychiat. 126:241–248.

Mendels, J., A. Frazer, J. Baron, A. Kukopulos, D. Reginaldi, L. Tondo, and B. Caliari. 1976. Intra-erythrocyte lithium ion concentration and long-term maintenance treatment. Lancet 1:966.

Mendels, J., J. L. Stinnett, D. Burns, and A. Frazer. 1975. Amine precursors and depression. Arch. Gen. Psychiat. 32:22–30.

Mendlewicz, J., and J. L. Fleiss. 1974. Linkage studies with X-chromosome markers in bipolar (manic-depressive) and unipolar (depressive) illnesses. Biol. Psychiat. 9:261.

Mendlewicz, J., J. L. Fleiss, and R. R. Fieve. 1972. Evidence for X-linkage in the transmission of manic-depressive illness. JAMA 222:1624.

Mendlewicz, J., J. L. Fleiss, and R. R. Fieve. 1975. Linkage studies in affective disorders. The Xg blood group and manic-depressive illness. In Genetics and Psychopathology, Fieve, R., D. Rosenthal, and H. Brill (Eds.). Baltimore, Johns Hopkins University Press.

Mendlewicz, J., and J. D. Rainer. 1974. Morbidity risk and genetic transmission in manic-depressive illness. Am. J. Hum. Genet. 26:692–701.

Mitsuda, H. 1967. In Clinical Genetics in Psychiatry, pp. 3–21. Kyoto, Bunko-sha Co., Ltd.

Molinoff, P. B., S. Brimijoin, R. Weinshilboum, and J. Axelrod. 1970. Neurally mediated increase in dopamine-β-hydroxylase activity. Proc. Nat. Acad. Sci. 66:453–458.

Morrison, J. R. 1975. The family histories of manic depressive patients with and without alcoholism. J. Nerv. Ment. Dis. 160:227–229.

Morton, N. E. 1955. Sequential tests for the detection of linkage. Am. J. Hum. Genet. 7:277–318.

Murphy, D. L. 1973. Technical Strategies for the Study of Catecholamines in Man. In Frontiers in Catecholamine Research, Usdin, E., and S. Snyder (Eds.), pp. 1077–1082. Oxford, Pergamon Press.

Murphy, D. L., M. Baker, F. K. Goodwin, H. Miller, J. Kotin, and W. E. Bunney, Jr. 1974. L-Tryptophan in affective disorders: Indoleamine changes and differential clinical effects. Psychopharmacologia 34:11–20.

Murphy, D. L., H. K. H. Brodie, F. K. Goodwin, and W. E. Bunney, Jr. 1971. Regular induction of hypomania by L-dopa in "bipolar" manic-depressive patients. Nature 229:135–136.

Murphy, D. L., and C. H. Donnelly. 1974. Monoamine oxidase in man: Enzyme characteristics in platelets, plasma, and other human tissues. Adv. Biochem. Psychopharmacol. 12:71–85.

Murphy, D. L., F. K. Goodwin, H. K. H. Brodie, and W. E. Bunney, Jr. 1973. L-Dopa, dopamine, and hypomania. Am. J. Psychiat. 130:79–82.

Murphy, D. L., and R. Weiss. 1972. Reduced monoamine oxidase activity in blood platelets from bipolar depressed patients. Am. J. Psychiat. 128:1351–1357.

Murphy, D. L., and R. J. Wyatt. 1975. Neurotransmitter-related enzymes in the major psychiatric disorders: I. Catechol-O-methyl transferase, monoamine oxidase in the affective disorders, and factors affecting some behaviorally correlated enzyme activities. Res. Publ. Assoc. Res. Nerv. Ment. Dis. 54:277–288.

Muscettola, G., T. Wehr, and F. K. Goodwin. 1976. Central norepinephrine responses in depression versus normals. New Research Abstracts, APA Meeting, Miami.

Nagatsu, T., and S. Udenfriend. 1972. Photometric assay of dopamine-β-hydroxylase activity in human blood. Clin. Chem. 18:980–983.

Nahunek, K., J. Svestka, V. Kamenicka, et al. 1972. Preliminary clinical experience with L-dopa in endogenous depressions. Acta Nerv. Super. 14:101–102.

Neff, N. H., and C. Goridis. 1972. Neuronal monoamine oxidase: Specific enzyme types and their rates of formation. Adv. Biochem. Pharmacol. 5:307–323.

Nies, A. Personal communication.

Nies, A., D. S. Robinson, L. S. Harris, and K. R. Lamborn. 1974. Comparison of monoamine oxidase substrate activities in twins, schizophrenics, depressives, and controls. Adv. Biochem. Psychopharmacol. 12:59–70.

Nies, A., D. S. Robinson, K. R. Lamborn, and R. P. Lampert. 1973. Genetic control of platelet and plasma monoamine oxidase activity. Arch. Gen. Psychiat. 28:834–838.

Nies, A., D. S. Robinson, C. L. Ravaris, and J. M. Davis. 1971. Amines and monoamine oxidase in relation to ageing and depression in man. Psychosomat. Med. 33:470.

Noyes, R., G. Dempsey, A. Blum, and G. Cavanaugh. 1974. Lithium treatment in depression. Comp. Psychiat. 15:187–193.

Nyhan, W. L., J. Pesek, L. Sweetman, D. G. Carpenter, and C. H. Carter. 1967. Genetics of an X-linked disorder of uric acid and metabolism and cerebral function. Pediat. Res. 1:5.

Ogihara, J., C. A. Nugent, S-W. Shen, and S. Goldfein. 1975. Serum dopamine-β-hydroxylase activity in parents and children. J. Lab. Clin. Med. 85:566–573.

Oka, M., K. Kajikawa, T. Ohuchi, H. Yoshida, and R. Imaizumi. 1967. Distribution of dopamine-β-hydroxylase in subcellular fractions of adrenal medulla. Life Sci. 6:461–465.

Overall, J. E., L. E. Hollister, M. Johnson, and V. Pennington. 1966. Nosology of depression and differential response to drugs. JAMA 195:946–948.

Parker, J. B., A. Theilie, and C. D. Spielberger. 1961. Frequency of blood types in a homogeneous group of manic-depressive patients. J. Ment. Sci. 107:936–942.

Pearson, P. L., R. Sanger, and J. A. Brown. 1975. Report of the Committee on the Genetic Constitution of the X-Chromosome. In Human Gene Mapping 2, Rotterdam Conference 1974; Second International Workshop on Human Gene Mapping, Birth Defects Original Article Series, 11:190.

Perris, C. 1966. A study of bipolar (manic-depressive) and unipolar recurrent depressive psychoses. Acta Psychiat. Scand. 42:Suppl. 194.

Perris, C. 1974a. A study of cycloid psychoses. Acta Psychiat. Scand. Suppl. 253.

Perris, C. 1974b. The Genetics of Affective Disorders. In Biological Psychiat., Mendels, J. (Ed.). New York, John Wiley & Sons, 385–415.

Perry, T. L., J. A. Bratty, S. H. Hansen, and J. Kennedy. 1975. Hereditary mental depression and parkinsonism with mental deficiency. Arch. Neurol. 32:108–113.

Post, R. M., and F. K. Goodwin. 1973. Simulated behavior states: An approach to specificity in psychobiological research. Biol. Psychiat. 7:237–254.

Post, R. M., and F. K. Goodwin. In press. Approaches to Brain Amines in Psychiatric Patients: A Re-evaluation of Cerebrospinal Fluid Studies. In Handbook of Psychopharmacology, Snyder, S., S. Iverson, and L. L. Iverson (Eds.). New York, Plenum Press.

Post, R. M., F. K. Goodwin, E. K. Gordon, and D. M. Watkin. 1973. Amine metabolites in human cerebrospinal fluid: Effects of cord transsection and spinal fluid block. Science 179:897–899.

Potter, L. T., and J. Axelrod. 1963. Properties of norepinephrine storage particles of the rat heart. J. Pharmacol. Exp. Ther. 142:299–305.

Price, J. 1968. The Genetics of Depressive Behavior. In Recent Developments in Affective Disorders, Coppen, A., and A. Walk (Eds.). Brit. J. Psychiat. Special Publication No. 2, pp. 37–54.

Prien, R. F., E. M. Caffey, Jr., and C. J. Klett. 1973. Lithium carbonate and imipramine in prevention of affective episodes. Arch. Gen. Psychiat. 29:420–425.

Ramsey, T. A., A. Frazer, W. L. Dyson, and J. Mendels. 1976. Intracellular lithium and clinical response. Brit. J. Psychiat. 128:103–104.

Reich, T., P. J. Clayton, and G. Winokur. 1969. Family history studies: V. The genetics of mania. Am. J. Psychiat. 125:1358.

Reich, T., J. W. James, and C. A. Morris. 1972. The use of multiple thresholds in determining the mode of transmission of semi-continuous traits. Ann. Hum. Genet. 36:163.

Reich, T., G. Winokur, and J. Mullaney. 1975. The Transmission of Alcoholism. In Genetic Research in Psychiatry, Fieve, R. R., D. Rosenthal, and H. Brill (Eds.), pp. 259–272. Baltimore, Johns Hopkins University Press.

Renwick, J. H., and J. Schulze. 1964. An analysis of some data on the linkage between Xg and color blindness in man. Am. J. Hum. Genet. 16:410.

Rieder, R. R., and E. S. Gershon. Unpublished data. Genetic strategies: Approaches to the biology of psychiatric disorders.

Rifkin, A., S. J. Levitan, J. Galewski, and D. Klein. 1972a. Emotionally unstable character disorder—a follow-up study. I. Description of patients and outcome. Biol. Psychiat. 4:65–79.

Rifkin, A., S. J. Levitan, J. Galewski, and D. Klein. 1972b. Emotionally unstable character disorder—a follow-up study. II. Prediction of outcome. Biol. Psychiat. 4:81–88.

Rifkin, A., F. Quitkin, C. Carrillo, A. Blumberg, and D. Klein. 1972c. Lithium carbonate in emotionally unstable character disorder. Arch. Gen. Psychiat. 27:519–523.

Roberts, J. M. 1959. Prognostic factors in the electroshock treatment of depressive states. J. Ment. Sci. 105:703–713.

Robins, E., and S. B. Guze. 1972. Classification of Affective Disorders: The Primary-Secondary, the Endogenous-Reactive, and the Neurotic-Psychotic Concepts. In Recent Advances in the Psychobiology of the Depressive Illnesses, Williams, T. A., M. M. Katz, and J. A. S. Shields (Eds.), DHEW Publ. No. (HSM) 70-9053, p. 283. Washington, D.C., U.S. Government Printing Office.

Rockson, S., R. Stone, M. Van Der Weyden, and W. N. Kelley. 1974. Lesch-Nyhan syndrome: Evidence for abnormal adrenergic function. Science 186:934–935.

Rosenthal, D. 1970. Genetic Theory and Abnormal Behavior. New York, McGraw-Hill Books, Inc.

Ross, S. B., L. Wetterberg, and M. Myrhed. 1973. Genetic control of plasma dopamine-β-hydroxylase. Life Sci. 12:529–532.

Roth, R. H., J. R. Walters, and G. K. Aghajanian. 1973. Effect of impulse flow on the release and synthesis of dopamine in the rat striatum. In Frontiers in Catecholamine Research, Usdin, E., and S. H. Snyder (Eds.), pp. 567–574. New York, Pergamon Press.

Rybakowski, J., M. Chlopocka, Z. Kapelski, B. Hernacka, Z. Szajnerman, and K. Kasprzak. 1974a. Red blood cell lithium index in patients with affective disorders in the course of lithium prophylaxis. Int. Pharmacopsychiat. 9:166–171.

Rybakowski, J., M. Chlopocka, J. Lisowska, and A. Czerwinski. 1974b. Badania nad skutecznoscia lecznicza weglanu litu w endogennych zespolach depresynych (The study of therapeutic efficacy of lithium carbonate in endogenous depression). Psychiat. Pol. 2:129–139.

Rybakowski, J., and W. Strzyzewski. 1976. Red blood cell lithium index and long-term maintenance treatment. Lancet 1:1408–1409.

Sachar, E. J., N. Altman, P. H. Gruen, A. Glassman, F. Halpern, and J. Sassin. 1975. Human growth hormone response to levodopa. Arch. Gen. Psychiat. 32:502–503.

Sachar, E. J., A. G. Frantz, N. Altman, and J. Sassin. 1973. Growth hormone and prolactin in unipolar and bipolar depressed patients, responses to hypoglycemia and L-dopa. Am. J. Psychiat. 130:1362–1367.

Sack, R. L., and F. K. Goodwin. 1974. Inhibition of dopamine β-hydroxylase in manic patients. Arch. Gen. Psychiat. 31:649–654.

Schildkraut, J. J. 1965. The catecholamine hypothesis of affective disorders: A review of supporting evidence. Am. J. Psychiat. 122:509–522.

Schildkraut, J. J. 1973. Catecholamine Metabolism and Affective Disorders: Studies of MHPG Excretion. In Frontiers in Catecholamine Research, Usdin, E., and S. Snyder (Eds.), pp. 1165–1171. New York, Pergamon Press.

Schildkraut, J. J., B. A. Keeler, E. L. Grob, J. Kantrowich, and E. Hartmann. 1973. MHPG excretion and clinical classification in depression. Lancet 1:1251–1252.

Schildkraut, J. J., and S. S. Kety. 1967. Biogenic amines and emotion. Science 156:21–37.

Schuckit, M., F. N. Pitts, Jr., T. Reich, L. J. King, and G. Winokur. 1969. Alcoholism I. Two types of alcoholism in women. Arch. Gen. Psychiat. 20:301–306.

Schulsinger, H. 1976. A ten-year follow-up of children of schizophrenic mothers; clinical assessment. Acta Psychiat. Scand. 53:371–386.

Shapiro, R. W., E. Bock, O. J. Rafaelsen, L. P. Ryder, and A. Svejgaard. 1976. Histocompatibility antigens and manic-depressive disorders. Arch. Gen. Psychiat. 33:823–825.

Shields, J. 1975. Some recent developments in psychiatric genetics. Arch. Psychiat. Nervenkr. 220:347–360.

Shih, J. H., and S. Eiduson. 1971. Multiple Forms of Monoamine Oxidase in Developing Tissues: The Implications for Mental Disorder. In Brain Chemistry and Mental Disease, Ho, B. J., and W. M. Isaac (Eds.), pp. 3–20. New York, Plenum Press.

Shokeir, M. H. 1975. Investigation on Huntington's disease: III. Biochemical observations, a possibly predictive test? Clin. Genet. 7:354–360.

Shopsin, B., L. S. Freedman, M. Goldstein, and S. Gershon. 1972. Serum dopamine-β-hydroxylase (DBH) activity and affective states. Psychopharmacologia 27:11–16.

Shopsin, B., E. Friedman, and S. Gershon. 1976. Parachlorophenylalanine reversal of tranylcypromine effects in depressed patients. Arch. Gen. Psychiat. 33:811–819.

Shopsin, B., E. Friedman, M. Goldstein, et al. 1975. The use of synthesis inhibitors in defining a role for biogenic amines during imipramine treatment in depressed patients. Psychopharmacol. Comm. 1:239–249.

Shore, P. A. 1962. Release of serotonin and catecholamines by drugs. Pharmacol. Rev. 14:531–550.

Smith, A. D., W. P. DePotter, E. J. Moorman, and A. F. DeSchaepdryver. 1970. Release of dopamine-β-hydroxylase and chromogranin upon stimulation of the splenic nerves. Tissue and Cell 2:547–568.

Squires, R. F. 1972. Multiple forms of monoamine oxidase in intact mitochondria as characterized by selective inhibitors and thermal stability: A comparison of eight mammalian species. Adv. Biochem. Psychopharmacol. 5:355–370.

Stember, R. H., and R. R. Fieve. 1976. Histocompatibility complex in affective disorders. Proceedings of the A.P.A., Miami.

Stendstedt, A. 1952. A study in manic-depressive psychosis. Acta Psychiat. Scand. Suppl. 79.

Stewart, J., and R. C. Elston. 1973. Biometrical genetics with one or two loci: The inheritance of physiological characters in mice. Genetics 73:675–693.

Stewart, M. A., and J. R. Morrison. 1973. Affective disorder among the relatives of hyperactive children. J. Child Psychol. Psychiat. 14:209–212.

Stoddard, F. J., R. M. Post, J. C. Gillin, M. S. Buchsbaum, J. S. Carman, and W. E. Bunney, Jr. 1974. Phasic changes in manic-depressive illness. Presented at annual meeting of A.P.A., Detroit.

Subrahmanyam, S. 1975. Role of biogenetic amines in certain pathological conditions. Brain Res. 87:355–362.

Svejgaard, A., M. Hauge, C. Jersild, P. Platz, et al. 1975. The HLA system: An introductory survey. Monographs in Human Genetics, 7. Basel, Karger.

Svejgaard, A., C. Jersild, L. S. Nielsen, and W. F. Bodmer. 1974. HLA antigens and disease—statistical and genetical considerations. Tissue Antigens 4:95–105.

Svejgaard, A., and L. P. Ryder. 1976. Interaction of HLA molecules with nonimmunological ligands as an explanation of HLA and disease associations. Lancet 2:547–549.

Tanna, V. L., and G. Winokur. 1968. A study of association and linkage of ABO blood types and primary affective disorder. Brit. J. Psychiat. 114:1175–1181.

Tanna, V. L., G. Winokur, R. C. Elston, and C. P. Rodney. 1976. A linkage study of depression spectrum disease. Presented at New Research of A.P.A., Miami.

Tecce, J. J., and J. O. Cole. 1974. Amphetamine effects in man: Paradoxical drowsiness and lowered electrical brain activity (CNV). Science 185:451–453.

Thoenen, H., and J. P. Tranzer. 1968. Chemical sympathectomy by selective destruction of adrenergic nerve endings with 6-hydroxydopamine. Naunyn-Schmeideberg's Arch. Exp. Path. Pharmacol. 281:271–288.

Thomas, J. C., and E. J. C. Hewitt. 1939. Blood groups in health and in mental disease. J. Ment. Sci. 85:667–688.

Tipton, K. F. 1973. Biochemical aspects of monoamine oxidase. Brit. Med. Bull. 29:116–119.

Trendelenburg, U., P. R. Draskoczy, and K. H. Graefe. 1972. The influence of intraneuronal monoamine oxidase on neuronal net uptake of noradrenaline and on sensitivity to noradrenaline. Adv. Biochem. Psychopharm. 5:371–377.

Tsuang, M. T. 1975. Schizophrenia and affective disorders: One illness or many? In

Freedman, D. X. (Ed.): Res. Publ. Assoc. Res. Nerv. Ment. Dis., Vol. 54. New York, Raven Press.

Tsuang, M. T., G. Dempsey, and F. Rauscher. 1976. A study of "atypical schizophrenia." Arch. Gen. Psychiat. 33:1157–1160.

Usdin, E. (Ed.) 1974. Neuropsychopharmacology of monoamines and their regulatory enzymes. Advances in Biochemical Psychopharmacology, Vol. 12. New York, Raven Press.

Usdin, E., and Bunney, W. E., Jr. (Eds.) 1975. Pre- and Post-synaptic Receptors. New York, Marcel Dekker.

van Eerdewegh, M., E. S. Gershon, and S. D. Targum. Unpublished data. H-LA and blood group associations in affective disorder.

van Eerdewegh, M., E. S. Gershon, and P. van Eerdewegh. 1976. X-chromosome threshold models of bipolar manic-depressive illness. Sci. Proc. Am. Psychiat. Assoc. 129:124–125 (summary).

van Kammen, D. P., W. E. Bunney, Jr., J. P. Docherty, D. C. Jimerson, R. M. Post, S. Siris, M. Ebert, and J. C. Gillin. Unpublished data. Amphetamine-induced catecholamine activation in schizophrenia and depression, behavioral and physiological effects.

van Praag, H. Unpublished data. Significance of biochemical parameters in the diagnosis, treatment and prevention of depressive disorders.

van Praag, H., and J. Korf. 1971. Endogenous depressions with and without disturbances in the 5-hydroxytryptamine metabolism: A biochemical classification? Psychopharmacologia 19:148.

van Praag, H., and J. Korf. 1974. Serotonin metabolism in depression: Clinical application of the probenecid test. Int. Pharmacopsychiat. 9:35–51.

van Praag, H., J. Korf, and D. Schut. 1973. Cerebral monoamines and depression. Arch. Gen. Psychiat. 28:827–831.

Viveros, O. H., L. Arqueros, and N. Krishner. 1968. Release of catecholamines and dopamine-β-oxidase from the adrenal medulla. Life Sci. 7:609–618.

Weil-Malherbe, H. 1976. The biochemistry of affective disorders. In Biological Foundations of Psychiatry, Grenell, R. G., and S. Gabay (Eds.), Vol. 2, pp. 683–728. New York, Raven Press.

Weiner, N., and R. Bjur. The role of intraneuronal monoamine oxidase in the regulation of norepinephrine synthesis. Adv. Biochem. Psychopharmacol. 5:409–419.

Weinshilboum, R. M., and J. Axelrod. 1971a. Reduced plasma dopamine-β-hydroxylase activity in familial dysautonomia. New Engl. J. Med. 285:938–942.

Weinshilboum, R. M., and J. Axelrod. 1971b. Serum dopamine-β-hydroxylase activity. Circ. Res. 28:307–315.

Weinshilboum, R. M., and J. Axelrod. 1971c. Serum dopamine-β-hydroxylase: Decrease after chemical sympathectomy. Science 73:931–934.

Weinshilboum, R. M., F. A. Raymond, L. R. Elveback, and W. H. Weidman. 1973. Serum dopamine-β-hydroxylase activity: Sibling-sibling correlation. Science 181: 943–945.

Weinshilboum, R. M., F. A. Raymond, L. R. Elveback, and W. H. Weidman. 1974. Correlation of erythrocyte catechol-O-methyltransferase activity between siblings. Nature 252:490–491.

Weinshilboum, R. M., H. G. Schrott, F. A. Raymond, W. H. Weidman, and L. R. Elveback. 1975. Inheritance of very low serum dopamine-β-hydroxylase activity. Am. J. Hum. Genet. 27:573–585.

Weinshilboum, R. M., N. B. Thoa, D. G. Johnson, I. J. Kopin, and J. Axelrod. 1971. Proportional release of norepinephrine and dopamine-β-hydroxylase from sympathetic nerves. Science 174:1349–1351.

Werdinius, B. 1967. Effect of probenecid on the levels of monoamine metabolites in the rat brain. Acta Pharmacol. Toxicol. 25:18–23.

Wetterberg, S., H. Aberg, S. B. Ross, and O. Froden. 1972a. Plasma dopamine-β-hydroxylase activity in hypertension and various neuropsychiatric disorders. Scand. J. Clin. Lab. Invest. 30:283–289.

Wetterberg, L., R. H. Gustavson, M. Backstrom, S. B. Ross, and O. Froden. 1972b. Low dopamine-β-hydroxylase activity in Down's syndrome. Clin. Genet. 3:152–153.

White, H. L., M. N. McLeod, and J. R. Davidson. 1976. Catechol-O-methyltransferase in red blood cells of schizophrenic, depressed and normal human subjects. Brit. J. Psychiat. 128:184–187.

Wilson, I. C., and A. J. Prange, Jr. 1972. Tryptophan and mania: Theory of affective disorders. Psychopharmacologia 26:1976 (Suppl.).

Wimmer, A. 1922. Sur la transmission hereditaire des maladies mentales. Encephale 17:129.

Winokur, G. 1972. Depression spectrum disease: Description and family study. Comp. Psychiat. 13:3–8.

Winokur, G. 1974. The division of depressive illness into depression spectrum disease and pure depressive disease. Int. Pharmacopsychiat. 9:5–13.

Winokur, G., W. R. Cadoret, M. Baker, and J. Dorzab. 1975. Depression spectrum disease vs. depressive disease: Some further data. Brit. J. Psychiat. 127:75–77.

Winokur, G., W. R. Cadoret, J. Dorzab, and M. Baker. 1971. Depressive disease. Arch. Gen. Psychiat. 24:135–144.

Winokur, G., and P. Clayton. 1967. Family history studies. I. Two types of affective disorders separated according to genetic and clinical factors. In Recent Advances in Biological Psychiatry, Wortis, J. (Ed.), Vol. 9, pp. 35–50. New York, Plenum Press.

Winokur, G., P. Clayton, and T. Reich. 1969. Manic-Depressive Illness. St. Louis, C. V. Mosby Co.

Winokur, G., J. Morrison, J. Clancy, and R. R. Crowe. 1972. The Iowa 500. Arch. Gen. Psychiat. 27:462–464.

Winokur, G., and F. N. Pitts, Jr. 1965. Affective disorder VI. A family history study of prevalences, sex differences and possible genetic factors. J. Psychiat. Res. 3:113–123.

Winokur, G., T. Reich, J. Rimmer, and F. N. Pitts, Jr. 1970. Alcoholism. III. Diagnosis and familial psychiatric illness in 259 alcoholic probands. Arch. Gen. Psychiat. 23:104–111.

Winokur, G., and V. L. Tanna. 1969. Possible role of X-linked dominant factor in manic-depressive disease. Dis. Nerv. Syst. 30:89.

Wooten, G. F., R. Eldridge, J. Axelrod, and R. S. Stern. 1973. Elevated plasma dopamine-β-hydroxylase activity in autosomal dominant torsion dystonia. New Eng. J. Med. 288:284–287.

Wurtman, R., and J. Fernstrom. 1976. Control of brain neural transmitter synthesis by precursor availability and nutritional state. Biochem. Pharmacol. 25:1691–1696.

Wyatt, R. J., and D. L. Murphy. 1975. Neurotransmitter-Related Enzymes in the Major Psychiatric Disorders: II. MAO and DBH in Schizophrenia. In Biology of the Major Psychoses: A Comparative Analysis. Freedman, D. X. (Ed.), pp. 289–298.

Wyatt, R. J., D. L. Murphy, R. Belmaker, S. Cohen, C. H. Donnelly, and W. Pollin. 1973. Reduced monoamine oxidase activity in platelets: A possible genetic marker for vulnerability to schizophrenia. Science 179:916–918.

Youdim, M. B. H. 1976. Unpublished data. Factors Influencing the Deamination and Functional Acitivity of Biogenic Monoamines in the Central Nervous System. In Impact of Biology on Modern Psychiatry, Gershon, E. S., R. H. Belmaker, S. S. Kety, and M. Rosenbaum (Eds.). New York, Plenum Press.

Youdim, M. B. H., and G. G. S. Collins. 1975. Properties and Physiological Significance of Multiple Forms of Mitochondrial Monoamine Oxidase. In Isozymes, Markert, C. L. (Ed.), pp. 619–639.

Youdim, M. B. H., G. G. S. Collins, M. Sandler, A. B. B. Jones, C. M. B. Pare, and W. J. Nicholson. 1972. Human brain monoamine oxidase: Multiple forms and selective inhibitors. Nature 236:225–228.

Zerbin–Rudin, E. 1969. Zur Genetik der depressiven Erkrankungen. In Das Depressive Syndrom, Hippius-Selbach (Ed.), Int. Symp. Berlin, pp. 37–56. Berlin, Urban and Schwarzenberg.

Zvolsky, P. 1973. A contribution to questions of genetics of mood disorders. Acta Univ. Carol. Med. 19:541–557.

4

The Mutational Basis of the Thalassemia Syndromes[*]

HAIG H. KAZAZIAN, JR.

SECHIN CHO

JOHN A. PHILLIPS, III

Department of Pediatrics, Johns Hopkins University School of Medicine, Baltimore, Maryland 21205.

[*]The authors are supported by the following National Institutes of Health grants and contracts: HHK—AM 13983, HB-1-2401, and AM 70669; SC—GM 00145; JAP— GM 00261.

165

INTRODUCTION AND GENERAL BACKGROUND

Inherited abnormalities of hemoglobin can serve as models of mutations that occur in man. Nearly all conceivable types of point mutations are among the causes of abnormal hemoglobins. Many of the same kinds of point mutations are being implicated as causes of the thalassemia syndromes, which are quantitative variants affecting globin chain synthesis (Benz and Forget, 1974; Nathan, 1972; Weatherall, 1974; Orkin and Nathan, 1976; Clegg and Weatherall, 1976). In this review of the thalassemia syndromes, we emphasize the potential role of mutations located in DNA nucleotides outside those whose messenger RNA is translated. These mutations can affect the early steps in gene action and thereby alter the production of the specified protein. As the mutational basis of the thalassemia syndromes is elucidated, further mutations of this type should be verified biochemically. Thus the thalassemias are presented here from a genetic point of view in order to concentrate on those aspects which can be generalized to mutations affecting the action of genes specifying other proteins. It is hoped that this approach will be helpful to medical geneticists in their thinking and teaching on this subject.

The Gene and Transcribed DNA

The definition of a mammalian gene has changed in recent years as our biochemical knowledge has grown. Bacterial geneticists call the DNA nucleotides encoding a polypeptide a "structural gene," whereas those nucleotides regulating its function are termed "regulatory genes." These regulatory genes may be either contiguous with or distant from the structural gene (Jacob and Monod, 1961). In bacterial operons, transcribed DNA, or that DNA from which the initial RNA transcript is produced, usually includes more than one gene (Adhya and Shapiro, 1969). In contrast, operons have not been described in mammalian cells. Since only a portion of the initial RNA transcript of mammals is translated, this transcribed DNA must contain nucleotide sequences important for both the structure of a polypeptide and the regulation of its synthesis (Proudfoot and Brownlee, 1976).

So, for purposes of this discussion, and in contrast to the convention employed by bacterial geneticists, we will arbitrarily equate the gene with transcribed DNA, although we are aware that some contiguous nucleotides important to gene expression may not be transcribed (Fig. 1).

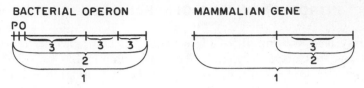

1 = Transcribed DNA
2 = Nucleotides encoding a single mRNA
3 = Nucleotides represented in protein

Figure 1.   The bacterial operon containing many genes and the mammalian gene are compared. Although our knowledge of the mammalian gene is somewhat insecure, a smaller fraction of its nucleotides encode polypeptide than the nucleotides of an operon. Certain evidence suggests that the DNA nucleotides whose information is decoded into protein structure lie at one end of the mammalian gene. (Darnell et al., 1973.)

Although the size of the initial RNA transcript corresponding to a gene specifying a protein is unknown, we have recently learned that it contains many more nucleotides than those required to encode the protein (Maroun et al., 1971; Williamson et al., 1973; Imaizumi et al., 1973). An unknown fraction of the sequences within transcribed DNA corresponds to cytoplasmic mRNA, and about two thirds of these mRNA nucleotides code for polypeptide structure (Proudfoot and Brownlee, 1976; Marotta et al., 1974; Forget et al., 1975b). Thus it is probable that regulatory elements reside within transcribed DNA in those nucleotides not encoding protein structure (Benz and Forget, 1974; Proudfoot and Brownlee, 1976).

Early Steps in Genetic Activity

In order to discuss regulatory mechanisms in general, and mutations affecting regulation of globin synthesis specifically, we will briefly discuss the early steps in eukaryotic protein synthesis. While bacterial DNA is transcribed into mRNA, and the mRNA is translated while it is still attached to the bacterial chromosome (Das et al., 1967), a number of processing steps occur after transcription in higher organisms (Fig. 2) (Watson, 1976; Lewin, 1974). These steps in mRNA processing suggest many possible sites and mechanisms for the regulation of genetic activity.

   mRNA Precursor.   Although the number and size of precursors for mammalian mRNAs remain in doubt, the weight of evidence indicates that the initial RNA transcript is much larger than its final product, cytoplasmic mRNA. A small pool of very large, rapidly turn-

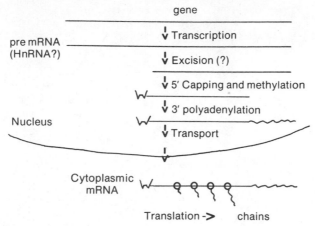

Figure 2. Early steps in genetic activity are diagrammed. Our present state of knowledge indicates that these steps in mRNA processing occur, but their order and function are not well understood. (From Kazazian, H. H., Jr.: Johns Hopkins Med. J., *139*:215–219, 1976. Reprinted by permission.)

ing-over RNA found in the nucleus is called heterogeneous nuclear RNA (HnRNA), and many investigators have suggested that HnRNA contains the initial RNA transcript (Darnell et al., 1971, 1973; Lewin, 1974). HnRNA of erythroid cells is greater than 30S in size, or at least ten times larger than cytoplasmic mRNA, and has been shown by more than one means to contain globin mRNA sequences (Williamson et al., 1973; Imaizumi et al., 1973). However, polymerization of cytoplasmic mRNA into very large molecules has not yet been completely excluded as an explanation for these findings. Recently other work using mouse spleen erythroblasts has suggested a 16S precursor for globin mRNA which is three times larger than cytoplasmic globin mRNA (Kwan et al., 1977). Since other eukaryotic RNAs, ribosomal RNA (rRNA) and transfer RNA (tRNA), are excised from larger precursor molecules, precedents exist for such processing (Das et al., 1970; Bernhardt and Darnell, 1969). Excision of mRNA from the initial transcript requires that at least one enzyme, probably an endonuclease, recognizes a specific site or sites within the mRNA precursor and excises the mRNA fragment. Whether mRNA is excised from the middle or one end of its precursor is unclear, but what data there are place mRNA at the extreme 3'-end of precursor RNA (Coutelli et al., 1970; Darnell et al., 1973). As soon as mRNA precursors are definitively identified, the discovery of excision enzymes and the length and location of their recognition sites on precursor mRNA should follow.

5'-End Modification. In contrast to rRNA and tRNA, mRNA is

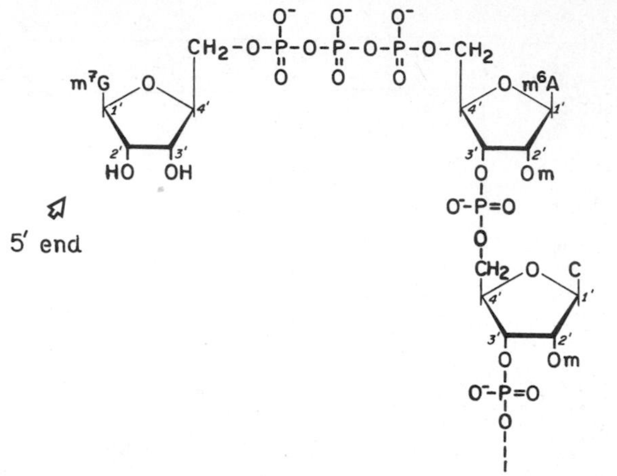

Figure 3.   The first three nucleotides at the 5'-end of the α and β globin mRNAs of mouse and rabbit are shown. Abbreviations used are as follows: m, methyl; G, guanosine; A, adenine; C, cytosine.

modified at both its 5'- and 3'-ends (Proudfoot and Brownlee, 1976; Darnell et al., 1973). The order in which these modifications take place in the nucleus is unsettled, but it is probably determined by the cellular localization and stability of the specific modification enzymes. Moreover, 5'-end modification goes on through much of the life of the erythroid cell, because it can be demonstrated in enucleated reticulocytes (Cheng et al., 1976).

The 5'-end modification is of great interest, because both transcription and translation of RNA proceed in the 5' to 3' direction. This means that the 5'-end of mRNA contains that portion which was transcribed first, along with the initiation site for translation of polypeptide chains. Modification of this 5'-end is called "capping and methylation," because mRNA is "capped" with 7-methyl guanosine-5'-triphosphate in a 5' linkage to the second nucleotide (Fig. 3). Thus, unlike bacterial mRNA, eukaryotic mRNA lacks a free phosphate at the 5'-end, and both the 5'- and 3'-ends terminate in 3'-OH groups. Studies of the pool of mRNAs from a variety of cell types have indicated that not only is the 5'-end "capped" but the second, and often the third, nucleotide is methylated in the 2' position of the ribose (Wei et al., 1975; Perry and Kelley, 1974; Wei et al., 1976; Rottman et al., 1974; Cory and Adams, 1975). We, and others, have recently reported that both α and β globin mRNAs of mouse have the same sequence in the first three nucleotides, highlighted by a 7-methylguanosine cap and four methyl groups (Cheng and Kazazian, in press; Heckle et al., in press). In contrast, although the α and β

mRNAs of man also contain N^6-2'-O-dimethyladenosine at the second position, it appears that one has 2'-O-methylcytidine and the other 2'-O-methyluridine at the third position (Cheng and Kazazian, unpublished data). Others have found that in rabbit globin mRNAs the first three nucleotides are identical to those of the α and β globin mRNAs of mouse, but that sequence differences between the α and β mRNAs occur between 8 and 10 nucleotides from the 5'-end (Lockard and RajBhandary, 1976). The significance of these differences is still to be discovered, but they may relate to observed differences in the rate of initiation of translation of rabbit and human α and β mRNAs.

The functional roles of these 5'-end methyl groups are not completely elucidated, but the 7-methylguanosine has been shown to be vital to initiation of translation of many mRNAs (Both et al., 1975; Hickey et al., 1976; Weber et al., 1976), including globin mRNA (Muthukrishnan et al., 1975). Moreover, although the globin mRNAs contain four methyl residues on the first three nucleotides, they have no other methyl groups in the entire molecule (Cheng and Kazazian, in press; Heckle et al., in press).

A number of enzymes are involved in 5'-end modification (Furuichi et al., 1976): a coupling enzyme joins guanosine triphosphate to the 5'-end, and at least three different methyl transferases methylate the 7 position of guanosine, the 6 position of adenosine, and the 2' position of the riboses. All these enzymes presumably recognize specific nucleotide sequences within excised mRNA as binding sites. Whether or not these recognition sites include the first few nucleotides at the 5'-end is unknown, but certain nucleotide sequences which act as binding sites for these enzymes may be common to all eukaryotic mRNAs. The order in which these enzymes act and their subcellular localization are also under investigation.

3'-End Modification. The 3'-end modification involves the addition of polyadenylic acid [poly(A)], which in the case of globin mRNA is 150 nucleotides in length in developing erythroblasts (Merkel et al., 1975). Since some HnRNA contains poly(A) (Darnell et al., 1973), it is possible that poly(A) is attached prior to excision of the 5'-end of precursor mRNA. However, other data suggest that poly(A) addition occurs after 5'-end modification and may be important in the transport of mRNA to the cytoplasm (Adesnik et al., 1972). Again, a specific enzyme, poly(A) synthetase, is required for this modification, and it presumably binds to specific nucleotides near the 3'-end of the mRNA. Globin mRNA lacking poly(A) can be translated without difficulty; but when this mRNA is translated in a cell-free system or is injected into *Xenopus laevis* oocytes, it is unstable relative to polyadenylated mRNA (Soreq et al., 1974; Marbaix et al., 1975). In reticulocytes of various species a variable fraction (29 to 74 percent) of α and β globin mRNAs contains poly(A) of 1 to 50 nucleotides in length, reflecting in part the reduction of poly(A) length which accompanies aging of globin mRNA (Cann et al., 1974; Lingrel et al., 1974).

How fully modified mRNA is finally transported to the cytoplasm is unclear, but the binding of two proteins at or near the poly(A) may play an important role in this transport (Blobel, 1972, 1973).

Once the excised and modified mRNA has been transported to the cytoplasm, ribosomes, amino-acyl tRNAs, and many proteins required for initiation, elongation, and termination of translation perform their task of protein assembly, utilizing the mRNA templates (Benz and Forget, 1974; Watson, 1976; Prichard et al., 1970). This important phase of protein synthesis has been extensively reviewed and continues to grow in complexity as more and more factors are discovered (Filipowicz et al., 1976; McKeehan, 1974; Hunt, 1976).

Although *only* 425 to 450 nucleotides are required to encode the globin chains in reticulocytes, α and β mRNA molecules contain about 650 and 720 nucleotides, respectively, of which polyadenylic acid comprises about 50 nucleotides on the average. The remaining 125 to 200 nucleotides of globin mRNAs are untranslated, and most of these lie between the COOH terminal amino acid codon and the poly(A) (Benz and Forget, 1974; Proudfoot and Brownlee, 1976; Marotta et al., 1974; Forget et al., 1975b; Clegg et al., 1971; Poon et al., 1974). Thus, although the exact size of the initial globin transcript is unknown, and it may exceed 2000 nucleotides, only about 450 nucleotides are translated into protein.

It is worth noting that the number of known loci whose products are involved in the transfer of information from DNA to protein structure is greater than 200. Most of these encode amino-acyl synthetases, ribosomal proteins, protein translation factors, tRNAs, and enzymes involved in tRNA and rRNA modification, all of which are crucial to translation (Watson, 1976). Many more loci whose products are involved in the processing of mRNA prior to translation are yet to be discovered. Although a mutation in any one of these genes may not be life threatening, because of the diploid nature of eukaryotes, homozygosity for any one of many such mutations would probably be a cause of premature death or developmental failure. On the other hand, a mutation in transcribed DNA which affects the way in which a protein synthesis factor interacts with that DNA or its RNA product may be expressed as a deficiency in the specified protein (Fig. 7, p. 194).

For example, homozygosity for a mutation in α or β globin transcribed DNA which affects the ability of poly(A) synthetase to attach to its nucleotide binding site on the RNA could lead to markedly reduced production of the encoded protein and result in a thalassemia condition.

The Structure-Function Hypothesis: Effects of Mutation

Over the past 20 years molecular biologists have successfully followed the hypothesis that the structure of a macromolecule determines its function. One corollary to this tenet is that all structure is nonrandom and plays a significant functional role. An obvious example is the relationship of the double helical structure of DNA to its function in replication and information transfer, but the close relationship of structure to function has also been well documented for proteins, most notably hemoglobin, and RNA molecules (Perutz, 1976; Watson, 1976; Rieder, 1974).

A logical extension of this basic doctrine is most important to geneticists: that altered structure of a macromolecule alters the function of that molecule in a biological system (Kirkman, 1972). We are now most familiar with the single nucleotide change in DNA which produces a single amino acid substitution in the encoded polypeptide chain (Hunt and Dayhoff, 1974). In the case of hemoglobin mutations, about 40 percent are detrimental to the function of the hemoglobin tetramer and produce illness in the individual in the heterozygous state (White, 1976; Bellingham, 1976; Lang and Lorkin, 1976). For the remaining hemoglobin mutations, the change in function, although present, is too small to produce significant deviation from normal or the change is in a portion of the protein sequence which is not of functional importance. However, since most of these mutations are quite rare, the clinical significance of the homozygous state is generally unknown.

Since mutation probably occurs at a constant rate and at random, all genetic material is at risk. This means that the large amount of untranslated DNA is also subject to mutation. Furthermore, the probability that such a mutation will alter function is the same as for a mutation in DNA whose information is later translated into protein. Mutations that alter the regulation of genetic activity as opposed to the amino acid sequence of a polypeptide are now beginning to be elucidated. The phenotypic expressions of mutations in this regulatory DNA may vary more than those of mutations affecting amino acid sequences.

In eukaryotic cells, mutations in DNA whose information is not subsequently translated into protein are now being elucidated in the thalassemia syndromes. Further studies of these particular syndromes should reveal the heterogeneity of mutations affecting genetic regulation in general. However, in order to discuss specifically the mutational basis of the thalassemia syndromes, it is necessary to review the hemoglobin wild-type states and to present selected examples of mutations which have their major effect on hemoglobin structure.

HEMOGLOBIN WILD-TYPE STATES

Globin Chain Structure

Hemoglobin A (Hb A), which accounts for 97 percent of the hemoglobin in the erythrocytes of the adult human being, is a tetramer composed of two α and two β globin subunits, each with its own heme group. The α chain, which is found in nearly all hemoglobins, contains 141 amino acids; and the β chain, 146 amino acids. Hb A_2 ($\alpha_2\delta_2$) comprises 2 percent, and Hb F ($\alpha_2\gamma_2$) makes up less than 1 percent of the hemoglobin of adults. δ and γ chains are more similar to the β than to the α chain; all three have 146 amino acids, and δ differs from β at 10 positions, whereas γ differs from β at 39 positions (Lang and Lorkin, 1976; Kazazian, 1974). Two other globins, ϵ and ζ, are found in embryonic erythrocytes, but knowledge of their primary structure is incomplete. However, partial sequences of the mouse and rabbit ϵ chains (Steinheider et al., 1975) and of the human ζ chain (Kamuzora and Lehmann, 1975) suggest that these chains are analogues of β and α chains, respectively (Wood, 1976).

The 3-dimensional structures of oxygenated and deoxygenated forms of Hb A and the mechanisms by which the structures influence the functions of Hb A have been elegantly solved in extensive studies. Moreover, knowledge of the 3-dimensional structure of Hb A has allowed precise delineation for many mutant hemoglobins of the functional abnormality as well as the prediction of sites and types of mutations affecting Hb A structure that would be well or poorly tolerated (Perutz, 1976).

Globin Chain Genetics

Numbers of Globin Loci. Evidence that the human genotype contains only one locus capable of specifying β chains consists of the absence of normal β chains in the erythrocytes of individuals homozygous for a mutant β chain and roughly 35 to 50 percent mutant β globin in the red cells of heterozygotes (Lehmann and Carrell, 1968; Lang and Lorkin, 1976). Similarly, heterozygotes for δ chain variants have roughly equal quantities of normal and variant δ chains, suggesting the presence of a single δ locus in man (Lang and Lorkin, 1976).

In contrast, it appears that some persons have two α chain loci, whereas others have only one (Rucknagel and Winter, 1974; Lang and Lorkin, 1976). Many observations support the existence of two α loci in certain racial groups. Three α chains differing in primary structure have been found in certain Hungarians, a Black American, and an Indian (Hollan et al., 1972; Bradley et al., 1975; DeJong et al., 1975). In addition, Malaysian individuals with a double dose of a common α gene variant along with normal α genes have been observed (Lie-Injo et al., 1974). Since no more than two different chains can be encoded by homologous loci, these findings indicate that the minimum number of α loci in these groups is two. Further evidence comes from Chinese with Hb H disease, who by molecular hybridization studies have one quarter, not one half, of the normal amount of DNA encoding the α chain in their genome (see Mutations Producing α-Thalassemia, p. 185) (Kan et al., 1975a). Similarly, variant α chains usually account for only 15 to 25 percent of the total α chains in individuals carrying a single variant α gene (Lehmann and Carrell, 1968). In addition, members of many other species, such as mouse and goat, have two different α chains, and therefore two functional α loci (Hilse and Popp, 1968; Adams et al., 1969).

On the other hand, some populations may have a single α locus. In Micronesia, a few "homozygotes" for Hb J-Tongariki, which contains an α chain variant, lacked *normal* α chains in their red cells, whereas heterozygotes for this variant had 45 to 50 percent of Hb J-Tongariki (Abramson et al., 1970). Moreover, no evidence of α-thalassemia was noted in any of these individuals, suggesting that these Micronesians have a single functional α locus (Lang and Lorkin, 1976).

The minimum number of γ loci in man is two. Two different γ chains, differing in that one contains glycine ($^{G}\gamma$) and the other alanine ($^{A}\gamma$) at residue 136, exist in all individuals studied to date (Schroeder et al., 1968). When a mutant γ chain is found, it contains either glycine or alanine at residue 136, indicating that the mutation is in a separate $^{G}\gamma$ or $^{A}\gamma$ gene, respectively (Schroeder et al., 1968; Kamuzora, 1975). These data provide conclusive evidence for the existence of two or more γ loci in man. Molecular hybridization studies also sup-

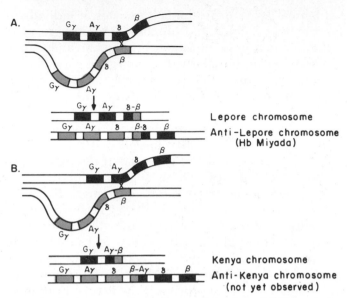

Figure 4. A, The Lepore and anti-Lepore (Miyada and P-Nilotic) chromosomes are produced by unequal crossing-over between closely linked and structurally similar δ and β genes. B, The Kenya and anti-Kenya chromosomes follow from unequal crossing-over between linked $^A\gamma$ and β genes. (From Kazazian, H. H., Jr.: Semin. Hematol. *11*:525–548, 1974. Reprinted by permission.)

port the concept of two γ loci (Williamson, 1976); other, less direct, evidence suggests the possibility of up to four γ loci (Huisman et al., 1972a; Schroeder and Huisman, 1974). The numbers of ε and ζ loci are unknown.

Gene Locations. We have known since 1958 that recombination between the α and β globin loci is random (Smith and Torbert, 1958), but recent evidence indicates that these loci are asyntenic (Deisseroth et al., 1976). Early in situ hybridization studies had suggested that these loci were on chromosomes 2 and 4 (Price et al., 1972), but these findings remain unconfirmed. Thus the chromosomal location of the globin loci is uncertain.

Considerable evidence indicates that the γ, δ, and β loci are closely linked. Moreover, the chromosomal order of these loci can be surmised from the existence of δβ and γβ fusion chains in Hbs Lepore and Kenya, respectively, and is most likely $^G\gamma$, $^A\gamma$, δ, β (Fig. 4) (Baglioni, 1962; Huisman et al., 1972b; Lang and Lorkin, 1976). The size of the transcribed DNA and the nature and size of regulatory elements within this cluster of globin genes are unknown.

Globin Gene Regulation: Selected Examples

Balanced α and β Production. Although most human beings have two α loci and one β locus, α and β chains are made at the same rate in their reticulocytes (Lang and Lorkin, 1976). Thus one may ask, How is balanced synthesis of α and β chains accomplished in the face of twice as many α loci as β loci? Although the process is not completely understood, regulation appears to occur at more than one point between the transcription of globin genes and the assembly of the polypeptide chains (Benz and Forget, 1974).

Lodish (1971) used inhibitors of polypeptide elongation in rabbit reticulocytes to demonstrate that α mRNA initiates protein synthesis 30 to 40 percent slower than β mRNA does. By further analysis, he suggested that the rates of translation and release of α and β chains are equal and that 30 to 40 percent more α than β mRNA is needed for balanced synthesis (Lodish and Jacobsen, 1972). Boyer has assayed the number of rabbit reticulocyte ribosomes on α and β mRNA molecules by immunoprecipitation of specific α and β polysomes and has calculated a 28 to 78 percent excess of functional α mRNA in his preparations (Boyer et al., 1974). In both these studies, the analyses were not dependent upon the presence of poly(A) in globin mRNA. A number of laboratories have attempted to quantify α and β mRNA containing poly(A) by formamide gel electrophoresis and have obtained α to β mRNA ratios in various species closer to 1 (Kazazian et al., 1975; Hamlyn and Gould, 1975). On the other hand, Forget et al. (1975a) found 25 to 50 percent more α mRNA in human reticulocytes by these same techniques.

Recently we have purified α and β mRNAs of rabbit, mice, and sheep and made complementary DNA probes specific for the individual mRNAs. Using these cDNA probes, we have assayed α and β mRNA concentrations in polysomes and found 1.2 to 1.4 times as much α as β mRNA in the reticulocyte polysomes of all three species (Phillips et al., 1976). Our assays measured both poly(A)-containing and poly(A)-lacking globin mRNA. Thus the weight of evidence suggests that the 2-fold excess of α genes is reduced to a 1.3-fold excess of α mRNA on cytoplasmic polysomes. Initiation of protein synthesis occurs 30 percent faster on β mRNA than on α mRNA to yield balanced globin synthesis (Lodish, 1971). The mechanism by which regulation from the level of the gene to that of cytoplasmic mRNA is achieved remains unknown, but it could occur at any of the steps in mRNA processing.

Deficient δ Chain Synthesis. Another question of normal globin regulation is, Why is the number of δ chains in erythroid cells one fiftieth the number of β chains even though δ and β genes are present in the same number? A number of steps have been implicated in δ chain regulation, including (1) marked deficiency of δ mRNA in reticulocytes (Kazazian and Itano, 1968), (2) instability of the δ mRNA produced (Clegg and Weatherall, 1974a), and (3) moderately reduced rate of translation of the δ mRNA as compared to the β mRNA (Winslow and Ingram, 1966). Again, the final answers to this question will be forthcoming.

Qualitative Changes in Hbs During Development. During fetal development, the changes in Hb phenotype are quite striking and of great interest (Kazazian, 1974; Wood, 1976). Embryonic ϵ chains of yolk cell origin are generally replaced by γ chains and small amounts of β chains beginning at 3 to 4 weeks of fetal life. These latter chains are present in cells of hepatic origin, and the production of small amounts of β chains by the early fetus makes possible the prenatal diagnosis of such hemoglobinopathies as β-thalassemia and sickle cell anemia (Kan et al., 1975b; Nathan and Alter, 1975; Kazazian and Woodhead, 1974).

At 32 to 34 weeks, the changeover from predominantly γ to predominantly β chain production begins, so that at birth (40 weeks of gestation) γ chains comprise 70 to 90 percent of non-α chains, whereas β chains make up 10 to 30 percent. This switching process continues through early childhood until Hb F accounts for 1 percent of the total hemoglobin at age 2 (Wood, 1976; Bard, 1975).

Recent interest has focused on molecular events leading to the increase in β chain production and the decrease in γ chain synthesis. Much of the molecular biology of this process remains to be discovered, but in erythroid cells of 14- to 20-week human fetuses, the concentration of poly(A)-containing β mRNA is deficient relative to that of γ and α mRNAs (Kazazian et al., 1975). Observations on erythrocytes of fetal sheep around the time of γ to β switching suggest that in erythroid polyribosomes a decrease in the ratio of γ/α poly(A)$^+$ mRNA occurs prior to the increase in β chain production (Kazazian et al., 1976).

In other experiments, it has been found that adult marrow cells in plasma clots make increased amounts of Hb F after several days in culture (Papayannopoulou et al., 1976). These results suggest that the normal process of globin chain switching may be deciphered and possibly controlled in the not-too-distant future. The ability to maintain Hb F at prenatal levels or induce its synthesis to high levels after birth would in all likelihood be an effective treatment for β-thalassemia and sickle cell anemia.

The mechanisms involved in balancing α and β chain synthesis, inhibiting δ chain synthesis, and switching hemoglobin types may differ one from another, but may be important to survival of the organism. In all these normal regulatory processes, DNA nucleotides not included among those encoding the globin chains must play important, but unknown, roles. A better understanding of these roles should help in deciphering regulatory mutations of globin synthesis and aid us in clarifying other normal regulatory processes in eukaryotes.

MUTATIONS AFFECTING THE HEMOGLOBIN CHAINS

At the DNA level, all mutations are structural in that they result in changes of sequence or number of nucleotides at a particular location in the genome. Yet mutations are still termed structural or regulatory according to their effect on the particular protein under observation; i.e., a structural mutation affects its structure, whereas a regulatory mutation affects the quantitative expression of the gene. Perhaps someday we will base the classification of mutation on its location within the genome; e.g., (1) within the "translated" DNA segment of transcribed DNA; (2) outside the "translated" DNA, but within the cytoplasmic mRNA region of transcribed DNA; (3) outside the "translated" and cytoplasmic mRNA regions of DNA, but still within transcribed DNA; or (4) within an untranscribed spacer region of DNA between two transcribed regions. Since this classification is still premature, we will discuss instead mutations that affect globin structure and mutations that affect the regulation of globin synthesis. This division is an oversimplification, because many mutations which affect the structure of a globin chain also affect, to some extent, its rate of synthesis.

Mutations Which Chiefly Affect Globin Structure

The purpose of this section is to review the various types of point mutations, point out examples of each known to affect chiefly globin structure, and indicate that some mutations which affect the rate of globin synthesis and which are responsible for the thalassemia syndromes may also be point mutations in similar locations within globin genes. In this vein, out of a large number of known mutations affecting globin structure, only a handful are chosen for illustrative purposes.

Substitutions in DNA Nucleotides Which Are Subsequently

Translated. SENSE TO SENSE MUTATIONS. A sense codon is defined as a nucleotide triplet that encodes the wild-type amino acid at a particular position in the protein being specified. In this type of mutation, one nucleotide is substituted for another, but because of degeneracy of the genetic code, no amino acid substitution occurs. Examples of this type of mutation are not yet known in eukaryotes, because specific nucleic acid sequences corresponding to globin, or other proteins, have not been studied in a number of individuals. It has been suggested that this type of mutation could result in a thalassemic syndrome if a deficiency of the tRNA whose anticodon is complementary to the mutant codon exists in erythroid cells (Itano, 1965). However, such a situation would alter the rate of β chain assembly in these syndromes because of the tRNA deficiency, but this rate has been normal in all individuals with β-thalassemia studied to date (Clegg et al., 1968; Rieder, 1972).

SENSE TO MISSENSE MUTATIONS. A sense to missense mutation is a nucleotide substitution in the wild-type codon which results in an amino acid substitution in the encoded polypeptide. About 230 mutations of this type are known to affect the various globin chains, and this number continues to increase at a rate of roughly 10 per year (Hunt and Dayhoff, 1974; Lang and Lorkin, 1976). Many of these mutations also lead to a mild decrease in the rate of synthesis of the mutant chain. For example, the rate of β^S synthesis is about 80 percent that of β^A in reticulocytes of sickle trait individuals (Boyer et al., 1964). Since conventional thalassemia mutations greatly reduce the synthesis of the affected globin chain, the mutant alleles producing β^S and other mutant β chains may be considered to be very mild "thalassemia" genes.

Mutations of this type can produce a variety of phenotypes, including methemoglobinemia, hemolytic anemia, polycythemia, anemia, and one unusual β-thalassemia syndrome (β^{KW}) (White, 1976; Bellingham, 1976; Lang et al., 1974). In many cases the nature of the resultant phenotype can be correlated with the change in the 3-dimensional structure of hemoglobin caused by the amino acid substitution (Perutz, 1976).

SENSE TO TERMINATOR MUTATIONS. A sense to terminator mutation is a nucleotide substitution which changes the wild-type codon to one of three terminator codons not represented by any tRNA anticodons. This mutation, which is well known in bacteria, leads to premature termination of polypeptide assembly. It has recently been observed in higher organisms as the probable cause of Hb McKees Rocks (Winslow et al., 1976). In this hemoglobin the last two residues of the β chain, tyrosine and histidine, are deleted. Since the tyrosine codons are UAU and UAC, the mutation is probably a nucleotide substitution to either UAA or UAG, both of which are terminator codons for polypeptide assembly.

It is likely that other mutations of this type occur with some frequency but lead to globin chains which have lost considerably longer sequences from their carboxyl ends and cannot function properly in Hb tetramers. The $\beta^{McKees\ Rocks}$ mutation, $\beta^{145\ Tyr\ \to\ term}$, is observed because it occurs in the β gene so near to those nucleotides which encode the carboxyl terminus of the β chain. Mutations of this type occurring in DNA nucleotides encoding the amino-terminal region of the β chain would produce thalassemia syndromes characterized by an absence of the full-length β chain in erythroid cells, but this mutational basis for thalassemia has not yet been observed.

TERMINATOR TO MISSENSE MUTATIONS: A NUCLEOTIDE SUBSTITUTION OUTSIDE DNA ENCODING GLOBIN CHAINS. These mutations occur in the "stop sign" codon for polypeptide assembly adjacent to the codon for the carboxyl-terminal amino acid. Known examples have occurred in the terminator codon of the α chains leading to α^{CS}, α^{Icaria}, $\alpha^{Koya\ Dora}$, and $\alpha^{Seal\ Rock}$, in which the 142nd amino acids are glutamine, lysine, serine, and glutamic acid, respectively (Clegg et al., 1971, 1974; Milner et al., 1971; DeJong et al., 1975; Bradley et al., 1975). These mutations allow one to deduce that a single triplet, UAA, designates termination of α chain synthesis and that single nucleotide substitutions of UAA to CAA, AAA, UCA, and GAA account for the new amino acids inserted in the mutant chains. They also demonstrate that the next terminator codon in phase is 93 nucleotides from this UAA, because in α^{CS} 31 amino acids are added to the normal α chain length of 141 residues. Since mutations of this type greatly decrease the synthesis of α chains (Clegg et al., 1971), they are causes of α-thalassemia (see Mutations Producing α-Thalassemia, p. 185), and they demonstrate how nucleotides close to those encoding polypeptide structures can greatly affect the regulation of globin synthesis.

Changes in Nucleotide Number. DELETIONS. Loss of DNA nucleotides, or deletions, may vary in size from a single nucleotide through a single codon, to whole genes, and finally to segments of chromosomes visible under the microscope. All types of fine deletion not visible microscopically have been observed in mutations affecting the globin molecules.

1. *Deletion of a single nucleotide.* Deletion of a single nucleotide leads to a "frameshift," because the codon reading frame for polypeptide assembly is altered. In the mutation leading to the abnormally long α chain, α^{Wayne}, an adenylic acid residue from the

codon for α 139 lysine is deleted (Seid-Akhanan et al., 1976). Thus the wild-type lysine codon, AAA, becomes changed to AAU, which is translated asparagine. Subsequent codons are also changed, and a terminator codon finally returns into phase after the α chain has elongated to 146 amino acids, or 5 more than α^A. Knowledge of the sequence of amino acids after α 141 arginine of α^{CS} and the last 8 amino acids of α^{Wayne} and the genetic code allows the deduction of the nucleotide sequence of the α gene from the codon for α 139 lysine through the first 20 untranslated nucleotides. Much of this sequence has now been directly confirmed by nucleotide sequencing of α mRNA (Marotta et al., 1974).

   2. *Deletions involving small numbers of nucleotides.* In the β^{Leiden} gene, three nucleotides in phase with the ribosome reading frame and designating glutamic acid at either the β 6 or β 7 position are deleted (De Jong et al., 1968). The resulting β chain is shortened by one amino acid. Examples of deletions of more than one triplet are found in individuals with Hb Gun Hill and Hb Tochigi, the β chains of which are missing amino acid residues 91 to 95 and 56 to 59, respectively (Bradley et al., 1967; Shibata et al., 1970). $\beta^{Gun\ Hill}$ originates in a deletion of 15 nucleotides coding for the 5 amino acids involved, and $\beta^{Tochigi}$ is the result of a deletion of 12 nucleotides. If these deletions were not multiples of three nucleotides, or were multiples of three nucleotides but were out of phase with the reading frame, the amino acid sequence distal to the mutation would be completely altered. With the exception of α^{Wayne}, deletions which change the reading frame have not been observed, suggesting that they usually produce a nonfunctional polypeptide and could be associated with a thalassemia syndrome in which a globin chain is lacking.

   3. *Deletions involving large numbers of nucleotides.* Deletions of most or all of the DNA encoding the α and β chains have been found in the α-thalassemias, hereditary persistence of fetal hemoglobin (HPFH), and $\delta\beta$ thalassemia (Ottolenghi et al., 1974, 1976; Kan et al., 1975c; Ramirez et al., 1976). These deletions will be discussed further under the molecular basis of thalassemias. Other deletions associated with thalassemia syndromes and presumed to occur by nonhomologous crossing-over between members of a chromosome pair have led to the Lepore globins ($\delta\beta$ chains) and Kenya globins ($\gamma\beta$ chains) (Baglioni, 1962; Huisman et al., 1972b). Deletions such as these provide important information on globin regulatory sites within the non-α gene cluster, and they also suggest that other smaller deletions of the α and β genes may be explained by nonhomologous crossing-over after mispairing in meiosis.

ADDITIONS.   Thalassemia syndromes could also be produced by additions which cause frameshifts in polypeptide assembly. The addition of two nucleotides at the β 145 tyrosine codon leads to an elongated β chain, $\beta^{Cranston}$ (Bunn et al., 1975). Nucleotide sequence studies of normal β mRNA indicate that two inserted nucleotides, AG, are identical to the two preceding nucleotides found normally in the translated DNA sequence of the β chain (Forget et al., 1975b). This addition alters the reading frame, and $\beta^{Cranston}$ reaches 157 amino acids, 11 more than β^A, before an in-phase termination codon interrupts polypeptide assembly. Another 157 amino acid chain, β^{TAK}, is derived from the addition of two nucleotides at the codon for β 146 histidine (Flatz et al., 1971). It is worth re-emphasizing that the only known additions and deletions of nucleotides, other than multiples of three, affect globin chains close to their COOH ends; i.e., codons for residue 139 in α (Seid-Akhanan et al., 1976) and residues 145 (Bunn et al., 1975) and 146 (Flatz et al., 1971) in the β chain. Although the examples given are not associated with thalassemias, some individuals with β^0-thalassemia whose erythrocytes carry β mRNA (Kan et al., 1975d) may have small additions or deletions in the DNA encoding the amino-terminal region of the β globin which drastically alter the primary structure of the chain.

Addition of large numbers of nucleotides. Larger additions of one or more genes have been observed only in individuals with Hb Miyada (Yanase et al., 1968) and Hb P-Nilotic (Dherte et al., 1959; Lehmann and Charlesworth, 1970), in whom $\beta\delta$ chains are found but Hb A and Hb A$_2$ levels are normal. These individuals are believed to carry the reciprocal chromosomes produced by a nonhomologous crossing-over of the type which leads to Hb Lepore. Thus individuals heterozygous for Hb Miyada or Hb P-Nilotic genes carry a chromosome with the non-α gene cluster composed of $^G\gamma$, $^A\gamma$, δ, $\beta\delta$, and β genes (Kazazian, 1974; Lang and Lorkin, 1976). Their extra genetic material is made up of the $\beta\delta$ gene and whatever nucleotides make up the spacer region between the δ and β genes. Since Hb Miyada and Hb P-Nilotic account for 15 to 20 percent of the total hemoglobin of heterozygotes (Yanase et al., 1968; Badr et al., 1973), the mechanism for balancing α and non-α chain synthesis in the face of an extra β gene in these individuals is worthy of study.

Mutations Which Chiefly Affect Globin Synthesis

The Thalassemias: General Descriptions. The thalassemias and their variations are single gene disorders caused by mutations

Globin Synthetic Ratios

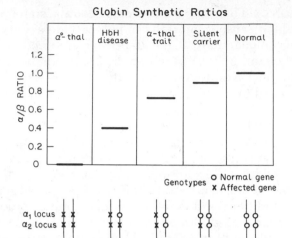

Figure 5. Chain synthesis ratios are correlated with the proposed genotypes in the α thalassemia states. (The chain synthesis portion of this figure is redrawn from Nathan, 1972.)

which affect the regulation of globin synthesis. In α-thalassemia there exists a relative deficiency of α chain synthesis, whereas in β-thalassemia, β chain production is deficient. We now realize that the number of different mutations in the population capable of producing these conditions is large. These mutations include gene deletions, terminator to missense changes, sense to missense changes, and many others presumed to lie in regulatory DNA, which must consist of nucleotide substitutions, additions, or deletions. In contrast to sickle cell anemia, in which a single high frequency mutant gene produces a frequent recessive disease in a particular ethnic group, in thalassemia many different mutations must account for the high frequency of this disease in Mediterranean people and Southeast Asians (Clegg and Weatherall, 1976; Lang and Lorkin, 1976). Why the frequency of β-thalassemia carrier status in Greeks and Italians has reached 2 to 5 percent of the population (Weatherall and Clegg, 1972; Malamos et al., 1962; Livingstone, 1967) and that of α-thalassemia is as frequent in Southeast Asia is not clear (Lopez and Eng, 1971), but a selective advantage for one or two mutants, together with many rare ones, could account for this frequency.

α-Thalassemia: Chain Synthesis and Genetics. The α-thalassemias have been observed to exhibit four different levels of severity: α°-thalassemia, or hydrops fetalis; Hb H disease; α-thalassemia trait; and the silent carrier. In these states, the α/β chain synthetic ratio in reticulocytes is 0, 0.4, 0.75, and 0.9, respectively (Fig. 5) (Nathan, 1972). The four states correspond to the number of functional α genes in most populations. Good evidence suggests that α°-thalassemia individuals have mutations affecting all four α genes (Ottolenghi et al., 1974; Taylor et al., 1974). Hb H disease individuals usually have mutations of three α genes, and so on (Kan et al., 1975a).

Individuals with α°-thalassemia die in utero, or very shortly after birth, with hydrops fetalis. These babies, generally of Chinese and Southeast Asian origin, lack Hb A or Hb F and have only Hb Barts (γ_4) and Hb Portland ($\zeta_2\gamma_2$) in their erythrocytes. Hb H disease is characterized by a mild hemolytic, hypochromic anemia and hepatosplenomegaly, with Hb H (β_4) comprising 5 to 15 percent of the hemoglobin (Weatherall and Clegg, 1972). This relatively benign condition is seen in high frequency in Southeast Asia and is also observed in Greeks and Italians. α-Thalassemia trait individuals are essentially normal, with a mild reduction in MCV and MCH in their red cells. The silent carrier is differentiated from normal only by genetic studies and chain synthesis analyses (Weatherall, 1974; Orkin and Nathan, 1976).

The genotype for a form of α-thalassemia which consists of mutations affecting two α loci on the same chromosome has been called α-thal 1. α-Thal 2 is the designation of a mutation affecting one of the two α loci. Thus an individual with Hb H disease usually carries the genotype for both α-thal 1 and α-thal 2. Two to 3 percent of Black babies in the United States have Hb Barts in moderately elevated concentrations (2 percent or more) at birth (Weatherall, 1963; Minnich et al., 1962), and at follow-up these infants have been found to have an α-thal 1 genotype, the phenotype of which is α-thalassemia trait (Friedman et al., 1974). Since Hb H disease is more frequent among Mediterranean and Southeast Asian peoples than among American Blacks, it is probable that α-thal 2 alleles are more common in the former groups (Friedman et al., 1974). Moreover, we now know of two common α-thal 2 alleles in Southeast Asia; an α gene deletion and an α^{CS} gene (Kan et al., 1975a; Lie-Injo et al., 1974). The absence of the α°-thalassemia phenotype in Black populations suggests that Blacks do not carry the same α-thal 1 genotype as that which is most common in Southeast Asians. Their α-thalassemia trait must be the result of a mutation whose molecular qualities are as yet unknown.

Mutations Producing α-Thalassemia. Three types of mutations causing α-thalassemia have been discovered to date. One is a deletion of α DNA nucleotide sequences (Ottolenghi et al., 1974; Taylor et al., 1974); another is a mutation involving DNA nucleotides coding for the terminator codon of α mRNA (Marotta et al., 1974); and a third

Table 1. Known Molecular Defects in the α-Thalassemias

Thalassemia Genes	Molecular Data
α-Thal 1 (Southeast Asia)	Deletion of both α-chain genes
α-Thal 1 (some Chinese)	Unknown
α-Thal 1 (Black)	Unknown
α-Thal 2 (Southeast Asia)	Deletion of one α-chain gene
	Terminator → missense mutations:
Hb Constant Spring	α 142 gln UAA → CAA
Hb Icaria	α 142 lys UAA → AAA
Hb Koya Dora	α 142 ser UAA → UCA
Hb Seal Rock	α 142 glu UAA → GAA

involves some other, as yet unknown, form of disordered regulation (Table 1) (Kan et al., 1976a; Friedman et al., 1974).

DELETIONS.   In the reticulocytes of Hb H disease individuals, α globin mRNA concentrations are one tenth to one fifth those of β mRNA. This relative deficiency of α mRNA has been observed in cDNA-RNA hybridization assays using DNA copies of rabbit and human α and β mRNAs and by formamide gel electrophoresis of the mRNAs (Housman et al., 1973; Kazazian et al., 1975; Forget et al., 1975a). Two groups have used relatively pure β mRNA (about 80 to 90 percent) derived from reticulocytes of Hb H disease patients to make β-specific cDNA and have purified further the α cDNA made using the predominantly α mRNA of β-thalassemia reticulocytes to assay the α and β gene sequences in various individuals by cDNA-DNA hybridization. Both groups found a virtual absence of the portions of α genes encoding cytoplasmic α mRNA in the DNA of patients with α°-thalassemia (Ottolenghi et al., 1974; Taylor et al., 1974).

Kan then used similar techniques to demonstrate that roughly one fourth of the α gene sequences encoding cytoplasmic α mRNA are present in most Hb H disease individuals (Kan et al., 1975a). This result suggests that these patients have two α loci and that the combination of two different deletions in the same individual, a deleted α allele at one α locus (α-thal 2 genotype) and a deletion of both α loci (α-thal 1 genotype) on the chromosomal homologue, is one cause of Hb H disease.

TERMINATOR TO MISSENSE MUTATIONS.   The chain terminator mutations which change α^A to α^{CS} and other similar variant α genes result in synthesis rates of these α chain variants that are about 1 to 2 percent that of α^A (Clegg and Weatherall, 1974b; Koler et al., 1971).

The frequency of the α^{CS} allele is roughly 0.02 in Southeast Asians (Clegg and Weatherall, 1974b), so that the combination of an α-thal 1 deletion and an α^{CS} allele accounts for a large fraction of Hb H disease cases in that area. The cause of the reduction in α^{CS} synthesis is unknown, but some investigators believe that α^{CS} mRNA is unstable (Clegg and Weatherall, 1976).

UNKNOWN MUTATIONS. Recently another α-thal 1 genotype has been found in Chinese patients which does not consist of a deletion of α nucleotide sequences in that the combination of two α-thal 1 genes in the same individual results in Hb H disease and not α°-thalassemia (Kan et al., 1976a). The site and type of this mutation are still unknown.

To summarize, the common α-thal 1 genotype of Southeast Asia consists of a deletion of most or all of the nucleotide sequences corresponding to the cytoplasmic mRNA encoded by two presumably tandem α loci. A second α-thal 1 genotype of Southeast Asia is not a deletion, and its mutational derivation is unknown. A third α-thal 1 genotype found in Black Americans is another mutation, but is also probably not a deletion of α nucleotide sequences. The known α-thal 2 alleles are (1) a deletion of nucleotide sequences encoding the cytoplasmic mRNA of a single α locus and (2) four chain terminator mutations, including the α^{CS} gene. Thus we now recognize at least eight different mutations in the etiology of α-thalassemia, and the list has just begun.

β-Thalassemia. GENETICS. Pedigree analyses to date have placed β-thalassemia genes very close to or allelic with the single β locus (Huisman et al., 1961; Pearson and Moore, 1965). In contrast with the α-thalassemia states in which there are four levels of severity, depending upon how many of the four α genes are affected, the β-thalassemias can be generally considered as having two degrees of severity: one, the β-thalassemia trait, is associated with a single β-thalassemia allele; the second, β-thalassemia major, or Cooley's anemia, is produced by the presence of two β-thalassemia alleles in an individual.

In β-thalassemia major, as in other inborn errors, the alleles may be identical, thereby producing a homozygous individual. Alternatively, two different thalassemia alleles may be present in a single individual. Since many β-thalassemia genes are present in diverse populations, it is likely that a large proportion of β-thalassemia major patients fall into the category of genetic compounds (Clegg and Weatherall, 1976). A few exceptional individuals are found with disease of intermediate severity, β-thalassemia intermedia, and they, too, may often be heterozygous for two different β-thalassemia alleles. β-Thalassemia intermedia is the predominant thalassemia in Blacks, but is infrequent in Mediterranean peoples (Charache et al., 1974; Schwartz, 1969).

CHAIN SYNTHESIS RATIOS. In β-thalassemia heterozygotes, the α/β synthetic ratio in reticulocytes is 1.5 to 2.0, in contrast to ratios around 1.0 in unaffected individuals. In β-thalassemia major individuals, the α/β synthetic ratio may vary from 4 to infinity in reticulocytes (Nathan, 1972). β-Thalassemia genes responsible for the synthesis of reduced numbers of β chains are called β^+, whereas those from which no β chains are synthesized are β°-thalassemia genes. These latter genes account for a minority of the β-thalassemia genes in man.

The clinical course of β-thalassemia major is not affected in any consistent manner by the type of β-thalassemia genes present, either β°-thalassemia or β^+-thalassemia. A compensatory increase in γ chain production occurs in these states, which usually results in an $\alpha/(\beta+\gamma)$ synthetic ratio of 2 to 3 when the α/β synthetic ratio is 4 to infinity (Weatherall and Clegg, 1972). This compensatory increase in γ-chain synthesis leads to similar $\alpha/(\beta+\gamma)$ ratios in β°-thalassemia and β^+-thalassemia individuals. The Hb F in β-thalassemia is distributed heterogeneously in the red cells (Sheppard et al., 1962).

CLINICAL STATES. The benign heterozygous state, β-thalassemia trait, is characterized by very mild anemia with some reduction in hemoglobin per red cell and reduced red cell volume, but an increase in the number of erythrocytes. The percentage of Hb A_2 in the total hemoglobin is usually elevated, and this finding, along with a mild hypochromic, microcytic anemia, is usually sufficient to diagnose the condition (Weatherall and Clegg, 1972).

In contrast, deficiency in β chain production in β-thalassemia major produces a hypochromic, hemolytic anemia, because reduced synthesis of hemoglobin leads to hypochromic cells, whereas precipitation of excess free α chains secondary to the imbalance in α and β globin synthesis produces hemolysis. After the first year of life, blood transfusions every 4 to 8 weeks are usually required. These children develop hepatosplenomegaly and an Oriental facial appearance produced by extramedullary and excessive intramedullary hematopoiesis of the maxillary bones, respectively. Patients with α-thalassemia genes in addition to β-thalassemia major do better because they have less globin synthetic imbalance and hemolysis than individuals with β-thalassemia major alone.

The major cause of mortality in β-thalassemia major is cardiac hemochromatosis secondary to excessive iron intake from blood transfusions and increased gastrointestinal absorption of iron. Since therapy is presently unsatisfactory, death often occurs in the third and fourth decades of life.

Although Greek and Italian homozygotes generally follow this course, Black Americans often have a very mild disease (β-thalassemia intermedia) in which transfusions are not required. Since these mildly affected Blacks have α/β synthetic ratios similar to those observed in severely affected Mediterranean peoples, the reasons for the difference in clinical course of these groups are unclear (Charache et al., 1974; Schwartz, 1969).

Prenatal diagnosis of hemoglobinopathies in general and of β-thalassemia in particular has recently been accomplished in a few centers; and although it is still experimental, the results have been generally promising (Kan et al., 1975b; Nathan and Alter, 1975; Kan et al., 1976b; Alter et al., 1976; Kazazian, Boyer, Park, Dover, and Lightbody, unpublished data). Its feasibility is based on a number of factors. First, β chains are synthesized by erythroid precursors as early as 6 weeks of fetal age (Hollenberg et al., 1971; Cividalli et al., 1974; Kazazian, 1974). Second, standards of normal β chain synthesis at 18 to 20 weeks of gestation have been obtained (Kazazian and Woodhead, 1973; Cividalli et al., 1974). Third, fetal cells can usually be obtained either by transabdominal placental puncture under ultrasonography or by fetoscopy (Hobbins and Mahoney, 1974; Kan et al., 1974). Fourth, small numbers of fetal reticulocytes can now be separated from large numbers of maternal erythrocytes (Boyer et al., 1976). Among the potential problems of prenatal diagnosis of β-thalassemia is the possibility of overlap in the β chain synthesis of β-thalassemia trait and β-thalassemia major fetuses. Recent observations suggest that this problem may not exist, because β-thalassemia major fetuses, even those with β^+-thalassemia, appear to lack β chain synthesis (Kan et al., 1976c). Another potential hazard, that of fetal mortality secondary to the procedure for obtaining fetal blood, has occurred in roughly 5 to 8 percent of the cases. Thus prenatal diagnosis of β-thalassemia major, although not completely perfected, offers an alternative to couples at risk for this disease.

β-THALASSEMIA VARIANTS. 1. $\delta\beta$-Thalassemia. Another β-thalassemia, $\delta\beta$-thalassemia, is characterized by an absence of δ and β chain synthesis in the homozygote, and yet this condition is often milder than the more common forms of β-thalassemia major. In $\delta\beta$-thalassemia heterozygotes, the red cells appear thalassemic; and the Hb F, which makes up 5 to 20 percent of the hemoglobin, is distributed heterogeneously within red cells (Weatherall and Clegg, 1972).

2. Hereditary persistence of fetal hemoglobin (HPFH). The HPFH syndromes are clinically mild variants of β-thalassemia and

Table 2. Types of Hereditary Persistence of Fetal Hemoglobin (HPFH)

γ Chain Type	Ethnic Group	Distribution of Hb F in Cells	% Hb F in Heterozygotes	cis β Chain Production
$G_\gamma A_\gamma$ (2:3)	Black	Equal	~30	No
$G_\gamma A_\gamma$ (1:10)	Black	Equal	~18	No
$G_\gamma A_\gamma$ (1:10)	English	Not equal	~ 7	Yes
$G_\gamma A_\gamma$ (1:1)	Black	Not equal	3–8	Yes°
G_γ	Black	Equal	~15	No
G_γ	Black	Equal	15–30	Yes
G_γ (+ Hb Kenya)	East African	Equal	~ 7	Deleted
A_γ	Greek	Equal	~15	Probable
A_γ	American	Equal	~ 5	Probable
?	European	Not equal	~ 2	Yes

°See Stamatoyannopoulos et al., 1975.

have recently been reviewed extensively (Clegg and Weatherall, 1976; Kazazian, 1976; Huisman et al., 1974). Presently at least ten different types of HPFH are known, and no single diagnostic criterion has remained common to all types. The classification in Table 2 is arbitrary and perhaps artificial, and the boundaries between the HPFH syndromes, $\delta\beta$-thalassemia, and other thalassemias have become blurred as the number of HPFH syndromes has increased. These syndromes are classified here on the basis of percentages of fetal hemoglobin present in the heterozygous state, the ratio of $^G\gamma$ to $^A\gamma$ chains in fetal hemoglobin of the heterozygote, the cellular distribution of fetal hemoglobin, and whether or not the β gene on the chromosome carrying the HPFH allele is active. In all HPFH types, the gene affects only the activity of the γ chain genes *cis* to it; i.e., on the same chromosome.

As Table 2 indicates, there is a $^G\gamma^A\gamma$ type of HPFH in which both $^G\gamma$ and $^A\gamma$ chains are produced, β chain synthesis does not occur in *cis*, and the Hb F distribution is homogeneous within the cells (Conley et al., 1963). Another $^G\gamma^A\gamma$ type occurs in which fetal hemoglobin contains mostly $^A\gamma$ chains, β chains are made from the β gene adjacent to the HPFH gene, and this hemoglobin is heterogeneously distributed within the cells (Weatherall et al., 1975). There also exist $^G\gamma$ types (no $^A\gamma$ chains are present in the Hb F in this condition) in which β chains are not made in *cis* (Huisman et al., 1969), along with $^G\gamma$ types in which β chain synthesis is directed by the β gene adjacent to the HPFH genes (Huisman et al., 1975; Friedman and Schwartz, 1976). In contrast, all $^A\gamma$ types of HPFH (no $^G\gamma$ chains are produced) are probably associated with B chain synthesis *cis* to the HPFH gene (Huisman et al., 1970a, b).

Hb Kenya trait seems also to belong to the HPFH syndromes. As mentioned earlier, in this condition a meiotic crossing-over event has occurred between an $^A\gamma$ gene and a β gene producing a $\gamma\beta$ fusion gene and a deletion spanning the δ gene and regions between the δ gene and the $^A\gamma$ and β genes (Fig. 4) (Clegg et al., 1973). Individuals with Hb Kenya trait are not anemic, have normal erythrocyte morphology with a slight reduction in MCH, and have an even distribution of Hb F in their red cells (Nute et al., 1976). Of the total hemoglobin in these individuals, 6 to 23 percent is Hb Kenya and 5 to 8 percent is Hb F, consisting solely of α and $^G\gamma$ chains (Clegg et al., 1973).

Therefore it becomes clear that neither a homogeneous distribution of Hb F in red cells nor the absence of β chain synthesis *cis* to the HPFH gene is an absolute criterion of these syndromes. Moreover, the percentage of Hb F in the total hemoglobin of heterozygotes may vary from 1 to 2 percent up to 30 percent (Clegg and Weatherall, 1976).

Although HPFH heterozygotes generally do not have an imbalance in α and non-α globin chain synthesis, an α/γ synthetic ratio of 1.4 has been found in the homozygous state along with some reduction in MCH and MCV in erythrocytes (Charache et al., in press). Thus the differentiation between homozygous $\delta\beta$-thalassemia and homozygous HPFH without Hb A production hangs precariously on the following features: (1) $\delta\beta$-thalassemia may have a somewhat worse clinical picture than HPFH; (2) in heterozygous relatives, the cellular distribution of Hb F in $\delta\beta$-thalassemia is heterogeneous, whereas it is often homogeneous in HPFH; and (3) red cell indices are more normal in $\delta\beta$-thalassemia heterozygotes than in heterozygotes for HPFH. How long these diagnostic criteria will remain valid in the face of the continued blurring between these syndromes remains to be seen.

Mutations Producing β-Thalassemia and Its Variants. More detailed biochemistry is known about the β-thalassemias than about any other inborn error of metabolism; yet we still know little about the nature or the location of mutations causing many of these conditions. Although there is a consensus that all the genes associated with β-thalassemia are allelic with β^A, we have no evidence that this is always so. Pedigree data are limited to a few families representing very few β-thalassemia genes. However, some mutations are known to involve the β locus (Table 3).

SENSE TO MISSENSE MUTATION. In β^{KW} carriers, the abnormal

Table 3. Known Molecular Defects in the β-Thalassemias and Variants

Thalassemia Gene	Molecular Data		
	β Gene	β mRNA	β Chain
$\beta°$-Thal	+	−	−
$\beta°$-Thal (other)	+	↓	−
$\beta°$-Catania	+	Sl. ↓	−
$\beta°$-Ferrara	+	Abnormal or −	−
β^{KW}	+	↓ (?)	↓
β^+-Thal(Mediterranean)	+	↓	↓
β^+-Thal (Black)	+	↓	↓
$\delta\beta$-Thal	−	−	−
Hb Lepore	−($\delta\beta$ gene)	−(↓ $\delta\beta$ mRNA)	−(↓ $\delta\beta$ chain)
Hb Kenya	−($\gamma\beta$ gene)	−(↓ $\gamma\beta$ mRNA)	−(↓ $\gamma\beta$ chain)
HPFH (common $G_\gamma A_\gamma$ type)	−	−	−

+ = Present.
− = Absent.
↓ = Decreased.

β chain is made at a rate of 50 percent of normal and a thalassemia-like condition is present. The β^{KW} chain contains a glutamine in place of lysine in residue 132 (Allan et al., 1965). Thus a simple A to C nucleotide substitution within the DNA encoding the β chain has led to a significant reduction in β globin synthesis (Lang et al., 1974). However, since most β chain variants, including β^S and β^C, are synthesized at about 80 percent the rate of β^A (Boyer et al., 1964), the defect in β^{KW} synthesis may merely represent an exaggeration of the defect in β chain synthesis which usually follows mutation in the translated region of the β gene. The assembly rates of a number of these variant β chains, including β^S, β^C, and β^{KW}, are normal (Rieder, 1972; Lang et al., 1974). Therefore a likely cause of decreased synthesis of these variants is decreased stability of the $\beta^{Variant}$ mRNA. Since the secondary structure of an RNA formed by hydrogen bonding between base pairs is probably vital to the molecule's resistance to ribonucleases, nucleotide substitutions which alter the normal base pairing arrangements within single or double stranded regions in mRNA may render it more susceptible to ribonuclease attack and premature degradation.

DELETIONS. In Hb Lepore traits, the $\delta\beta$ chains are made at 20 percent the rate of the normal β chain, again producing a β-type thalassemia (White et al., 1972). A number of Lepore deletions have been described, and each is characterized by the loss of the δ and β genes and all the regulatory DNA between these genes (Labie et al., 1966; Curtain, 1964). Presumably, those mechanisms which regulate downward the synthesis of normal δ chains decrease the synthesis of Lepore chains. Since Lepore chains are translated at a normal rate, it is probable that Lepore mRNA is unstable in individuals with Lepore trait (White et al., 1972).

In the Hb Kenya trait, the deletion is larger, removing the DNA from the middle of the $^A\gamma$ gene through to the middle of the translated region of the β gene, leading to the synthesis of a γβ chain. This deletion produces an HPFH syndrome in the heterozygote (Huisman et al., 1972b; Clegg et al., 1973).

In the few individuals homozygous for δβ-thalassemia who have been studied, cDNA/RNA hybridization has indicated a marked deficiency of cytoplasmic β mRNA (Forget et al., 1974; Ramirez et al., 1976) and cDNA/DNA hybridization has suggested deletions of both the β and δ genes (Ramirez et al., 1976; Ottolenghi et al., 1976). The extent of this deletion is not known, but it must also include regions of DNA between the deleted δ and β loci.

Using cDNA/DNA hybridization methods, a similar deletion has been found in American Blacks with the $^G\gamma^A\gamma$ type of HPFH (Kan et al., 1975c; Forget et al., 1976). This deletion presumably spans the δ and β genes, but it is postulated that, unlike the deletion of δβ-thalassemia, it includes nucleotides between the $^A\gamma$ and δ loci which may play a regulatory role in γ chain synthesis (Huisman et al., 1974).

In addition, Huisman has postulated that the $^G\gamma$ type of HPFH in which no β chains are made in *cis* is due to a deletion which spans the $^A\gamma$, δ, and β genes. On the other hand, a smaller deletion could account for the $^G\gamma$ type of HPFH in which the *cis* β gene is active (Huisman et al., 1974).

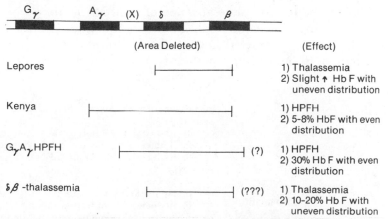

Figure 6. Deletions in the non-α gene cluster on an autosome. Data suggest one regulator region for suppression of γ chain synthesis at (X). (Modified from Kazazian, H. H., Jr.: Johns Hopkins Med. J., *139*:215–219, 1976.)

All these deletions or postulated deletions suggest the existence of a regulatory region between the $^A\gamma$ and δ genes, the absence of which leads to persistent synthesis of γ chains (Fig. 6) (Huisman et al., 1974). An unconventional feature of this postulated regulatory region is that it lies distal to the genetic material, the γ loci, on which it acts. In addition, this single regulatory region cannot explain the findings in other HPFH syndromes, especially the $^A\gamma$ types, in which this region is presumably intact.

UNKNOWN MUTATIONS.   In other β-thalassemia cases, the type and site of mutation are unknown (Fig. 7). In all the β°-thalassemias studied to date by cDNA/DNA hybridization methods, gene sequences are present in normal quantities (Table 3) (Kan et al., 1975d; Tolstoshev et al., 1976). However, β mRNA levels appear to vary in these patients. In one variety, β°-Catania, β mRNA is present in reticulocyte RNA but is slightly reduced relative to α mRNA levels (Ramirez et al., 1976). In another type, β°-Ferrara, β mRNA is either absent or structurally abnormal, because it hybridizes in an unusual fashion with β cDNA (Ramirez et al., 1976). In a third group of β°-thalassemia patients, β mRNA is absent in reticulocytes (Forget et al., 1974; Tolstoshev et al., 1976). In all three of these groups, β chain synthesis is lacking in erythroid cells.

Although the sites of mutations leading to these β°-thalassemias are unknown, our knowledge of the early steps in gene activity allows some reasonable speculations (Figs. 4 and 7). In β°-thalassemias in which β mRNA is lacking, the mutation may alter the RNA polymerase binding site and completely block transcription of β mRNA precursor. Alternatively, mutation might affect any of the steps by which mRNA is processed, but whether processing mutations could produce complete absence of β mRNA is unknown. The mutation causing β°-Catania might be deletion or addition of nucleotides within the β translated DNA sufficient to produce a frameshift in translation. Should such a mutation occur near the initiation site

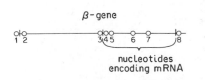

β-gene

1 2   3,4 5   6   7   8

nucleotides
encoding mRNA

Figure 7. Postulated defects in β-thalassemia:

1. Reduced RNA polymerase binding.
2. Reduced binding of regulatory protein(s).
3. Reduced excision of mRNA from precursor.
4. Deficient 5'-"capping."
5. Deficient 5'-end methylation.
6. Reduced rate of translation.
7. Nonsense or frameshift mutation leading to absence of normal polypeptide.
8. Deficient polyadenylation.

for translation, it could result in a completely nonfunctional β chain but nearly normal amounts of β mRNA in the cell. Another possibility is that the mutation affects the binding of the methyltransferase which adds a methyl group to the 7 position of guanosine at the 5'-end of β globin mRNA. The lack of this methyl group or 7-methylguanosine-5'-triphosphate on β globin mRNA may completely eliminate β chain synthesis in vivo (Muthukrishnan et al., 1975; Hickey et al., 1976).

In β°-Ferrara individuals, the abnormal mRNA could result from any one of a number of mutations (Ramirez et al., 1976). One possibility is a small deletion of nucleotides encoding the 3'-end of β mRNA, rendering polyadenylation impossible and altering β cDNA hybridization characteristics in vitro. Other data have indicated that some β chain synthesis can be induced by adding supernatant from normal reticulocytes to ribosomes of β°-Ferrara patients (Conconi et al., 1972). How this effect occurs is unclear. However, since many different mutations lead to an absence of β chain synthesis in β°-thalassemia, it is not surprising that other mutations, in addition to deletions, are now being implicated in the causation of α°-thalassemia.

Although the mutational basis of nearly all β^{+}-thalassemia is not understood, the β^{+}-thalassemia of both Greeks (Housman et al., 1973; Kacian et al., 1973) and American Blacks (Kazazian et al., 1975) is associated with a β mRNA deficiency commensurate with the reduction in β chain synthesis. Since the degree of deficiency of β chain synthesis varies from family to family in the β^{+}-thalassemias, we presume that many different causes, perhaps related to defects in the various steps in mRNA processing, will be found in these syndromes also. Since the various enzymes which modify mRNA after transcription must recognize specific nucleotide sequences on the RNA, mutation in these sequences in the β gene could result in a defect in mRNA modification, even though the enzyme doing the modifying is normal. A defect at any of the steps in mRNA processing after transcription could result in reduced quantities of β mRNA through increased degradation of the mRNA. Alternatively, moderate deficiencies in transcription of the β gene may underlie many of the β^{+}-thalassemias.

SUMMARY

The next 5 years should bring a great unraveling of the many mutations that produce the α and β thalassemia syndromes. We postulate that many of these mutations occur outside the DNA whose information is subsequently translated into globin and that they involve regulatory DNA. Presumably, these mutations are either in or near the globin genes and affect the interaction of proteins, such as an RNA polymerase, a methyltransferase, or poly(A) synthetase with nucleotide sequences at either the DNA or the RNA level.

To generalize from the β-thalassemia experience is tempting. Many rare inborn errors of metabolism could be the result of the inheritance of two different alleles for the disease. As in the thalassemias, mutations of both regulatory DNA and DNA whose mRNA is subsequently translated could combine in the same individual to produce an enzyme deficiency. Such individuals would be CRM-positive, making the comparison of the quantity of CRM protein in the affected individual with that in controls very important. Although mutations of DNA encoding a protein may result in the reduced production of the specified protein, as in the β^{KW} mutation, the experience with thalassemia indicates that deletions and other mutations in regulatory DNA are more likely causes of the numerous CRM-negative disorders. Thus as our knowledge of the mutations producing the thalassemia syndromes increases, it should help us to understand the mutational basis of other inborn errors of metabolism. In the process, we will also discover just how little we presently know about the normal regulation of genetic activity in eukaryotes.

ACKNOWLEDGMENT

The authors thank Drs. Barton Childs, Barbara R. Migeon, and Samuel Charache for helpful criticism of the manuscript.

References

Abramson, R. K., D. L. Rucknagel, D. C. Shreffler, and J. J. Suave. 1970. Homozygous Hb J Tongariki: Evidence for only one alpha chain structural locus in Melanesians. Science 169:194–196.

Adams, H. R., R. N. Wrightstone, A. Miller, and T. H. J. Huisman. 1969. Quantitation of hemoglobin α chains in adult and fetal goats; gene duplication and the production of polypeptide chains. Arch. Biochem. Biophys. 132:223–236.

Adesnik, M., M. Salditt, W. Thomas, and J. E. Darnell. 1972. Evidence that all messenger RNA molecules (except histone messenger RNA) contain poly(A) sequences and that the poly(A) has a nuclear function. J. Molec. Biol. 71:21–30.

Adhya, S. L., and J. A. Shapiro. 1969. The galactose operon of E. coli K-12. 1. Structural and pleiotrophic mutations of the operon. Genetics 62:231–247.

Allan, N. D., D. Beale, D. Irvine, and H. Lehmann. 1965. Three hemoglobins K: Woolwich, an abnormal, Cameroon and Ibadan, two unusual variants of human hemoglobin A. Nature 208:658–661.

Alter, B. P., S. Friedman, J. C. Hobbins, M. J. Mahoney, A. S. Sherman, J. F.

McSweeney, E. Schwartz, and D. G. Nathan. 1976. Prenatal diagnosis of sickle cell anemia and alpha G-Philadelphia. New Eng. J. Med. 294:1040–1041.

Badr, F. M., P. A. Lorkin, and H. Lehmann. 1973. Haemoglobin P-Nilotic containing a β-δchain. Nature New Biol. 242: 107–110.

Baglioni, C. 1962. The fusion of two peptide chains in hemoglobin Lepore and its interpretation as a genetic delection Proc. Nat. Acad. Sci. U.S.A. 48:1880–1886.

Bard, H. 1975. The postnatal decline of hemoglobin F synthesis in normal full-term infants. J. Clin. Invest. 55:395–398.

Bellingham, A. J. 1976. Hemoglobins with altered oxygen affinity. Brit. Med. Bull. 32:234–238.

Benz, E. J., Jr., and B. G. Forget. 1974. The biosynthesis of hemoglobin. Semin. Hematol. 11:463–523.

Bernhardt, D., and J. E. Darnell. 1969. tRNA synthesis in Hela cells: A precursor to tRNA and the effects of methionine starvation on tRNA synthesis. J. Molec. Biol. 42:43–56.

Blobel, G. 1972. Protein tightly bound to globin mRNA. Biochem. Biophys. Res. Commun. 47:88–95.

Blobel, G. 1973. A protein of molecular weight 78,000 bound to the polyadenylate region of eukaryotic messenger RNAs. Proc. Nat. Acad. Sci. U.S.A. 70:924–928.

Both, G. W., A. K. Banerjee, and A. J. Shatkin. 1975. Methylation-dependent translation of viral messenger RNAs in vitro. Proc. Nat. Acad. Sci. U.S.A. 72:1189–1193.

Boyer, S., P. Hathaway, and M. D. Garrick. 1964. Modulation of protein synthesis in man: An in vitro study of hemoglobin synthesis by heterozygotes. Cold Spring Harbor Symp. Quant. Biol. 29:333–346.

Boyer, S. H., A. N. Noyes, and M. L. Boyer. 1976. Enrichment of erythrocytes of fetal origin from adult-fetal blood mixtures via selective hemolysis of adult blood cells: An aid to antenatal diagnosis of hemoglobinopathies. Blood 47:883–897.

Boyer, S. H., K. D. Smith, A. N. Noyes, and M. A. Mullen. 1974. Immunological characterization of rabbit hemoglobin α and β chain–synthesizing polysomes (estimation of relative numbers of active α- and β-messenger ribonucleic acid). J. Biol. Chem. 249:7210–7219.

Bradley, T. B., R. C. Wohl, and R. F. Rieder. 1967. Hemoglobin Gun Hill: Deletion of five amino acid residues and impaired heme-globin binding. Science 157:1581–1583.

Bradley, T. B., R. C. Wohl, and G. J. Smith. 1975. Elongation of the α globin chain in a black family: Interaction with Hb G Philadelphia (abstract). Clin. Res. 23:131A.

Bunn, H. F., G. J. Schmidt, D. N. Haney, and R. G. Dluhy. 1975. Hemoglobin Cranston, an unstable variant having an elongated β chain due to nonhomologous crossover between two normal β chain genes. Proc. Nat. Acad. Sci. U.S.A. 72:3609–3613.

Cann, A., R. Gambino, J. Banks, and A. Bank. 1974. Polyadenylate sequences and biologic activity of human globin messenger ribonucleic acid. J. Biol. Chem. 249:7536–7540.

Charache, S., J. B. Clegg, and D. J. Weatherall. In press. The Negro variety of hereditary persistence of fetal hemoglobin is a mild form of thalassemia. Brit. J. Haematol.

Charache, S., C. L. Conley, T. D. Doeblin, and M. Bartalos. 1974. Thalassemia in Black Americans. Ann. N.Y. Acad. Sci. 232:125–134.

Cheng, T-c., and H. H. Kazazian, Jr. In press. The 5'-terminal structures of murine α and β globin messenger RNA. J. Biol. Chem.

Cheng, T-c., B. J. Thompson, and H. H. Kazazian, Jr. 1976. Methylated 5'-terminal structures of human α and β globin (abstract). Abs. Annual Meeting of Am. Soc. Hematol., p. 92.

Cividalli, G., D. G. Nathan, Y. W. Kan, B. Santamarina, and F. Frigoletto. 1974. Relation of beta to gamma synthesis during the first trimester: An approach to prenatal diagnosis of thalassemia. Pediat. Res. 8:553–560.

Clegg, J. B., and D. J. Weatherall. 1974a. β° thalassemia—Time for a reappraisal? Lancet 2:133–135.

Clegg, J. B., and D. J. Weatherall. 1974b. Hemoglobin Constant Spring, an unusual α chain variant involved in the etiology of hemoglobin H disease. Ann. N.Y. Acad. Sci. 232:168–178.

Clegg, J. B., and D. J. Weatherall. 1976. Molecular basis of thalassemia. Brit. Med. Bull. 32:262–269.

Clegg, J. B., D. J. Weatherall, T. Contopolou-Griva, K. Caroutsos, P. Poungouros, and H. Tsevrenis. 1974. Haemoglobin Icaria, a new chain-termination mutant which causes α thalassemia. Nature 251:245–247.

Clegg, J. B., D. J. Weatherall, and H. M. Gilles. 1973. Hereditary persistence of foetal haemoglobin associated with a γβ fusion variant, Haemoglobin Kenya. Nature New Biol. 246:184–186.

Clegg, J. B., D. J. Weatherall, and P. F. Milner. 1971. Hemoglobin Constant Spring—a chain terminator mutant? Nature 234:337–340.

Clegg, J. B., D. J. Weatherall, S. Na-Nakorn, and P. Wasi. 1968. Hemoglobin synthesis in β thalassemia. Nature 220:664–668.

Conconi, F., P. T. Rowley, L. Del Senno, and S. Pontremoli. 1972. Induction of β-globin synthesis in the β-thalassemia of Ferrara. Nature New Biol. 238:83–87.

Conley, C. L., D. J. Weatherall, S. N. Richardson, M. K. Shepard, and S. Charache. 1963. Hereditary persistence of fetal hemoglobin: A study of 79 affected persons in 15 Negro families in Baltimore. Blood 21:261–281.

Cory, S., and J. M. Adams. 1975. The modified 5'-terminal sequences in messenger RNA of mouse myeloma cells. J. Molec. Biol. 99:519–547.

Coutelli, C., A. P. Ryskov, and G. P. Giorgiev. 1970. Localization of messenger RNA near the 3'-end of the dRNA precursor molecule. FEBS Let. 12:21–23.

Curtain, C. C. 1974. A structural study of abnormal haemoglobins occurring in New Guinea. Aust. J. Exp. Biol. Med. Sci. 42:89–97.

Darnell, J. E., W. R. Jelinek, and G. R. Malloy. 1973. Biogenesis of mRNA: Genetic regulation in mammalian cells. Science 181:1215–1221.

Darnell, J. E., L. Phillipson, R. Wall, and M. Adesnik. 1971. Polyadenylic acid sequences: Role in conversion of nuclear RNA into messenger RNA. Science 174:507–510.

Das, N. K., A. Goldstein, and L. I. Lowney. 1967. Attachment of ribosomes to nascent messenger RNA in *Escherichia coli.* J. Molec. Biol. 24:231–245.

Das, N. K., J. Micou-Eastwood, G. Ramamurthy, and M. Alfert. 1970. Sites of synthesis and processing of ribosomal RNA precursors within the nucleolus of *Urechis caupo* eggs. Proc. Nat. Acad. Sci. U.S.A. 67:968–975.

Deisseroth, A., R. Velez, and A. W. Niehuis. 1976. Hemoglobin synthesis in somatic cell hybrids: Independent segregation of the human alpha- and beta-globin genes. Science 191:1262–1263.

DeJong, W. W., P. M. Khan, and L. F. Bernini. 1975. Hemoglobin Koya Dora: High frequency of a chain termination mutant. Am. J. Hum. Genet. 27:81–90.

DeJong, W. W., L. N. Went, and L. F. Bernini. 1968. Hemoglobin Leiden: Deletion of β 6 or 7 glutamic acid. Nature 220:788–790.

Dherte, P., H. Lehmann, and J. Vandepitte. 1959. Haemoglobin P in a family in the Belgian Congo. Nature 184:1133–1135.

Filipowicz, W., J. M. Sierra, C. Nombela, S. Ochoa, W. C. Merrick, and W. F. Anderson. 1976. Polypeptide chain initiation in eukaryotes. Initiation factor requirements for translation of natural messengers. Proc. Nat. Acad. Sci. U.S.A. 73:44–48.

Flatz, G., J. L. Kinderlerer, J. V. Kilmortin, and H. Lehman. 1971. Haemoglobin TAK: A variant with additional residues of the end of the β chains. Lancet 1:732–733.

Forget, B. G., E. J. Benz, A. Skoultchi, C. Baglioni, and D. Housman. 1974. Absence of messenger RNA for beta globin chain in β°-thalassemia. Nature 247:379–381.

Forget, B. G., D. G. Hillman, H. Lazarus, E. F. Barell, E. J. Benz, C. T. Caskey, T. H. J. Huisman, W. A. Schroeder, and D. Housman. 1976. Absence of messenger RNA and gene DNA for β-globin chains in hereditary persistence of fetal hemoglobin. Cell 7:323–329.

Forget, B. G., D. Housman, E. J. Benz, Jr., and R. P. McCaffrey. 1975a. Synthesis of

DNA complementary to separated human alpha and beta globin messenger RNAs. Proc. Nat. Acad. Sci. U.S.A. 72:984:988.

Forget, B. G., C. A. Marotta, S. M. Weissman, and M. Cohen-Solal. 1975b. Nucleotide sequences of the 3'-terminal untranslated region of messenger RNA for human beta globin chain. Proc. Nat. Acad. Sci. U.S.A. 72:3614–3618.

Friedman, S., J. Atwater, F. M. Gill, and E. Schwartz. 1974. α-Thalassemia in Negro infants. Pediat. Res. 8:955–959.

Friedman, S., and E. Schwartz. 1976. Hereditary persistence of foetal haemoglobin with β-chain synthesis in cis position ($^G\gamma$-β^+-HPFH) in a Negro family. Nature 259:138–140.

Furuichi, Y., S. Muthukrishnan, J. Tomasz, and A. J. Shatkin. 1976. Mechanism of formation of reovirus mRNA 5'-terminal blocked and methylated sequence, m[7]-GpppG^{m}pC. J. Biol. Chem. 251:5043–5053.

Hamlyn, P. H., and H. J. Gould. 1975. Isolation and identification of separated messenger RNAs for rabbit α and β globin. J. Molec. Biol. 94:101–109.

Heckle, W. L., R. G. Fenton, T. G. Wood, C. G. Merkel, and J. B. Lingrel. In press. Methylated nucleosides in globin mRNA from mouse nucleated erythroid cells. J. Biol. Chem.

Hickey, E. D., L. A. Weber, and C. Baglioni. 1976. Inhibition of protein synthesis by 7-methyl guanosine 5'-monophosphate. Proc. Nat. Acad. Sci. U.S.A. 73:19–23.

Hilse, K., and R. A. Popp. 1968. Gene duplication as the basis for amino acid ambiguity in the alpha-chain polypeptides of mouse hemoglobins. Proc. Nat. Acad. Sci. U.S.A. 61:930–936.

Hobbins, J. C., and M. J. Mahoney. 1974. In utero diagnosis of hemoglobinopathies: Technic for obtaining fetal blood. New Eng. J. Med. 290:1065–1067.

Hollan, S. R., J. G. Szelenyi, B. Brimhall, M. Duerst, R. T. Jones, R. D. Koler, and Z. Stocklen. 1972. Multiple alpha chain loci for human hemoglobins: Hb J-Buda and Hb G-Pest. Nature 235:47–50.

Hollenberg, M. D., M. M. Kaback, and H. H. Kazazian, Jr. 1971. Adult hemoglobin synthesis by reticulocytes from the human fetus at midtrimester. Science 174:698–702.

Housman, D., B. G. Forget, A. Shoultchi, and E. J. Benz, Jr. 1973. Quantitative deficiency of chain-specific globin messenger ribonucleic acid in the thalassemia syndromes. Proc. Nat. Acad. Sci. U.S.A. 70:1809–1813.

Huisman, T. H. J., A. Miller, and W. A. Schroeder. 1975. A $^G\gamma$ type of hereditary persistence of fetal hemoglobin with β chain production in cis. Am. J. Hum. Genet. 27:765–777.

Huisman, T. H. J., K. Punt, and J. D. G. Schaad. 1961. Thalassemia minor associated with hemoglobin B₂ heterozygosity. A family report. Blood 17:747–757.

Huisman, T. H. J., W. A. Schroeder, H. R. Adams, J. R. Shelton, J. B. Shelton, and G. Apell. 1970a. A possible subclass of the hereditary persistence of fetal hemoglobin. Blood 36:1–9.

Huisman, T. H. J., W. A. Schroeder, W. H. Bannister, and J. L. Grech, 1972a. Evidence for four nonallelic structural genes for the γ chain of human fetal hemoglobin. Biochem. Genet. 7:131–139.

Huisman, T. H. J., W. A. Schroeder, A. M. Dozy, J. R. Shelton, J. B. Shelton, E. M. Boyd, and G. Apell. 1969. Evidence for multiple structural genes for the gamma-chain of human fetal hemoglobin in hereditary persistence ·of fetal hemoglobin. Ann. N.Y. Acad. Sci. 165:320–331.

Huisman, T. H. J., W. A. Schroeder, G. D. Efremov, H. Duma, B. Mladenovski, C. B. Human, E. A. Rachmilewitz, N. Bouver, A. Miller, A. Brodie, J. R. Shelton, J. B. Shelton, and G. Apell. 1974. The present status of the heterogeneity of fetal hemoglobin in β-thalassemia: An attempt to unify some observations in thalassemia and related conditions. Ann. N.Y. Acad. Sci. 232:107–124.

Huisman, T. H. J., W. A. Schroeder, G. Stamatoyannopoulos, N. Bouver, J. R. Shelton, J. B. Shelton, and G. Apell. 1970b. Nature of fetal hemoglobin in the Greek type of hereditary persistence of fetal hemoglobin with and without concurrent β-thalassemia. J. Clin. Invest. 49:1035–1040.

Huisman, T. H. J., R. N. Wrightstone, J. B. Wilson, W. A. Schroeder, and A. G. Kendall. 1972b. Hemoglobin Kenya, the product of fusion of γ and β polypeptide chains. Arch. Biochem. Biophys. 153:850–853.

Hunt, L. T., and M. O. Dayhoff. 1974. Table of abnormal human globins. Ann. N.Y. Acad. Sci. 241:722–735.

Hunt, T. 1976. Control of globin synthesis. Brit. Med. Bull. 32:257–261.

Imaizumi, T., H. Diggelmann, and K. Scherrer. 1973. Demonstration of globin messenger sequences in giant nuclear precursors of messenger RNA of avian erythroblasts. Proc. Nat. Acad. Sci. U.S.A. 70:1122–1126.

Itano, H. A. 1965. The synthesis and structure of normal and abnormal hemoglobins. In Abnormal Hemoglobins in Africa, Jonxis, J. H. P. (Ed.), pp. 3–16. Oxford, Blackwell.

Jacob, F., and J. Monod. 1961. Genetic regulatory mechanisms in the synthesis of proteins. J. Molec. Biol. 3:318–356.

Kacian, D. L., R. Gambino, L. W. Dow, E. Grossbard, C. Natta, F. Ramirez, S. Spiegelman, P. A. Marks, and A. Bank. 1973. Decreased globin messenger RNA in thalassemia detected by molecular hybridization. Proc. Nat. Acad. Sci. U.S.A. 70:1886–1890.

Kamuzora, H. 1975. Recent developments in foetal haemoglobin research. Humangenetik 30:197–205.

Kamuzora, H., and H. Lehmann. 1975. Human embryonic haemoglobins including a comparison by homology of the human ζ and α chains. Nature 256:511–513.

Kan, Y. W., A. M. Dozy, R. F. Trecartin, and D. Todd. 1976a. Identification of a non-deletion type of α thalassemia-1 defect (abstract). Abs. Annual Meeting of Am. Soc. Hematol., p. 93.

Kan, Y. W., A. M. Dozy, H. E. Varmus, J. M. Taylor, J. P. Holland, L. E. Lie-Injo, J. Ganesan, and D. Todd. 1975a. Deletion of α-globin genes in hemoglobin-H disease demonstrates multiple α-globin structural loci. Nature 255:255–256.

Kan, Y. W., M. S. Golbus, P. Klein, and A. M. Dozy. 1975b. Successful application of prenatal diagnosis in a pregnancy at risk for homozygous β-thalassemia. New Eng. J. Med. 292:1096–1099.

Kan, Y. W., M. S. Golbus, and R. Trecartin. 1976b. Prenatal diagnosis of sickle cell anemia. New Eng. J. Med. 294:1039–1040.

Kan, Y. W., M. S. Golbus, R. F. Trecartin, A. M. Dozy, and H. M. Koenig. 1976c. Prenatal diagnosis of hemoglobin disorders (abstract). Abs. Annual Meeting Am. Soc. Hematol., p. 158.

Kan, Y. W., J. P. Holland, A. M. Dozy, S. Charache, and H. H. Kazazian, Jr. 1975c. Deletion of the β-globin structure gene in hereditary persistence of foetal haemoglobin. Nature 258:162–163.

Kan, Y. W., J. P. Holland, A. M. Dozy, and H. E. Varmus. 1975d. Demonstration of non-functional β-globin mRNA in homozygous β°-thalassemia. Proc. Nat. Acad. Sci. U.S.A. 72:5140–5144.

Kan, Y. W., C. Valenti, V. Carnazza, R. Guidotti, and R. F. Rieder. 1974. Fetal blood-sampling in utero. Lancet 1:79–80.

Kazazian, H. H., Jr. 1974. Regulation of fetal hemoglobin production. Semin. Hematol. 11:525–548.

Kazazian, H. H., Jr. 1976. The hereditary persistence of fetal hemoglobin syndromes: Variations on the thalassemia theme. Johns Hopkins Med. J. 139:215–219.

Kazazian, H. H., Jr., G. D. Ginder, P. G. Snyder, R. J. Van Beneden, and A. P. Woodhead. 1975. Further evidence of a quantitative deficiency of chain-specific globin mRNA in the thalassemia syndromes. Proc. Nat. Acad. Sci. U.S.A. 72:567–571.

Kazazian, H. H., Jr., and H. A. Itano. 1968. Studies on the quantitative control of polypeptide synthesis in human reticulocytes. J. Biol. Chem. 243:2048–2055.

Kazazian, H. H., Jr., A. M., Silverstein, P. G. Snyder, and R. J. Van Beneden. 1976. Increasing haemoglobin β-chain synthesis in foetal development is associated with a declining γ- to α-mRNA ratio. Nature 260:67–70.

Kazazian, H. H., Jr., and A. P. Woodhead. 1973. Hemoglobin A synthesis in the developing fetus. New Eng. J. Med. 289:58–62.

Kazazian, H. H., Jr., and A. P. Woodhead. 1974. Adult hemoglobin synthesis in the human fetus. Ann. N.Y. Acad. Sci. 241:691–698.

Kirkman, H. N. 1972. Enzyme defects. Prog. Med. Genet. 8:125–168.

Koler, R. D., R. T. Jones, P. Wasi, and S. Pootrukul. 1971. Genetics of hemoglobin H and α-thalassemia. Ann. Hum. Genet. 34:371–377.

Kwan, S-P., T. G. Wood, and J. B. Lingrel. 1977. Purification of a putative globin messenger RNA precursor from mouse nucleated erythroid cells. Proc. Nat. Acad. Sci. U.S.A. 74:178–182.

Labie, D., W. A. Schroeder, and T. H. J. Huisman. 1966. The amino acid sequence of the delta-beta chains of haemoglobin = Lepore Washington. Biochim. Biophys. Acta 127:428–437.

Lang, A., H. Lehmann, and P. A. King-Lewis. 1974. Hb K Woolwich, the cause of a thalassemia. Nature 249:467–469.

Lang, A., and P. A. Lorkin. 1976. Genetics of human haemoglobins. Brit. Med. Bull. 32:239–245.

Lehmann, H., and R. W. Carrell. 1968. Differences between α- and β-chain mutants of human haemoglobin and between α- and β-thalassemia. Possible duplication of the α-chain gene. Brit. Med. J. 4:748–750.

Lehmann, H., and D. Charlesworth. 1970. Observations on haemoglobin P (Congo type). Biochem. J. 119:43p.

Lewin, B. 1974. Gene Expression—2 Eukaryotic Chromosomes, pp. 229–319. New York, John Wiley & Sons.

Lie-Injo, L. E., J. Ganesan, J. B. Clegg, and D. J. Weatherall. 1974. Homozygous state for Hb Constant Spring (slow-moving Hb x components). Blood 43:251–259.

Lingrel, J. B., M. Morrison, J. Gorski, and C. G. Merkel. 1974. Various size classes of polyadenylic acid in mouse α and β globin mRNAs and their significance. Ann. N.Y. Acad. Sci. 241:156–169.

Livingstone, F. B. 1967. Abnormal Hemoglobins in Human Population. Chicago, Aldine Publishing Company.

Lockard, R. E., and U. L. RajBhandary. In press. Nucleotide sequences at the 5′-termini of rabbit α and β globin mRNA. Cell.

Lodish, H. F. 1971. Alpha and beta globin messenger ribonucleic acid. Different amounts and rates of initiation of translation. J. Biol. Chem. 246:7131–7138.

Lodish, H. F., and M. Jacobsen. 1972. Regulation of hemoglobin synthesis. J. Biol. Chem. 247:3622–3629.

Lopez, C. G., and L-I. L. Eng. 1971. Alpha-thalassemia in newborns in West Malaysia. Hum. Hered. 21:185–191.

Malamos, B., P. Fessas, and G. Stamatoyannopoulos. 1962. Types of thalassemia-trait carriers as revealed by a study of their incidence in Greece. Brit. J. Haematol. 8:5–14.

Marbaix, G., G. Huez, A. Burny, Y. Clentis, E. Hubert, M. Leclerco, H. Chantrenne, H. Soreq. U. Nudel, and U. Z. Littauer. 1975. Absence of polyadenylate segment in globin messenger RNA accelerates its degradation in Xenopus oocytes. Proc. Nat. Acad. Sci. U.S.A. 72:3065–3067.

Marotta, C. A., B. G. Forget, S. M. Weissman, I. M. Verma, R. P. McCaffrey, and D. Baltimore. 1974. Nucleotide sequences of human globin messenger RNA. Proc. Nat. Acad. Sci. U.S.A. 71:2300–2304.

Maroun, L. E., B. F. Driscoll, and R. M. Nardone. 1971. Possible cytoplasmic precursor of haemoglobin messenger RNA. Nature New Biol. 231:270–271.

McKeehan, W. L. 1974. Regulation of hemoglobin synthesis. Effect of concentration of messenger ribonucleic acid, ribosome subunits, initiation factors, and salts on ration of α and β chains synthesized in vitro. J. Biol. Chem. 249:6517–6526.

Merkel, C. G., S-P. Kwan, and J. B. Lingrel. 1975. Size of the polyadenylic acid region of newly synthesized globin messenger ribonucleic acid. J. Biol. Chem. 250:3725–3728.

Milner, P. F., J. B. Clegg, and D. J. Weatherall. 1971. Hemoglobin-H disease due to a unique hemoglobin variant with an elongated α chain. Lancet 1:729–732.

Minnich, V., J. K. Cordonnier, W. J. Williams, and C. V. Moore. 1962. Alpha, beta, and gamma hemoglobin polypeptide chains during the neonatal period with description of fetal form of D₂ St. Louis. Blood 19:137–167.

Muthukrishnan, S., G. W. Both, Y. Furuichi, and A. J. Shatkin. 1975. 5′-Terminal 7-methylguanosine in eukaryotic mRNA is required for translation. Nature 255:33–37.

Nathan, D. G. 1972. Thalassemia. New Eng. J. Med. 286:586–594.

Nathan, D. G., and B. P. Alter. 1975. Antenatal diagnosis of the hemoglobinopathies. Brit. J. Haematol. 31(Suppl):145–154.

Nute, P. E., W. G. Wood, G. Stamatoyannopoulos, C. Olweny, and P. J. Fialkow. 1976. The Kenya form of hereditary persistence of fetal haemoglobin: Structural studies and evidence for homogeneous distribution of haemoglobin F using fluorescent anti-haemoglobin F antibodies. Brit. J. Haematol. 32:55–63.

Orkin, S. H., and D. G. Nathan. 1976. The thalassemias. New Eng. J. Med. 295:710–714.

Ottolenghi, S., P. Comi, B. Giglioni, P. Tolstoshev, W. G. Lanyon, G. J. Mitchell, R. Williamson, G. Russo, S. Musumeci, G. Schiliro, G. A. Tsistrakis, S. Charache, W. G. Wood, J. B. Clegg, and D. J. Weatherall. 1976. δβ-Thalassemia is due to a gene delection. Cell 9:71–80.

Ottolenghi, S., W. G. Lanyon, J. Paul, R. Williamson, D. J. Weatherall, J. B. Clegg, J. Pritchard. S. Pootrakul, and W. H. Boon. 1974. Gene deletion as the cause of α-thalassemia. Nature 251:389–391.

Papayannopoulou, Th., M. Brice., and G. Stamatoyannopoulos, 1976. Stimulation of fetal hemoglobin synthesis in bone marrow cultures from adult individuals. Proc. Nat. Acad. Sci. U.S.A. 73:2033–2037.

Pearson, H. A., and M. M. Moore. 1965. Human hemoglobin gene linkage. Report of a family with hemoglobin B₂, hemoglobin S and β-thalassemia, including a probable crossover between thalassemia and delta loci. Am. J. Hum. Genet. 17:125–132.

Perry, R. P., and D. E. Kelley. 1974. Existence of methylated messenger RNA in mouse L cells. Cell 1:37–42.

Perutz, M. F. 1976. Structure and mechanism of haemoglobin. Brit. Med. Bull. 32:195–208.

Phillips, J. A., P. G. Snyder, and H. H. Kazazian, Jr. 1976. Quantitation of α and β globin mRNA sequences in total and ribosomal RNA of reticulocytes (abstract). Abs. Annual Meeting of Am. Soc. Hematol., p. 163.

Poon, R., G. V. Paddock, H. Heindell, P. Whitcome, W. Salser, D. Kacian, A. Bank. R. Gambino, and F. Ramirez. 1974. Nucleotide sequence analysis of RNA synthesized from rabbit globin complementary DNA. Proc. Nat. Acad. Sci. U.S.A. 71:3502–3506.

Price, P. M., J. H. Conover, and K. Hirschhorn. 1972. Chromosomal localization of human hemoglobin structural genes. Nature 237:340–342.

Prichard, P. M., J. M. Gilbert, D. A. Shafritz, and W. F. Anderson. 1970. Factors for the initiation of haemoglobin synthesis by rabbit reticulocyte ribosomes. Nature 226:511–514.

Proudfoot, N. J., and G. G. Brownlee. 1976. Nucleotide sequences of globin messenger RNA. Brit. Med. Bull. 32:251–256.

Ramirez, F., J. V. O'Donnell, P. A. Marks, A. Bank, S. Musumeci, S. Schiliro, G. Pizzarelli, G. Russo, B. Luppis, and R. Gambino. 1976. Abnormal or absent β mRNA in β°-Ferrara and gene deletion in δβ thalassemia. Nature 263:471–475.

Rieder, R. F. 1972. Translation of β-globin mRNA in β-thalassemia and the S and C hemoglobinopathies. J. Clin. Invest. 51:364–372.

Rieder, R. F. 1974. Human hemoglobin stability and instability: Molecular mechanisms and some clinical correlations. Semin. Hematol. 11:423–440.

Rottman, F., A. J. Shatkin, and R. P. Perry. 1974. Sequences containing methylated nucleotides at the 5' termini of messenger RNAs: Possible implications for processing. Cell 3:197–199.

Rucknagel, D. L., and W. P. Winter. 1974. Duplication of structural genes for hemoglobin α and β chains in man. Ann. N.Y. Acad. Sci. 241:80–89.

Schroeder, W. A., and T. H. J. Huisman. 1974. Multiple cistrons for fetal hemoglobin in man. Ann. N.Y. Acad. Sci. 241:70–79.

Schroeder, W. A., T. H. J. Huisman, J. R. Shelton, J. B. Shelton, E. F. Kleihauer, A. M. Dozy, and B. Robberson. 1968. Evidence for multiple structural genes for the γ chain of human fetal hemoglobin. Proc. Nat. Acad. Sci. U.S.A. 60:537–544.

Schwartz, E. 1969. The silent carrier of beta thalassemia. New Eng. J. Med. 281:1327–1333.

Seid-Akhanan, M., W. P. Winter, R. K. Abramson, and D. L. Rucknagel. 1976. Hemoglobin Wayne: A frameshift mutation detected in human hemoglobin alpha chains. Proc. Nat. Acad. Sci. U.S.A. 73:882–886.

Sheppard, M. K., D. J. Weatherall, and C. L. Conley. 1962. Semi-quantitative estimation of the distribution of fetal hemoglobin in red cell populations. Bull. Johns Hopkins Hosp. 110:293–310.

Shibata, S., T. Miyaji, S. Ueda, M. Matsuoka, I. Iuchi, K. Yamada, and N. Shinkai. 1970. Hemoglobin Tochigi (β 56–59 deleted). A new unstable hemoglobin discovered in a Japanese family. Proc. Japan Acad. 46:440–445.

Smith, E. W., and J. V. Torbert. 1958. Study of two abnormal hemoglobins with evidence for a new genetic locus for hemoglobin formation. Bull. Johns Hopkins Hosp. 102:38–45.

Soreq, H., U. Nudel, R. Solomon, M. Revel, and U. Z. Littauer. 1974. In vitro translation of polyadenylic acid–free rabbit globin messenger RNA. J. Molec. Biol. 88:233–245.

Stamatoyannopoulos, G., W. G. Wood, Th. Papayannopoulou, and P. E. Nute. 1975. A new form of hereditary persistence of fetal hemoglobin in Blacks and its association with sickle cell trait. Blood 46:683–692.

Steinheider, G., H. Melderis, and W. Ostertag. 1975. Embryonic ϵ chains of mice and rabbits. Nature 257:714–716.

Taylor, J. M., A. M. Dozy, Y. W. Kan, H. E. Varmus, and L. F. Lie-Injo. 1974. Genetic lesion in homozygous α thalassemia (hydrops fetalis). Nature 251:392–393.

Tolstoshev, P., J. Mitchell, G. Lanyon, R. Williamson, S. Ottolenghi, P. Comi, B. Giglioni, G. Masera, B. Modell, D. J. Weatherall, and J. B. Clegg. 1976. Presence of gene for β globin in homozygous β° thalassemia. Nature 259:95–98.

Watson, J. D. 1976. Molecular Biology of the Gene, 3rd ed., pp. 129–410. Menlo Park, California, W. A. Benjamin, Inc.

Weatherall, D. J. 1963. Abnormal haemoglobins in the neonatal period and their relationship to thalassemia. Brit. J. Haematol. 9:265–277.

Weatherall, D. J. 1974. Molecular basis for some disorders of haemoglobin synthesis – II. Brit. Med. J. 4:516–519.

Weatherall, D. J., R. Cartner, J. B. Clegg, W. G. Wood, I. A. Macrae, and A. MacKenzie. 1975. A form of hereditary persistence of fetal haemoglobin characterized by uneven cellular distribution of haemoglobin F and the production of haemoglobins A and A_2 in homozygotes. Brit. J. Haematol. 29:205–220.

Weatherall, D. J., and J. B. Clegg. 1972. The Thalassemia Syndromes, 2nd ed. Oxford, Blackwell Scientific Publications.

Weber, L. A., E. R. Ferman, E. D. Hickey, M. C. Williams, and C. Baglioni. 1976. Inhibition of HeLa cell messenger RNA translation by 7-methylguanosine 5'-monophosphate. J. Biol. Chem. 251:5657–5662.

Wei, C-M., A. Gershowitz, and B. Moss. 1975. Methylated nucleotides block 5' terminus of HeLa cell messenger RNA. Cell 4:379–386.

Wei, C-M., A. Gershowitz, and B. Moss. 1976. 5'-Terminal and internal methylated nucleotide sequences in HeLa cell mRNA. Biochemistry 15:397–401.

White, J. M. 1976. The unstable hemoglobins. Brit. Med. Bull. 32:219–222.

White, J. M., A. Lang, P. A. Lorkin, H. Lehman, and J. Reeve. 1972. Synthesis of hemoglobin Lepore. Nature New Biol. 235:208–210.

Williamson, R. 1976. Direct measurement of the number of globin genes. Brit. Med. Bull. 32:246–250.

Williamson, R., C. E. Drewienkiewicz, and J. Paul. 1973. Globin messenger sequences in high molecular weight RNA from embryonic mouse liver. Nature New Biol. 241:66–68.

Winslow, R. M., and V. M. Ingram. 1966. Peptide chain synthesis of human hemoglobins A and A_2. J. Biol. Chem. 241:1144–1149.

Winslow, R. M., M. L. Swenberg, E. Gross, P. Chervenick, R. R. Buchman, and W. F. Anderson. 1976. Hemoglobin McKees Rocks ($\alpha_2\beta_2^{145\ tyr \rightarrow term}$). A human "nonsense" mutation leading to a shortened β chain. J. Clin. Invest. 57:772–781.

Wood, W. G. 1976. Haemoglobin synthesis during human fetal development. Brit. Med. Bull. 32:282–287.

Yanase, T., M. Hanada, M. Seita, I. Ohya, Y. Ohta, T. Imamura, T. Fijimura, K. Kawasaki, and K. Yamaoka. 1968. Molecular basis of morbidity from a series of studies of hemoglobinopathies in Western Japan. Jap. J. Hum. Genet. 13:40–53.

5

The Human Lactase Polymorphism: Physiology and Genetics of Lactose Absorption and Malabsorption

GEBHARD FLATZ

Institut für Genetik, Medizinische Hochschule Hannover, Hannover, Federal Republic of Germany

HANS WERNER ROTTHAUWE

Universitäts-Kinderklinik Bonn, Bonn, Federal Republic of Germany

205

INTRODUCTION

Lactose is the only nutritionally important carbohydrate in milk. Contrary to the α-glycosidic disaccharides maltose and sucrose, the two sugar moieties of lactose, glucose and galactose, are linked by a β-glycosidic bond. In order to be effectively absorbed in the small intestine, lactose must first be hydrolyzed by a specific enzyme, lactase, that is located in the brush border of small intestinal epithelial cells. The milk of almost all mammals contains lactose, and small intestinal lactase activity is high during the newborn and suckling period when milk is the prime nutriment. It is characteristic of most mammals that lactase activity declines at the physiologic time of weaning. Thereafter, lactase activity is maintained at low levels, usually less than 10 percent of the activity in the newborn. Man is an exception to this rule: although lactase activity is low in the majority of human adults, subjects with high lactase activity, comparable with that found in healthy infants, are frequent in certain populations, notably in Europeans and their descendants on other continents. Subjects with high lactase activity can tolerate large amounts of lactose without untoward symptoms. After a lactose load they show a considerable rise in blood glucose (and galactose) concentration. In contrast, the increase of glucose concentration is absent or small in persons with low lactase activity, and symptoms of lactose intolerance may develop. Enzyme activity determinations in mucosal homogenates and standardized lactose tolerance tests permit the differentiation of two nonoverlapping phenotypes, lactose absorbers and lactose malabsorbers. Lactase phenotype nomenclature will be discussed later in this review.

Considerable differences in distribution of the two lactase phenotypes first became evident during comparative studies of lactose tolerance and intestinal lactase activity in American blacks and whites (Cuatrecasas et al., 1965; Bayless and Rosensweig, 1966). The interpretation of these population differences remained controversial for many years. The question of whether lactose absorption and high intestinal lactase activity in the adult are due to a substrate-specific induction of enzyme activity by dietary lactose or due to a genetic control mechanism of lactase production seems to have been settled recently in favor of the genetic hypothesis. However, the nature of the genetic mechanism underlying the persistence of high intestinal lactase activity remains to be clarified. If the lactase phenotypes have a hereditary basis, their presence in human populations may be considered a genetic polymorphism which is most likely the result of natural selection over many generations.

The purposes of this review are (1) to describe the physiology of the two human lactose phenotypes in contrast to pathologic deficiency states of lactase; (2) to examine the evidence for substrate-induced adaptation of lactase; (3) to delineate the formal genetics and the distribution of the lactase phenotypes; and (4) to discuss the hypotheses that have been put forth to explain the vast differences of the frequency of the lactase phenotypes in human populations.

PHYSIOLOGY AND PATHOPHYSIOLOGY OF LACTOSE ASSIMILATION

Number and Properties of Human Intestinal β-Galactosidases

Independently and using different separation methods, two groups (Gray and Santiago, 1969; Asp and Dahlqvist, 1968, 1971a, and Asp et al., 1969, 1971) have demonstrated three different β-galactosidases in extracts of human small intestinal mucosa. These three enzymes are now usually named lactase (brush border lactase, "neutral" lactase, enzyme I), "acid" β-galactosidase (enzyme II) and hetero-β-galactosidase (enzyme III). Although the acid β-galactosidase hydrolyzes lactose in vitro, only the brush border lactase seems to be responsible for the hydrolysis of dietary lactose. Gray and Santiago (1969) separated the β-galactosidases of mucosal preparations by ultracentrifugation in a density gradient, whereas Dahlqvist and coworkers achieved the separation of the three enzymes by gel filtration. The results of the two methods are similar; they were confirmed with modified techniques by Rotthauwe et al. (1972b) and Lebenthal et al. (1974). The properties of the β-galactosidases of the human small intestinal mucosa are summarized in Table 1.

Table 1. Properties of the β-Galactosidases of Human Small Intestinal Mucosa*

Enzyme	Subcellular Localization	pH Optimum	Substrates Hydrolyzed†	Reaction with 0.2 mM PCMB†
Lactase	Brush border	5.5–6	Lactose, ONPG, PNPG	Not inhibited
Acid β-galactosidase	Lysosomes	4–4.5	Lactose, PG, ONPG, PNPG, NG, BNG	Inhibited
Hetero-β-galactosidase	Presumably cytoplasmic	5.5–6	PG, ONPG, PNPG, BNG	Inhibited

*From Asp and Dahlqvist (1972).
†ONPG, PNPG = ortho- and para-nitrophenyl β-galactoside; PG = phenyl β-galactoside; NG = 2-naphthyl β-galactoside; BNG = 6-bromo-2-naphthyl β-galactoside; PCMB = para-chloromercuribenzoate.

Only a small part of the lactase of mucosa homogenate is soluble; the major portion sediments with the particulate fraction. The enzyme can be solubilized with Papain (Gray and Santiago, 1969) and with the detergent Triton X-100 (Eggermont and Hers, 1969). The molecular weight was determined to be 280,000 ± 4000 (Gray and Santiago, 1969). Of all known substrates, lactose is hydrolyzed most rapidly. Lactase has also β-glucosidase activity; cellobiose is hydrolyzed in comparison with lactose in a ratio of 1:5.

Phlorizin hydrolase (=glycosylceramidase; Leese and Semenza, 1973) is closely associated with the brush border lactase (Malati and Crane, 1969). Lactase and phlorizin hydrolase conform to the same or similar biologic control mechanisms. In rats, phlorizin hydrolase shows the same age-dependent decrease of activity as lactase. In human adults with selectively low lactase activity the activity of phlorizin hydrolase is also markedly low or absent (Lorenz-Meyer et al., 1972).

Acid β-galactosidase is a lysosomal enzyme which is present in the small intestine of all mammals so far examined. The enzyme seems to occur in three forms with different molecular weights (Asp, 1971). The physicochemical properties are similar to the lysosomal acid β-galactosidases of other tissues (Alpers, 1969).

Hetero-β-galactosidase, the third enzyme with β-galactosidase activity in the small intestine of several species, including man (Gray and Santiago, 1969; Swaminathan and Radhakrishnan, 1969; Johnson, 1973), does not hydrolyze lactose, but numerous artificial hetero-β-galactosides are split with a pH optimum of about 6. Gray et al. (1969) proposed that hetero-β-galactosidase is a precursor of lactase, because the activity of both enzymes was lacking in some of the subjects with lactose malabsorption. Similarities in the pH-dependent activity of both enzymes and a low inhibitory effect of lactose on hetero-β-galactosidase seemed to favor this assumption. More recent examinations, however, do not lend support to this hypothesis (Johnson, 1973).

Determination of Activity of the β-Galactosidases of the Small Intestinal Mucosa

Several methods with and without prior separation of the enzymes were devised for the quantitative determination of the β-galactosidase activities in small intestinal biopsy material (Gray and Santiago, 1969; Asp and Dahlqvist, 1972). For the demonstration of a selectively low activity of the brush border lactase it is sufficient to measure the hydrolysis of lactose with inhibition of the acid β-galac-

Table 2. Activities of Three Small Intestinal Disaccharidases in Subjects from Four Different Populations (Mean and Range)

Population and Number of Subjects	Suedes, 37	Americans—LA,° 22	Americans—LM,° 12	Americans,† 23	Thai,‡ 74	Americans,†§ 30	Indians,†§ 38
Maltase	258 100–560	266 111–420	234 94–505	375 124–600	292 87–566	363 ±244	224 ±126
Sucrase	69 20–158	87 26–138	77 19–194	108 34–231	79 14–149	88 ±59	81 ±46
Lactase	29 6–56	44 9–98	2 0–6	37.5 2.5–129	2.1 0–58.3	36 ±36	3.4 ±5.8
Reference	Berg et al. (1970)	Dunphy et al. (1965)		Keusch et al. (1969b)		Swaminathan et al. (1970)	

°LA = Lactose absorbers; LM = lactose malabsorbers.
†Group contains a few lactose malabsorbers.
‡Group contains a few lactose absorbers.
§Standard deviations are given by the authors, although the enzyme activities do not seem to be normally distributed. McMichael et al. (1966) and Berg et al. (1970) reported a log-normal distribution of disaccharidase activities.

tosidase by PCMB. Applying this method, two nonoverlapping phenotypes with high and low lactase activity can be distinguished in healthy human adults. The activity ranges of lactase and two other disaccharidases in the intestinal mucosa of man are shown in Table 2.

Localization of the Intestinal β-Galactosidases

The vertical distribution of the intestinal β-galactosidases from the basis of the crypts to the tip of the villi was examined in human biopsy material by Nordström and Dahlqvist (1973). Lactase activity was found only in the villi, with a maximum in the intermediate and upper parts. At the tip of the villi lactase activity was somewhat lower. Similar patterns of distribution of the β-galactosidases were described in other species (Johnson, 1973). These findings support the hypothesis of Rey et al. (1971) that an accelerated cellular migration from the crypts to the villi lowers the activity of the brush border enzymes. According to Silverblatt et al. (1974) and Dubs et al. (1975), the sucrase-isomaltase complex is present in the crypt cells of human intestinal mucosa as an enzymatically inactive precursor that is activated during the differentiation of the cells and their migration to the villi. It is unknown whether or not a similar mechanism applies to lactase.

Disaccharidases are present along the entire length of the small intestine (Auricchio et al., 1963b; Newcomer and McGill, 1966). The activity of these enzymes is relatively low in the duodenum and exhibits a sudden increase in the proximal jejunum. In human adults, lactase activity reaches its maximum approximately 30 cm distal to the Treitz ligament, then remains constant over approximately 1 meter and decreases toward the ileum.

Differences between lactase activity in young and in adult mammals have been known since the investigations of Mendel and Mitchell (1907). A specific developmental pattern of lactase activity was proved by examinations in many mammalian species. The highest lactase activities are observed in the perinatal period. At the time of weaning there is a fairly rapid decrease of activity. When weaning is complete, lactase activity has fallen to the low levels typical of adult animals. Lactase activity at the time of birth is correlated to the developmental maturity of the newborn animals in different species. Exceptions to this rule are several species of Pacific pinnipedia whose milk lacks lactose (Sunshine and Kretchmer, 1964), and man with his high proportion of high adult lactase activity. In the human fetus lactase activity develops at the end of the first trimester of pregnancy. The activity of the enzyme then continually increases during intrauterine life and reaches its maximum at birth. In premature infants lactase activity may be low and symptoms of lactose intolerance may develop when milk feeding is begun (Boellner et al., 1965; Jarrett and Holman, 1966; Lifshitz et al., 1971).

Physiologic and Pathologic Variability of Intestinal Lactase Activity

In contrast to other attempts at classification (McCracken, 1971; Johnson et al., 1974), we propose to separate the two physiologic lactase phenotypes of adults from pathologic forms which are characterized either by a decreased lactase activity at a developmental stage in which it is normally high or by a pathologic lowering of lactase activity owing to gastrointestinal disease.

1. In analogy with other mammals, selectively low lactase activity is the usual human adult phenotype. Since the absorption of lactose in these individuals is low, it seems justified to denote this phenotype as "lactose malabsorption." If the intestinal enzyme activity is to be described, "hypolactasia" appears appropriate, whereas "lactase deficiency" should be avoided, because it implies a pathologic condition. Similarly, the expression "lactose intolerance" is misleading, because not all persons with lactose malabsorption develop symptoms of intolerance after a lactose load.

2. High intestinal lactase activity in the adult was considered "normal" until the examination of non-European populations proved that only a minority of humans, mainly Europeans and their descendants on other continents ("Europoids"), belong to this lactase phenotype. The regular decline of lactase activity in most mammals suggests that selective adult hypolactasia is the more ancient type in the evolution of man and that high adult lactase activity is the unusual phenotype (Simoons, 1970).

The nomenclature of the two physiologic lactase phenotypes reflects the changing concepts in this field of nutritional research. A selection of descriptive terms for the two "physiologic" lactase phenotypes, collected from the medical literature, is shown in Table 3.

The most frequent pathologic lactase type is secondary lactase deficiency resulting from damage to the small intestinal mucosa in various diseases. Acute and chronic gastroenteritis, protein-joule malnutrition, celiac disease, tropical sprue, cystic fibrosis of the pancreas, and extensive gastrointestinal operations are common causes

Table 3. Descriptive Terms for the Two Physiologic Lactase Phenotypes

Lactose tolerance	Lactose intolerance
Lactose absorption, absorber	Lactose malabsorption, malabsorber
Lactose digester	Lactose nondigester
Lactase sufficiency	(Acquired, adult, isolated, primary,
Adult lactase production	selective, specific) lactase deficiency
Lactase persistence	or hypolactasia
"Healthy," "normal"	

of secondary lactase deficiency. Usually, this type of deficiency is accompanied by distinct histologic changes in the intestinal mucosa and low activities of other brush border enzymes. The activity of lactase is often selectively reduced in the phase of restitution, after the primary disease has abated. The differentiation of this pathologic lactase deficiency from selective hypolactasia of healthy adults may be difficult if the personal history is not sufficiently considered and if the activity of the intestinal disaccharidases before the onset of the primary disease is not known. In the past, numerous cases of "secondary" lactase deficiency have been described, resulting from the erroneous assumption that high adult lactase activity is normal in man. If there were no symptoms of lactose intolerance during infancy, it was assumed that lactase activity must have been "normal" (i.e., high) before the onset of the disease. The present knowledge of the physiologic lactase phenotypes of adults suggests that many of these cases do not represent secondary lactase deficiency but rather a coincidence of gastrointestinal disease and primary selective hypolactasia that existed before the onset of the disease. The problems of interpreting apparently secondary lactase deficiency are illustrated by the report of Gray et al. (1968).

Hereditary congenital lactase deficiency is a rare condition that was first described by Holzel et al. in 1959. Only a few of the cases reported under this heading satisfy strict diagnostic criteria (Holzel, 1967). Infants with this type of lactase deficiency develop severe diarrhea and malnutrition after feeding with milk has begun. Symptoms are abolished by a lactose-free diet. Although definite proof is lacking, it is usually assumed that congenital lactase deficiency is due to homozygosity for an autosomal recessive gene.

The pathologic forms of low lactase activity are not subjects of this review.

Molecular Mechanism of Selectively Low Lactase Activity in Healthy Adults

The investigation of the "residual" activity of the brush border lactase in adults with selectively low lactase activity is of importance for the clarification of the molecular mechanisms responsible for the physiologic decrease of lactase activity. Gray et al. (1969) found no residual brush border lactase activity in lactose malabsorbers after the separation of the β-galactosidases by ultracentrifugation in a density gradient. In contrast, Rotthauwe et al. (1972b) and Lebenthal et al. (1974) demonstrated a distinct residual activity of lactase in the same phenotype. Similarly, determinations of lactase activity with differential inhibition (PCMB) in mucosal homogenates showed residual activity of brush border lactase in many persons with lactose malabsorption from different ethnic groups (Finns, Africans, Eskimos) (Asp et al., 1971; Cook et al., 1973; Asp and Dahlqvist, 1974). According to Asp (1971) and Lebenthal et al. (1974), the residual lactase has the same chromatographic characteristics, kinetic properties and pH dependent activity as the lactase from adults with high specific activity.

Recently, further progress on the molecular level was achieved; Crane et al. (cited by Freiburghaus et al., 1976) found a faint protein band with the mobility of brush border lactase on electrophoresis of isolated brush border proteins from lactose malabsorbers. Freiburghaus et al. (1976) actually measured disaccharidase activities in single gel fractions after electrophoretic separation of brush border proteins. These workers demonstrated a protein fraction with lactase activity and electrophoretic mobility identical with that of brush border lactase from adults with high enzyme activity in both congenital lactase deficiency and selective adult hypolactasia. These findings are compatible with a regulatory incomplete repression of lactase synthesis in lactose malabsorbers. Recently, however, Seetharam and Alpers (1976) reported marked differences in proteolytic degradation between lactase from subjects with high activity and that of persons with hypolactasia, a finding that favors a molecular difference of lactase in the two physiologic phenotypes. Since the concept of a "fetal lactase," as suggested by Elliot and Maxwell (1967) and Huang and Bayless (1967), is not supported by more recent evidence (Asp et al., 1969; Hore et al., 1972), it is difficult to explain the postweaning switch of lactase activity in lactose malabsorbers by an unstable structural "adult" enzyme variant. In addition, the normal vertical distribution of residual lactase activity (accumulation toward the tip of the villus) speaks against an increased catabolic rate as the cause of low enzyme activity. One may suspect that a solution to these problems will become possible only when purified enzyme preparations are available.

DIAGNOSIS OF THE LACTASE PHENOTYPES IN HEALTHY ADULTS

The best method for discriminating between the two lactase phenotypes is the determination of enzyme activity in intestinal biopsy material. As this method is not suitable for population studies, various tests causing less discomfort to the proband have been devised.

The personal history can give a hint to the presence of lactose malabsorption. If an otherwise healthy adult develops symptoms of lactose intolerance (watery, acid diarrhea; colicky abdominal pain; flatulence and borborygmi) after the intake of a large amount of milk, selective hypolactasia is probably present. Since not all persons with lactose malabsorption have symptoms after a lactose load, the history is an uncertain method for the diagnosis of lactose malabsorption. The same may be said of the examination of stools for pH and reducing substances after lactose administration.

The radiologic method for the diagnosis of the lactase phenotype, first described by Laws and Neale (1967), is based on the dilution of the jejunal contents by the osmotic effect of unabsorbed lactose. This test is mainly applied in clinical studies of lactose absorption. A detailed evaluation revealed a satisfactory correlation with the results of lactose tolerance tests (Morrison et al., 1974).

The standardized lactose tolerance test (LTT) is a relatively simple and reliable method for the diagnosis of the lactase phenotype. At a symposium on "Intestinal enzyme deficiencies and their nutritional implications," held in Sweden in 1972, recommendations for the LTT were proposed (Dahlqvist, 1974). The LTT should be performed in the morning after a fasting period of at least 6 hours. The dose of lactose is 50 gm for adults and 2 gm per kg of body weight (maximum, 50 gm) for children. The lactose should be taken as a 10 percent solution at room temperature. The following times for the collection of blood samples for glucose determination are recommended: (1) Fasting value: two samples with an interval of 5 or 10 minutes. (2) After lactose administration, at 15, 30, 45, 60, and, if possible, 90 minutes.

The glucose determinations must be performed on capillary blood (McGill and Newcomer, 1967). A glucose-specific method should be applied; the glucose oxidase method is recommended. In automated laboratories other enzymatic or nonenzymatic methods may have to be used. An increase of blood glucose concentration of 1.4 mmol per liter (25 mg per dl) or more over the fasting value is indicative of high lactase activity and lactose absorption. In lactose malabsorbers the rise of blood glucose is usually less than 1.1 mmol per liter (20 mg per dl); an increase between 1.1 and 1.4 mmol per liter (20 to 25 mg per dl) is considered ambiguous. In these cases a repeat LTT, if possible with intraduodenal administration of lactose, is recommended. If the increase of blood glucose concentration in the LTT is less than 1.1 mmol per liter ("flat LTT), the examination should be supplemented by a loading test with an equimolar mixture of glucose and galactose (GGTT) in order to exclude a disturbance in monosaccharide absorption.

In an abbreviated form of the LTT which is useful in field studies, the basic parameters (fasting period, lactose load, and administration) remain the same as in the standard method, but only three blood samples are taken, one before lactose and the others at t = 20 and 40 minutes.

Several modifications of the LTT were developed. In the lactose tolerance tests with ethanol (LTTE) (Fischer and Zapf, 1965; Kern and Heller, 1968; Jussila, 1969a) the conversion of galactose to glucose in the liver is inhibited by administration of ethanol (0.3 gram per kg of body weight) before the test. Two "bloodless" methods, the $^{14}CO_2$ breath test (Sasaki et al., 1970) and the H_2 breath test (Calloway et al., 1969), are based on the measurement of gaseous metabolites of lactose in expired air. Newcomer et al. (1975) and Bond and Levitt (1976) have compared variants of the LTT with the result that the LTTE and the H_2 breath test offer the best discrimination between the two physiologic lactase phenotypes. The characteristics of commonly used methods are summarized in Table 4.

CLINICAL SIGNIFICANCE OF LACTOSE MALABSORPTION

The severity of symptoms of lactose malabsorption depends on the amount of milk or lactose administered and on the speed of intake. More than half the persons with selective hypolactasia develop symptoms of intolerance after consuming 25 to 50 gm of lactose or the equivalent amount of milk (1 liter of cow's milk contains 45 to 50 gm of lactose), but symptoms of intolerance are usually absent when modest quantities of milk are ingested in small portions distributed over the whole day. However, marked individual differences of the

Table 4. Indirect Methods for the Diagnosis of the Lactase Phenotypes*

Test	Substances Administered	Laboratory Determination	Rationale of Test	Comment
Simple lactose tolerance test (LTT)	Lactose	Capillary plasma (or blood) glucose	Increase of plasma (blood) glucose dependent on hydrolysis of lactose	Capillary blood must be used to correct for peripheral tissue utilization; test is influenced by velocity of gastric emptying and by glucose metabolism
LTT with ethanol (LTTE)	Ethanol, lactose	Capillary plasma (blood) glucose and galactose	As above, and block of hepatic conversion of galactose to glucose by ethanol	Improved differentiation of the two lactase phenotypes; not applicable to children and in countries or groups with prohibition of alcohol consumption
$^{14}CO_2$ breath test	^{14}C-lactose and lactose	$^{14}CO_2$ specific activity in breath	$^{14}CO_2$ concentration in breath dependent on the rate of lactose hydrolysis	Unabsorbed lactose may be converted to $^{14}CO_2$ by colonic bacteria and appear in breath; differentiation of the lactase phenotypes not better than with simple LTT
Hydrogen (H_2) breath test	Lactose	Breath H_2 by gas chromatography	Unabsorbed lactose is converted to H_2 by colonic bacteria and appears in breath	Requires colonic bacteria capable of forming H_2 from unabsorbed lactose; best differentiation of the lactase phenotypes; ca. 2 percent false negatives in subjects with selective hypolactasia

*Adapted from Newcomer et al. (1975).

response of lactose malabsorbers to milk and lactose have been observed (Bayless and Huang, 1971; Gudmand-Höyer, 1971; Paige et al., 1971; Bedine and Bayless, 1973; Cook, 1973; Stephenson and Latham, 1974; Bayless et al., 1975; Mitchell et al., 1975; Garza and Scrimshaw, 1976). Bedine and Bayless (1973) observed symptoms of intolerance in some lactose malabsorbers after as little as 3 gm of lactose. The following factors are thought to be responsible for the variability of tolerance in subjects with low lactase activity: (1) velocity of gastric emptying, (2) speed of passage through the small intestine, (3) variability of intestinal secretion in response to an osmotic challenge, (4) individual differences of the intestinal kinetic response to an increased volume of fluid, and (5) irritability of the small and large intestines.

The symptoms of marked lactose intolerance and surprising psychologic sequelae are vividly described in a personal report by a Sudanese physician (Ahmed, 1975). However, severe clinical disturbances are not the rule. In self-chosen nutritional conditions, most persons with lactose malabsorption rarely have symptoms of lactose intolerance. They seem to subconsciously adjust milk consumption to their individual tolerance threshold, especially in countries with a high proportion of milk in the normal diet. The unconscious adaptation of nutritional habits to inherent abilities or disabilities to assimilate foodstuffs would appear to be an interesting field for behavioral research.

The clinical implications of low lactase activity are obviously relevant to the question of whether it is advisable to propagate the consumption of fresh milk and lactose-containing milk products in countries with a high proportion of lactose malabsorbers. A heated discussion concerning this question has been going on over the last years (McGillivray, 1968; Alford, 1969; Flatz and Saengudom, 1969; McCracken, 1970; Kretchmer and Ransome-Kuti, 1970; Dahlqvist and Lindquist, 1971; Paige and Graham, 1971; Paige et al., 1972a; Almy, 1975; Bradfield et al., 1975; Editorial, 1975; Mitchell et al., 1975; Stoopler et al., 1974). Official statements advocating a judicious continuation of "milk programs" in underprivileged societies with a high prevalence of lactose malabsorption have been issued (Protein Advisory Group, 1972; American Academy of Pediatrics, 1974) and deplored (Graham, 1975). An appraisal of the arguments forwarded suggests that aid programs for children with lactose malabsorption should make "a distinction between a possible diet in survival conditions and an optimum diet in affluent conditions" (Alford, 1969). Milk administration may aggravate the condition of a child with severe secondary lactase deficiency caused by protein malnutrition and/or gastroenteritis, but it may improve the nutritional status of a healthy child with lactose malabsorption despite causing some discomfort. Observations in Thai dairy workers support the contention that consumption of moderate amounts of milk by lactose malabsorbers over many years is innocuous (Flatz and Rotthauwe, 1971). The experimental evidence is not sufficient, however, to permit a conclusive answer to this problem. Despite an apparently adequate utilization of protein and energy from milk by lactose malabsorbers (Calloway and Chenoweth, 1973), the possibility must be considered that the upper intestinal fluid loss induced even by small amounts of lactose has detrimental effects, e.g., by inhibiting the absorption of water-soluble essentials (Bedine and Bayless, 1973). The hydrolytic reduction of the lactose content of milk is still technically cumbersome and hardly economical for application in large-scale food programs (Dahlqvist and Lindquist, 1971; Paige et al., 1975b; Bradfield et al., 1975).

Some earlier publications advocating global milk consumption betray a sense of nutritional mission based on the unfounded conviction that what is good for "whites" is good for everybody. One should also be aware of the economic interests at stake, and it seems appropriate to quote a cautioning note by Bradfield et al. (1975): "Some of the more widely cited work minimizing the problem [disadvantages of milk consumption in lactose malabsorbers] has been sponsored by grants from the dairy industry, and the possibility of unconscious bias should not be ruled out." Powdered milk is useful in aid programs because of its high protein content, relatively low cost, and long shelf life. However, since lactose may act as a strong laxative in lactose malabsorbers, the administration of reconstituted powdered milk with its high lactose content has not only nutritional advantages but also pharmacologic implications. Therefore judicious control of the application of milk products in populations with a high prevalence of hypolactasia is required, and the benefit of the recipients should be the prime consideration.

EFFECTS OF LACTOSE ON INTESTINAL LACTASE ACTIVITY

The Adaptive Hypothesis of the Lactase Phenotypes

Research on the physiology and pathophysiology of lactose assimilation has mostly been carried out in countries with predominantly Europoid populations. Therefore it is understandable that the lactase phenotype prevalent in Europeans was designed as normal, and all deviations from this type were considered abnormal or pathologic. Damage to the intestinal mucosa by malnutrition and parasites (secondary lactase deficiency) or the low or absent milk consumption after weaning in most people of non-European extraction (lack of adaptation = substrate specific induction of lactase production) was often cited as the cause of the high incidence of lactose malabsorption outside Europe, North America, and Australia. Secondary lactase deficiency was excluded as the cause of lactose malabsorption in the majority of the affected people by a normal nutritional status, normal absorption of monosaccharides and other disaccharides, and a normal morphology of the intestinal mucosa.

The "adaptive hypothesis," mainly advocated by an Australian group of workers (Bolin and Davis, 1969, 1970a, b; Bolin et al., 1968, 1969, 1970a, b, 1971), received wide recognition. Animal experiments designed to test the adaptive hypothesis and relevant observations in man will be summarized under the following two headings.

Lactase Activity After Lactose Administration in Animals

The animal experiments concerning the influence of lactose on lactase activity were usually performed on rats, but also on rabbits, pigs, and calves. The results are conflicting. No influence of lactose feeding on intestinal lactase activity of adult animals could be found by Plimmer (1906), Heilskov (1951), Fischer (1957), DeGroot and Hoogendoorn (1957), Doell and Kretchmer (1962), Siddons (1968), Powell et al. (1969), Leichter (1973), or Ekström et al. (1975). On the other hand, a significant rise of lactase activity in response to a lactose-rich diet was observed by Girardet et al. (1964), Huber et al. (1964), Reddy et al. (1968), Broitman et al. (1968), Bolin et al. (1969, 1971), Cain et al. (1969), Jones et al. (1972), Ekström et al. (1976), and Lifrak et al. (1976). Some of these studies must be criticized, because the methods used do not differentiate between neutral lactase and acid β-galactosidase. Others leave the impression of an inappropriate use of the word "significant." An increase of lactase activity after lactose feeding of 100 percent may be statistically significant; but nutritionally it may be meaningless if the lactase activity in newborns of the same species is 20- or 30-fold higher than the level in adult animals. In addition, it is noteworthy that an increase of lactase activity was also achieved by feeding other sugars and that in most examinations the concentration of lactose in the diet was unphysiologically high.

Experiments with a lactose diet given beyond the normal time of weaning are perhaps more important than examinations on adult animals. Sriratanaban et al. (1971) observed no effect of lactose-enriched feed on the activity of lactase, sucrase, and maltase in rats. In contrast, Lebenthal et al. (1973) found that rats who were suckled up to the thirtieth day of life (i.e., 2 weeks beyond the normal time of weaning), although showing the expected decrease of lactase activity, had a specific lactase activity "significantly" higher than in control animals. Special interest was aroused by the examinations of Wen et al. (1973) who studied the influence of lactose administration on the lactase activity of monkeys. Lactose absorption and relatively high lactase activities were present in some species, irrespective of the amount of lactose in the diet. Since monkeys are not known to have access to animal milk as adults, these findings, if confirmed, would have obvious implications for the evolution of high adult lactase activity in man.

Lactose Administration and Lactase Activity in Man

In several independent studies, no influence of lactose administration in form of milk or pure lactose on the intestinal lactase activity could be demonstrated. Daily consumption of 250 to 750 ml of milk or corresponding amounts of lactose during periods between 3 months and 20 years by persons with lactose malabsorption did not change the result of the LTT or increase the lactase activity (Cuatrecasas et al., 1965; Keusch et al., 1969b; Flatz and Rotthauwe, 1971; Gilat, 1971; Rosensweig, 1971; Gilat et al., 1972; Chua and Seah, 1973). In populations with a high incidence of selective hypolactasia, lactose malabsorption developed at the usual age in children who had continuously consumed animal milk after infancy (Cook, 1967; Huang and Bayless, 1967; Keusch et al., 1969a; Flatz and Rotthauwe, 1971; Gilat et al., 1972; Kretchmer et al., 1971; Sahi et al., 1972). Cuatrecasas et al. (1965), Knudsen et al. (1968), and Rosensweig and Herman (1969a) examined the effect of a lactose-free diet on lactase activity in adults with high lactase activity. Whereas Cuatrecasas et al. found a decrease, though not to the low levels of lactose malabsorbers, the other two studies did not reveal a significant effect on lactase activity.

The concept that "lactase deficiency" is caused by a lack of lactose in the diet is based on the idea of substrate-specific enzyme induction. However, experiments on mammalian tissues have shown that enzyme production is rarely regulated by substrates. The activity of intestinal enzymes can be influenced by various sugars but also by drugs, hormones, vitamins, and other compounds. (Rosensweig and Herman, 1968, 1969a, b, 1970; Stifel et al., 1968, 1969; Rosensweig et al., 1969, 1971; Zakim et al., 1969; Lufkin et al., 1972; Rosensweig, 1974). Yeh and Moog (1974) found the decrease of lactase activity in animals to be dependent on thyroid hormones. In summary, there is evidence for a general promotion of disaccharidase activity by carbohydrates, but the differences between the two physiologic lactase phenotypes cannot be abolished by lactose feeding. In view of the established genetic determination of the lactase phenotypes (see below), it is probable that lactase activity—like that of other enzymes—can be influenced by environmental factors in only a relatively narrow, genetically determined range.

FORMAL GENETICS OF THE LACTASE PHENOTYPES

Although a hereditary origin of adult "lactase deficiency" was often suspected, reports supporting the genetic hypothesis were scarce until 1973. The segregation of the lactase phenotypes had been studied in a few isolated families, and several observations concerning the incidence of the lactase phenotypes in racially mixed populations were interpreted in the sense of the genetic hypothesis. A summary of these reports will be given, followed by an appraisal of the work of Sahi and coworkers, who clarified the genetics of the lactase phenotypes in man.

Family Studies

The first family studies were reported by Fischer and Zapf (1965), Klaus and Siebner (1966), and Ferguson and Maxwell (1967). The last of these was particularly revealing because a complete family was examined by LTT and intestinal biopsy. Besides a child with severe gastrointestinal disease, the parents and three of their children were lactose absorbers, and two other children were lactose malabsorbers with selectively low lactase activity. Ferguson and Maxwell concluded that lactose malabsorption in this family was caused by an autosomal recessive gene. They proposed a genetic notation with 3 alleles at an autosomal locus: a dominant allele L, determining high lactase activity in adults, an allele l_1, responsible for selective hypolactasia, and an allele l_2, causing congenital lactase deficiency in the homozygous state. Further family studies were reported from the USA (Welsh et al., 1968; Welsh, 1970), England

(Neale, 1968), Ireland (Fine et al., 1968), Greenland (Gudmand-
Höyer et al., 1973), Thailand (Flatz and Saengudom, 1969), Nigeria
(Ransome-Kuti et al., 1972), Germany (Rotthauwe et al., 1972a), and
Israel (Gilat et al., 1973). Based on the distribution of the phenotypes
in these families, all authors concluded that genetic factors determine the lactase phenotypes. In some families the segregation was
compatible with autosomal recessive inheritance of lactose malabsorption. In others, the distribution did not fit a simple Mendelian
transmission. The main difficulties were posed by families in which
both parents were lactose malabsorbers but one child or more were
lactose absorbers. In the light of recent knowledge concerning the
sources of error in the LTT and the age dependence of lactose
malabsorption, one may suspect that the inclusion of young children
and false negative results of the LTT in lactose malabsorbers caused
the deviations from the expectation for autosomal recessive inheritance in these families. Sahi (1974b) remarked that until 1973 only
five families were examined with methods adequate for a reliable
diagnosis of the lactase phenotype.

Studies in Racially Mixed Populations

If the lactase phenotypes are genetically determined, the distribution among the offspring of parents belonging to populations
with markedly differing prevalence of lactose absorption and malabsorption may serve to test the genetic hypothesis. First suggestions
for an intermediary distribution of phenotypes in the offspring of
racially mixed groups of probands were provided by the studies of
McMichael et al. (1966), Cook and Kajubi (1966), and Gudmand-
Höyer and Jarnum (1969). In 1969, Bayless et al. compared the
results of LTT in the American black population (70 percent lactose
malabsorbers) with the population of coastal West Africa (nearly 100
percent lactose malabsorbers) and the white population of the USA
(8 percent lactose malabsorbers). Assuming a white admixture of 30
percent and autosomal recessive inheritance of lactose malabsorption, the observed incidence in the black American population fitted
well with the expectation. In Thailand, Flatz and Rotthauwe (1971)
examined persons with one European and one East Asiatic
parent—six lactose absorbers and three malabsorbers. The observations corresponded well with the expected frequencies calculated
from 10 percent lactose malabsorbers in northern Europe and 100
percent in the Southeast Asian population and autosomal recessive
inheritance of lactose malabsorption. Ransome-Kuti et al. (1972)

reported examinations on racially mixed families in Nigeria. All African parents, 22 percent of the European parents, and 44 percent of the children, were lactose malabsorbers. The results within the families were compatible with autosomal recessive inheritance of lactose malabsorption. Further evidence for the validity of the genetic hypothesis can be derived from the reports by Gudman-Höyer et al. (1973) and by Newcomer et al. (1977).

Formal Genetic Analysis of the Lactase Phenotypes

It is the merit of a group of Finnish workers (Sahi et al., 1973; Sahi, 1974b) to have first applied the classic methods of formal genetic analysis to a sufficiently large body of observations concerning the segregation of the lactase types in families. From a large Finnish population sample, 11 probands with lactose malabsorption (proved by LTT and intestinal biopsy) were selected according to family size and the number of generations available for study. A total of 371 family members were ascertained; more than 90 percent participated in the tests. Nearly all probands were examined by the LTT with ethanol (LTTE) and by the GGTT with ethanol. Persons under 20 years were excluded because the full expression of lactose malabsorption does not develop before the age of 15 to 20 years in the Finnish population. The sum of the maximal increase of blood glucose and blood galactose yielded a nonoverlapping bimodal distribution suggesting a single gene effect. The analysis of the family pedigrees excluded X-chromosomal and simple dominant inheritance of lactose malabsorption. For the test of autosomal recessive inheritance, families with at least one child with lactose malabsorption were selected and grouped according to three types: (1) both parents lactose absorbers; (2) one parent a lactose absorber, the other a malabsorber; and (3) both parents lactose malabsorbers.

In two families of type 3 all six children were lactose malabsorbers, as expected in the case of autosomal recessive inheritance. In the two other family types, the theoretical expectation for children with lactose malabsorption, assuming autosomal recessive inheritance, is 0.25 for type 1 and 0.5 for type 2. Both hypotheses were tested in nine families of each type for complete and single selection. The results, summarized in Table 5 (adapted from Sahi, 1974b), are in full agreement with autosomal recessive inheritance of lactose malabsorption. In addition, the expectation for lactose absorption and malabsorption for more distant relatives of lactose malabsorbers was calculated considering the gene frequency of the "lactose malab-

Table 5. Analysis of the Proportion of Lactose Malabsorption in Sibships in Which at Least One Child Had Lactose Malabsorption*

Mating Type 1 (LA × LA):†

	Observed Values			A Priori Correction for Truncate Complete Ascertainment			Correction for Truncate Single Ascertainment	
Size of Sibship s	Number of Sibships n_s	Total Number of Children $t_s = sn_s$	Number of Children with LM r_s	Theoretical Total Number of Children $c_s = \dfrac{t_s}{1-(3/4)^s}$	Corrected Proportion of Children with LM $B = \dfrac{R}{C}$	Standard Error	Corrected Proportion of Children with LM $B = \dfrac{R-N}{T-N}$	Standard Error
2	1	2	1	4.6				
3	3	9	5	15.6				
4	3	12	5	17.6				
5	1	5	1	6.6				
6	1	6	3	7.3				
Total	N = 9	T = 34	R = 15	C = 51.7	0.290	0.052	0.240	0.085

Mating Type 2 (LA × LM):†

s	n_s	t_s	r_s	$c_s = \dfrac{t_s}{1-(1/2)^s}$	$B = \dfrac{R}{C}$		$B = \dfrac{R-N}{T-N}$	
2	3	8	5	10.7				
3	2	6	4	6.9				
4	0	0	0	–				
5	2	10	5	10.3				
6	1	6	5	6.1				
Total	N = 9	T = 30	R = 19	C = 34.0	0.559	0.053	0.476	0.109

*Adapted from Sahi (1974b) with the author's permission. Calculations according to Neel and Schull (1954).

†LA = Lactose absorber; LM = lactose malabsorber.

sorption gene" in the Finnish population. The comparison with the observations is also fully compatible with autosomal recessive inheritance of lactose malabsorption (see Sahi, 1974b, Table 13).

The results of Sahi and coworkers leave no doubt that the human adult lactase phenotypes are due to different alleles at an autosomal locus and that the effect of the gene responsible for the switch-off of lactase production in childhood is recessive to that of the alleles causing high adult lactase activity. A comparison of the study of Sahi and coworkers with earlier controversial results of family studies shows that diagnostic reliability is the crux of such examinations. The ideal method in family studies would be the determination of lactase activity in intestinal biopsies. Since this method is obviously not applicable in large numbers of healthy probands, the utilization of the technical improvements of the LTT is mandatory in family studies. Although diagnostic difficulties are mentioned in the report by Lisker et al. (1975) from Mexico, this family study confirms the formal genetic analysis of the lactase phenotypes. Further confirming evidence was reported by Ransome-Kuti et al. (1975) from Nigeria. These examinations show that autosomal recessive inheritance of lactose malabsorption is not an isolated property of the Northern European population.

Hereditary Persistence of High Intestinal Lactase Activity

As mentioned before, a marked and lasting decrease of intestinal lactase activity after the physiologic period of weaning is characteristic of mammals. Although man is an exception to this rule, human adult lactose malabsorbers are far more frequent than lactose absorbers. These observations support the contention of Simoons (1970) that lactose malabsorption is the normal state in human adults ("wild type," in genetic terminology) and adult lactose absorption is the unusual type whose frequency in some populations requires explanation. In children who develop selective hypolactasia, lactase activity seems to decrease gradually; a structural difference between lactase in lactose absorbers and lactose malabsorbers is not very likely. Therefore the genetic mechanism underlying selective adult hypolactasia is perhaps not dissimilar to the switch-off of the production of hemoglobin γ-chains during the first year of life. In analogy with a genetically determined failure of this switch mechanism (hereditary persistence of fetal hemoglobin), we propose the term "hereditary persistence of high intestinal lactase activity," or, for short, "persistence of lactase activity" (PLA) for the phenotype "lactose absorption" and "PLA gene" for the responsible allele.

Differentiation of Homozygous and Heterozygous Lactose Absorbers

The genetic hypothesis implies that the phenotype "lactose absorption" comprises two genotypes, homozygotes and heterozygotes for the PLA gene. In analogy with other enzyme variants, one would expect that the metabolic performance and the enzyme activity of heterozygotes are intermediary between those of the two homozygotes. The expected trimodality of lactase activities was reported by Rosensweig et al. (1967), but this has not been confirmed in other studies. Sahi (1974b) found marked overlapping of the lactase activities and the results of LTTs between a group of certain heterozygotes and a group of lactose absorbers of undefined genotype. The lack of differentiation between homozygous and heterozygous lactose absorbers can be explained by factors which are independent of the physiologically active gene product, lactase, e.g., velocity of gastric emptying or mixed cell populations in intestinal biopsy material.

Multiple Allelism of Lactose Malabsorption?

The low lactase activities characteristic for the human wild type are apparently not attained at the same age in different populations. In Thailand, Keusch et al. (1969a) and Flatz et al. (1969) found that all children above the age of 4 years had flat LTTs. Similarly, in Bantu children in East Africa, lactose malabsorption seems to be fully developed before the age of 4 years (Cook, 1967). In contrast, the proportion of lactose malabsorbers increases up to 14 years in black American children (Huang and Bayless, 1967). In Finland, the full expression of hypolactasia is delayed to the period between the fifteenth and twentieth years of life in some lactose malabsorbers (Sahi et al., 1972). Paige et al. (1975a) reported a higher rise of blood glucose in the LTT of black American children with lactose malabsorption and substantial milk consumption in comparison with a control group with lactose malabsorption and low milk consumption. At present, it cannot be decided whether this phenotypic variability is due to multiple alleles with differing regulation characteristics or to environmental factors, e.g., differences in the amount and type of milk consumed during childhood.

THE DISTRIBUTION OF THE LACTASE PHENOTYPES

In Table 6 examinations relevant for the distribution of the lactase phenotypes are listed with pertinent references. Before a summarized description of the distribution of the lactase phenotypes is given, it must be emphasized that the available distribution data are very heterogeneous. The criteria for the selection of the probands differ widely, and the methods for the determination of the lactase phenotype are of varying quality. Owing to the inconveniences of the LTT for both the examiner and the proband, the number of subjects is often so small that large chance deviations from the true incidence are to be expected. Nevertheless, the published population studies show certain characteristic trends of distribution. Persistence of lactase activity (PLA) is very rare or absent in most Mongoloid populations, including American Indians and Eskimos. A similarly low incidence of PLA is observed in the populations of tropical Africa and also in the Khoisan peoples of Southern Africa. The same applies to Australian aborigines and to the people of Melanesia. In Arabian populations on the east and south shores of the Mediterranean Sea the frequency of PLA is very low. In Israel, PLA is rare both in Israelis and Arabs. The Bedouin population of Saudi Arabia makes an exception by showing a high proportion of PLA in a recently studied sample.

A consistently high incidence of PLA (over 75 percent) is found only in northern and central Europe and in descendants of Europeans in other continents, e.g., in the white population of the USA and Canada, in white Australians, and in New Zealand. In addition, high frequencies of PLA were found in few groups of nomadic pastoralists in Africa (Hima, Tussi, Fulani). Between the African and southwest Asian populations with a low frequency of PLA on the one side and the population of Northern Europe with a high frequency of PLA on the other lies a belt of intermediary distribution of the lactase phenotypes; in Spain, Italy, and Greece incidences of PLA between 30 and 70 percent were observed. A highly variable distribution of the lactase phenotypes was reported from southern Asia. A recent study in Afghanistan casts doubt on the previously reported high incidence of PLA in northwest India and Pakistan. Since the Indo-European groups of Afghanistan contain less than 20 percent of lactose absorbers, the contention that the PLA gene has been introduced to India by Aryan migration (Simoons, 1973) must be re-examined. The revealing intermediary distribution of the lactase phenotypes in the black American population was mentioned before. Differences within the white population of the USA may reflect the variable incidence of the lactase phenotypes in the original European populations. In Latin America the incidence of PLA seems to be correlated to the degree of European admixture to the original Indian population. "Pure" American Indians exhibit only a very low incidence of PLA.

MILK NUTRITION AND NATURAL SELECTION

The regularity of selective adult hypolactasia in other mammals and its predominance in human adults suggest that the gene responsible for persistence of lactase activity (PLA) emerged by mutation in the evolution of man and that natural selection in its favor has caused the present high frequencies in some populations. Chance deviations in isolates or founder groups can hardly explain the distinctively high PLA gene frequencies in Europe. The formal genetics of the lactase phenotypes implies that a selective advantage of lactose absorbers favors both homozygotes and heterozygotes for the PLA gene. In a two-allele system, advantage of one homozygote and the heterozygote results in a transient polymorphism with a final replacement of the allele present in the other homozygote who is at a selective disadvantage. For the human lactase polymorphism a tendency for elimination of the "adult hypolactasia gene" can be predicted for populations in which a selective advantage of the lactose absorbers exists. What is the nature of the hypothetical selective advantage of the lactose-absorbing genotypes? Almost all authors who have supported the genetic hypothesis postulated a direct relation between the selective advantage of the lactose absorbers and the physiologic activity of lactase. Johnson et al. (1974) mentioned the possibility that the distribution of the lactase phenotypes could be due to selective factors that are not associated with the function of brush border lactase. Such selection mechanisms are not known at present, although it may be appropriate to quote the interesting hypothesis of Semenza et al. (1975), who suggest a mutative origin of the lactase molecule from the evolutionary more ancient enzyme phlorizin hydrolase. Since there is no evidence for a selective advantage connected with phlorizin hydrolase, high frequencies of PLA cannot be explained as concomitant increase. The high incidence of PLA in populations with high fresh milk consumption throughout life is persuasive evidence for a correlation between selection and lactose nutrition.

The Culture Historical Hypothesis

A general nutritional advantage mediated by the ability to tolerate large amounts of fresh milk without gastrointestinal disturbances
is the basis of the culture historical hypothesis, first put forward by
Simoons (1970) and elaborated by Johnson et al. (1974). Other authors expressed similar views on the anthropologic implications of
lactose assimilation (Shatin, 1968; McCracken, 1971; Cook, 1973).
The culture historical hypothesis is based on the principle that
paleolithic man corresponded to the wild type of other mammals
with respect to intestinal brush border lactase; i.e., selective adult
hypolactasia was predominant. The domestication of milking animals
in the Neolithic era must not have necessarily resulted in a selective
advantage for the lactose absorber. Persons with lactose malabsorption can avoid the untoward side effects of milk by limiting the
amount consumed at one time or by preparing fermented milk products with a low lactose content. The culture historical hypothesis
explains the increase of the frequency of the PLA gene with a selective advantage of lactose absorbers "among peoples, whether farmers
or pastoralists, who had a plentiful milk supply, who did not process
their milk into products that were low in lactose, and for whom milk
provided essential nutrients that could not readily be obtained in the
other foods available" (Johnson et al., 1974).

Not all milking societies, in particular nomads, may have developed refined methods for the fermentation of milk, and because of
difficulties with storage these people may have taken to consuming
large amounts of fresh milk. In the absence of artificial refrigeration
in a settled community, no special skill is required for the preparation of sour milk, which has a low lactose content. Like present-day
milk drinkers in India, the ancient lactose malabsorber may be expected to have easily recognized the wholesomeness of sour milk in
contrast to the unfermented product. It seems unlikely therefore that
large segments of mankind have ever been dependent on the intake
of large amounts of fresh milk.

Therefore, the culture historical hypothesis may be well suited to
explain high frequencies of the PLA gene in small populations under
extreme environmental conditions; but its general validity may be
questioned. Contrary to the expectation, there is no parallelism between the milking habit and the prevalence of lactose absorption.
Large populations in Africa and Asia are milk consumers but have a
very low incidence of lactose absorption, comparable with that in the
nonmilking area. The argument that the PLA gene was not introduced into all populations of the milking area is invalidated by the

Table 6. Geographical Distribution of the Lactase Phenotypes and PLA Gene Frequencies

Country, Region, or Population	Group or Location	Number Examined	Number of Lactose Absorbers	Number of Lactose Malabsorbers	PLA Gene Frequency	References
Australia	White Australians	122	116	5	0.797	Bolin et al., 1968
						Bryant et al., 1970
						Davis and Bolin, 1967
	Aborigines	100	41	59	0.232	Bolin et al., 1970b
Fiji Islands	Fijians	12	0	12	0	Masarei et al., 1972
New Guinea		8	0	8	0	Bolin et al., 1968
Indonesia	Physicians, students	53	5	48	0.048	Surjono et al., 1973
East Asia	Chinese, Koreans, and Filipinos in USA	31	2	29	0.033	Chung and McGill, 1968 Huang and Bayless, 1968
Chinese	Australian-born	44	18	26	0.231	Bolin and Davis, 1970a
						Bryant et al., 1970
						Davis, 1969
	China-born in Australia	61	7	54	0.059	
	Hong Kong, Singapore	45	1	44	0.011	Bolin and Davis, 1969 Davis and Bolin, 1967
Singapore	Chinese, Malays, Indians	103	7	96	0.035	Bolin and Davis, 1970a Davis and Bolin, 1967
Japan	Japanese patients	25	1	24	0.020	Sasaki et al., 1970
Thailand	Northern Thai	149	0	149	0	Flatz et al., 1969 and unpublished
						Rotthauwe et al., 1971b
	Central Thailand	279	8	271	0.014	Flatz and Saengudom, 1969
						Keusch et al., 1969b
						Troncale et al., 1967
India	Indians in Delhi	70	50	20	0.465	Desai et al., 1967, 1970 Gupta et al., 1970
	Indians in other parts of India and overseas	197	94	103	0.277	Murthy and Haworth, 1970 Neale, 1968 Reddy and Pershad, 1972
Pakistan	Various ethnic groups	55	52	3	0.766	Rab and Baseer, 1976
Afghanistan	Tajik	79	14	65	0.093	Rahimi et al., 1976
	Pashtun	71	15	56	0.112	
	Pasha-i	60	8	52	0.069	
	Uzbek	16	0	16	0	
	Others	44	10	34	0.121	
Saudi Arabia	Bedouin and Saudi	22	16	6	0.478	Cook and Al-Torki, 1975
	Other Arabs	18	8	10	0.255	
Lebanon	Arabs	151	32	119	0.112	Loiselet and Jarjouhi, 1974
Syria, Egypt	Arabs	81	8	73	0.051	Bolin et al., 1970b El-Schallah et al., 1973 Rotthauwe et al., 1971a
Israel	Arabs	67	13	54	0.102	Gilat et al., 1971
Israel	Sephardim	68	20	48	0.160	Gilat et al., 1970
	Ashkenazim	53	8	45	0.079	
	Orientals and others	94	28	66	0.162	
	Mixed group	93	36	57	0.217	Rozen and Shafrir, 1968
Cyprus	Greeks	17	2	15	0.061	McMichael et al., 1966

Table continued on following page

Table 6. Geographical Distribution of the Lactase Phenotypes and PLA Gene Frequencies (*Continued*)

Country, Region, or Population	Group or Location	Number Examined	Number of Lactose Absorbers	Number of Lactose Malabsorbers	PLA Gene Frequency	References
Uganda	Bantu	64	8	56	0.065	Cook and Dahlqvist, 1968
	Hamitic groups	39	36	3	0.723	Cook and Kajubi, 1966
	Mixed group	28	18	10	0.402	
Ruanda	Bantu	50	6	44	0.062	Cox and Elliott, 1974
	Hamitic group	27	25	2	0.728	
	Mixed group	47	21	26	0.256	
Central Africa	Bantu	51	3	48	0.030	Elliott et al., 1973
	Hamitic group	14	13	1	0.733	
	Others (Cameroons, Sudan, Nigeria)	15	0	15	0	
Southern Africa	Bantu, mixed group	60	6	54	0.051	Jersky and Kinsley, 1967
	Bantu, Zambia	26	1	25	0.019	Cook et al., 1973
	!Kung Bushmen	40	1	39	0.013	Jenkins et al., 1974
Nigeria	Yoruba, Ibo, and related groups	109	11	98	0.052	Kretchmer et al., 1971 Olatunbosun and Adadevoh, 1971
	Haussa/Fulani	32	10	22	0.171	
	Fulani (town)	24	7	17	0.158	
	Fulani (nomads)	9	7	2	0.529	
Spain	Spaniards	267	209	58	0.534	Garcia et al., 1974 Vaquez et al., 1976
	Gypsies	40	18	22	0.258	Vazquez et al., 1976
Italy	Naples area	9	0	9	0	DeRitis et al., 1970
	Liguria	40	28	12	0.452	Marenco et al., 1970
Greece	Greeks	16	10	6	0.388	Spanidou and Petrakis, 1972
		250	192	58	0.518	Zografos et al., 1973
		700	371	329	0.314	Kanaghinis et al., 1974
Czechoslovakia	Czechs	104	76	28	0.481	Madžarovová-Nohejlová, 1972
Switzerland		64	54	10	0.605	Auricchio et al., 1963a Haemmerli et al., 1965 Kistler, 1966
Germany		67	59	8	0.654	Flatz et al., 1969 Rotthauwe et al., 1972a
Netherlands	Dutch soldiers in Surinam	14	14	0	–	Luyken et al., 1971
Denmark	Mostly patients	155	139	16	0.679	Balslev et al., 1971 Busk et al., 1975
Sweden	Patients	700	679	21	0.827	Gudmand-Höyer et al., 1969
Finland	Finns	953	784	169	0.579	Jussila, 1969b Jussila et al., 1970
	Swedish-speaking	91	84	9	0.723	Sahi, 1974a
England	Mixed group	44	30	14	0.440	McMichael et al., 1966
Greenland	Eskimo	32	9	23	0.152	Gudmand-Höyer, 1971
	"Greenlanders" (partially with Danish ancestry)	123	58	68	0.256	Gudmand-Höyer et al., 1973
Canada	Northern European extraction	16	15	1	0.750	Leichter, 1972
	Slavic extraction	38	29	9	0.513	Leichter and Lee, 1971
	Jewish extraction	32	10	22	0.171	Leichter, 1971
	Canadian Indians	30	11	19	0.204	Leichter and Lee, 1971

Table 6. Geographical Distribution of the ʟᴀctase Phenotypes and PLA Gene Frequencies (*Continued*)

Country, Region, or Population	Group or Location	Number Examined	Number of Lactose Absorbers	Number of Lactose Malabsorbers	PLA Gene Frequency	References
United States of America	Alaska (Eskimos and Indians)	36	6	30	0.087	Duncan and Scott, 1972
	Whites of Northern European extraction	188	174	14	0.727	Bayless and Rosensweig, 1966 Bayless et al., 1975 Bedine and Bayless, 1973
	Whites	771	592	179	0.518	Birge et al., 1967
	Blacks	349	76	273	0.116	Cady et al., 1967 Cuatrecasas et al., 1965 Duncan and Scott, 1972 Gray and Santiago, 1966 Huang and Bayless, 1968 Knudsen et al., 1968 Littman et al., 1968 McGill and Newcomer, 1967 Newcomer and McGill, 1967 Paige et al., 1975a Sasaki et al., 1970 Sheehy and Anderson, 1965 Spanidou and Petrakis, 1972 Welsh, 1970 Welsh et al., 1967
	American Indians	36	7	29	0.102	Bose and Welsh, 1973
		75	26	49	0.192	Newcomer et al., 1977
	Mexican Americans	28	14	14	0.293	Dill et al., 1972 Sowers and Winterfeldt, 1975
	Mixed groups	92	66	26	0.468	Dunphy et al., 1965 Keusch et al., 1969b
Mexico	Rural areas	401	105	296	0.141	Lisker et al., 1974
Curaçao	"Negroes"	35	0	35	0	Erkelens et al., 1972
Colombia	Mixed group	54	33	21	0.376	Alzate et al., 1968
	Chami Indians	24	10	14	0.236	Alzate et al., 1969
Surinam	Mixed group	60	0	60	0	Luyken et al., 1971
Peru	Rural group	50	10	40	0.106	Figueroa et al., 1971

Table 6 contains data from 8907 subjects over 15 years old. Children were excluded because of late onset of lactose malabsorption in some populations and because of the unreliability of simple LTTs in children (Krasilnikoff et al., 1975; Stoopler et al., 1974). Different studies in the same population were pooled when PLA gene frequencies differed by less than 15 percent. Studies on patients with severe gastrointestinal disease were excluded.

presence of small percentages of lactose absorbers in most populations, even in the nonmilking area (cf. Table 6). Figure 1 delineates the milking and nonmilking areas in the Old World according to the data of Simoons (1970). In Figure 2 the populations with a PLA gene frequency above 0.5 (i.e., more than 75 percent lactose absorbers) are

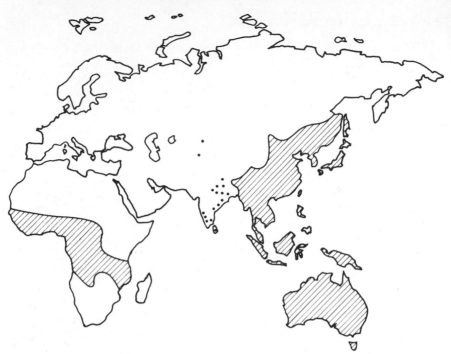

Figure 1. Milking and nonmilking areas in the Old World (drawn according to Simoons, 1970). Hatched areas: nonmilking predominant; open areas: milking predominant; dots: nonmilking locations in the milking area.

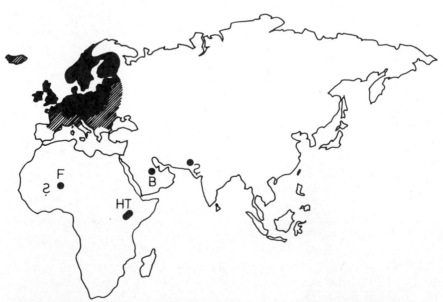

Figure 2. Populations with a frequency of the "persistence of lactase activity" (PLA) gene of more than 0.5 (certain in black areas, probable in hatched areas). Outside Europe only a few ethnic groups have high PLA gene frequencies. With the exception of the Hamitic groups in East Africa (HT), only very small numbers of subjects were examined in the non-European groups (F = Fulani, B = Bedouins).

shown. In the Old World, the only large population with a consistently high incidence of PLA is found in Northern Europe (Europe north of the Alps).

The distribution within Europe suggests a gradient of the PLA gene frequencies with the center of high frequencies (0.7 to 0.75) in southern Scandinavia. These PLA gene frequencies are higher than in any other population, including the nomadic groups of Africa and Southwest Asia, the areas where the milking habit is presumed to have originated some 7000 to 8000 years ago (Simoons, 1970, 1971). Cavalli-Sforza (1973) has calculated that 10,000 years, i.e., 350 to 400 generations in human terms, is sufficient to raise the frequency of the PLA gene, introduced by mutation, to the present European levels with a selection disadvantage of the lactose malabsorbers of only 2 to 3 percent. The dynamic model presented in Figure 3 shows that under these conditions the rise of the PLA gene frequency is minimal during the first 100 to 150 generations, followed by a more rapid sinusoidal increase. It is tempting to try to explain the differences of the PLA gene frequencies in the milking area by differences in the length of the selection period. However, this concept does not seem to be applicable to the population of Scandinavia, where a relatively late introduction of dairying is probable because of the unfavorable climatic conditions in the postglacial period. Stronger selection, e.g., an advantage of lactose absorbers of 5 percent, would result in an accelerated rise of PLA gene frequencies compatible with the findings in Northern Europe (see Fig. 3), but one may question whether more milk in the diet could explain the higher selection coefficient. Con-

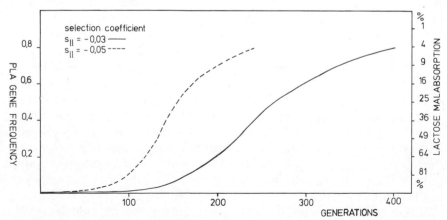

Figure 3. Simulation of the rise of the PLA gene frequency, assuming equal selective advantage of the homozygote and the heterozygote, after its introduction into an infinite population at a frequency on 10^{-4}. s_{II} refers to the selective disadvantage of the (homozygous) lactose malabsorbers.

sidering the long tradition of agriculture in Europe, the relatively low yield of milking animals before the introduction of systematic breeding, and the obvious limitations of daily milk intake, selection in favor of the PLA gene, increased over that in nomadic pastoralists, can hardly be explained by a higher milk consumption. A specific advantage of milk in the environmental conditions in Northern Europe is more likely.

Lactose and Calcium Absorption

With these objections to an unspecific selective advantage of milk as the sole cause of high PLA gene frequencies in mind, the authors of this review have put forward a hypothesis postulating a selective advantage for the lactose absorber in the environment of Northern Europe that is specifically connected with lactose, the substrate of the variant enzyme (Flatz and Rotthauwe, 1973). This hypothesis is based on the promotion of calcium absorption by lactose that has led a number of authors to conclude that lactose can replace vitamin D in restoring calcium balance in rickets (Lengemann et al., 1959; Lengemann and Comar, 1961; Dupuy et al., 1962; Nordio et al., 1966; Au and Raisz, 1967; Bernier et al., 1967; Pansu and Chapuy, 1970; Fournier et al., 1971; Leichter and Tolensky, 1975). Late rickets and osteomalacia are diseases of an age group in which selective hypolactasia has already developed. They are expected to reduce the fitness of affected individuals as a consequence of bone deformations, especially pelvic deformations in females. Several authors have contended that the conspicuous depigmentation of the Northern European is the result of selection through rickets in favor of "low pigment genes," permitting increased cutaneous formation of cholecalciferol in an environment characterized by low UV irradiation and insufficient dietary supply of vitamin D (Reche and Lehmann, 1959; Jonxis, 1961; Loomis, 1967). If this selective mechanism is accepted, it is reasonable to assume that any gene effective in the prevention of late rickets and osteomalacia would convey a selective advantage in the environmental conditions of Northern Europe before the improvement of public health care during the last decades. This selection model could explain the singularly high frequency of the PLA gene in "white" people originating in Northern Europe.

The crucial problem of the calcium absorption hypothesis is the mechanism of the surmised protective effect of the PLA gene. Is the positive calcium balance in lactose absorbers on a lactose diet, as evident from the study by Condon et al. (1970), merely a quantitative improvement resulting from slower passage of milk through the small intestine, or is there a specific enhancement of calcium absorption connected with the hydrolysis of lactose? The observed effect of lactose on calcium absorption in adult laboratory animals (Lengemann et al., 1959; Dupuy et al., 1962; Au and Raisz, 1967; Fournier et al., 1971) seems to disprove a role of lactose hydrolysis because lactase activities are presumably low. The very similar effect of lactose and galactose on the calcium and phosphorus content of animals (Scheunert and Sommer, 1956) may, on the other hand, indicate that lactose hydrolysis is essential and that galactose is the active metabolite. So far, calcium absorption has not been studied in intestinal preparations with differing levels of lactase activity.

The interesting study reported by Kocián et al. (1973) should not be construed as evidence against a possible beneficial effect of lactose on calcium metabolism in subjects with PLA. Calcium retention was measured in subjects presumably in calcium balance. Therefore it is not surprising that the 7-day retention of calcium did not significantly differ in lactose absorbers and malabsorbers. Short-term calcium absorption from lactose-rich milk was much higher in lactose absorbers than in malabsorbers, and this may improve retention if the calcium metabolism is not in balance. Likewise, the contention of Cook and Al-Torki (1975) that the calcium absorption hypothesis is untenable because "childhood malnutrition, especially marasmus, is common in many areas where adult hypolactasia is prevalent" misses the target because rickets and osteomalacia are specific disturbances of bone formation resulting from lack of activated cholecalciferol, and are not due to general protein-joule malnutrition, which, in addition, may cause secondary lactase deficiency.

CONCLUDING REMARKS

The lactose polymorphism is one of the few genetic polymorphisms of man for which plausible hypotheses connecting the function of the biologically active gene product and the distribution of the genotypes have been put forward. In further research on the lactase polymorphism it would perhaps be useful to heed the lessons taught by etiologic studies on the polymorphism at the human hemoglobin β-chain locus (particularly sickle-cell hemoglobin). A threefold approach to the open problems by population studies and on physiologic and molecular levels seems judicious.

Distribution studies of the lactase phenotypes in the Old World are of particular interest, because the populations of this region have been exposed to the environmental conditions of their present habitats for a long time. With the possible exception of Finland, no European country has been adequately examined. The existence of the genetic cline in Europe, with a center of high PLA gene frequencies in Scandinavia, has not been sufficiently demonstrated. In Africa and Asia, valuable information with respect to the culture historical hypothesis may be expected from further examinations of nomadic pastoralists. Distribution studies in delimited ethnic groups in America may permit conclusions concerning populations of the Old World which cannot be examined at present (cf. Leichter, 1972). Population studies should be designed to include a number of probands sufficient for a valid comparison between different populations. The inconveniences of the standard LTT limit the number of volunteering probands. Adaptation of the H_2 breath analysis to field conditions would provide a more convenient method for population studies.

On the physiologic level, many questions concerning the effect of lactose in subjects of the two lactase phenotypes remain open. Very little is known about the long-term effect of lactose in malabsorbers, in particular about the sequelae of a chronically increased acidity of the lower intestinal tract. Further studies concerning the long-term effect of lactose on the calcium balance in lactose absorbers and lactose malabsorbers seem indicated. An in vitro model suitable for the examination of the effect of lactose hydrolysis on calcium absorption would be of particular value.

On the molecular level, technical difficulties resulting from the instability of the intestinal disaccharidases and the cumbersome isolation of mucosa cells and cell organelles must be overcome. The recent studies of Freiburghaus et al. (1976) and Seetharam and Alpers (1976) perhaps show the way to a further elucidation of the molecular differences between the two lactase phenotypes. Possibly, a differentiation between homozygous and heterozygous lactose absorbers could be achieved by determining lactase activity in isolated brush border membranes. Genetic switch mechanisms similar to that of lactase production—e.g., that of the hemoglobin γ-chains—may provide heuristic models for the study of the lactase polymorphism.

Further research on the variation of human lactose assimilation would be facilitated by an agreement on nomenclature that clearly distinguishes between the physiologic and the pathologic lactase phenotypes. Selective adult hypolactasia, present in the majority of healthy human adults, should not be described with the terms "deficiency," "abnormal," or "intolerant." Likewise, persistence of lactase activity does not deserve the contradistinctive designations "healthy," "normal," or "tolerant." This is not a matter of semantic pedantry. The conceptual approach to the problems posed by the human lactase polymorphism is impeded by a nomenclature based on the unjustified assumption that conditions prevailing in European or "white" populations are the yardstick of normality.

References

Ahmed, H. F. 1975. Irritable-bowel syndrome with lactose intolerance. Lancet 2:319–320.

Alford, S. C. 1969. Lactose intolerance in Asians. Nature 221:562–567.

Almy, T. P. 1975. Evolution, lactase levels and global hunger. New Eng. J. Med. 292:1183–1184.

Alpers, D. H. 1969. Separation and isolation of rat and human intestinal β-galactosidase. J. Biol. Chem. 244:1238–1246.

Alzate, H., H. Gonzalez, and I. Guzman. 1969. Lactose intolerance in South American Indians. Am. J. Clin. Nutr. 22:122–123.

Alzate, H., E. Ramirez, and M. T. Echeverria. 1968. Intolerancia a la lactosa en un grupo de estudiantes de medicina. Antioquia Med. 18:237–246.

American Academy of Pediatrics. 1974. Committee on Nutrition (Holliday, M. A., Chairman). Should milk drinking by children be discouraged? Pediatrics 53:576–582.

Asp, N. G. 1971. Human small intestinal β-galactosidases. Separation and characterization of three forms of an acid β-galactosidase. Biochem. J. 121:299–308.

Asp, N. G., N. O. Berg, A. Dahlqvist, J. Jussila, and H. Salmi. 1971. The activity of three different small-intestinal β-galactosidases in adults with and without lactase deficiency. Scand. J. Gastroenterol. 6:755–762.

Asp, N. G., and A. Dahlqvist. 1968. Rat small-intestinal β-galactosidases. Kinetic studies with three separated fractions. Biochem. J. 110:143–150.

Asp, N. G., and A. Dahlqvist. 1971a. Assay of 2-naphthyl-β-galactosidase activity. Anal. Biochem. 42:275–280.

Asp, N. G., and A. Dahlqvist. 1971b. Multiplicity of intestinal β-galactosidases. Contribution of each enzyme to the total lactase activity in normal and lactose-intolerant patients. Acta Paediat. Scand. 60:364–365.

Asp, N. G., and A. Dahlqvist. 1972. Human small intestine β-galactosidases. Specific assay of three different enzymes. Anal. Biochem. 47:527–538.

Asp, N. G., and A. Dahlqvist. 1974. Intestinal β-galactosidases in adult low lactase activity and in congenital lactase deficiency. Enzyme 18:84–102.

Asp, N. G., A. Dahlqvist, and O. Koldovsky. 1969. Human small-intestinal β-galactosidases. Separation and characterization of one lactase and one hetero β-galactosidase. Biochem. J. 114:351–359.

Asp, N. G., A. Dahlqvist, and O. Koldovsky. 1970. Small intestinal β-galactosidase activity. Gastroenterology 58:591–593.

Asp, N. G., A. Dahlqvist, P. Kuitunen, K. Launiala, and I. K. Visakorpi. 1973. Complete deficiency of brush border lactase in congenital lactose malabsorption. Lancet 2:329–330.

Au, W. Y. W., and L. G. Raisz. 1967. Restoration of parathyroid responsiveness in vitamin D deficient rats by parenteral calcium or dietary lactose. J. Clin. Invest. 44:1572–1578.

Auricchio, S., A. Rubino, G. Semenza, M. Landolt, and A. Prader. 1963a. Isolated intestinal lactase deficiency in the adult. Lancet 2:324–326.

Auricchio, S., A. Rubino, R. Tosi, G. Semenza, M. Landolt, H. Kistler, and A. Prader.

1963b. Disaccharidase activities in human intestinal mucosa. Enzymol. Biol. Clin. 3:193–208.

Balslev, I., J. Kramhöft, and O. G. Backer, 1971. Lactose malabsorption before and after truncal and selective vagotomy. Scand. J. Gastroenterol. 6 (suppl. 9):71–74.

Bayless, T. M., N. L. Christopher, and S. H. Boyer. 1969. Autosomal recessive inheritance of intestinal lactase deficiency: Evidence from ethnic differences. J. Clin. Invest. 48:6a.

Bayless, T. M., and S.-S. Huang. 1969. Inadequate intestinal digestion of lactose. Am. J. Clin. Nutr. 22:250–256.

Bayless, T. M., and S.-S. Huang. 1971. Recurrent abdominal pain due to milk and lactose intolerance in school-aged children. Pediatrics 47:1029–1032.

Bayless, T. M., and N. S. Rosensweig. 1966. A racial difference incidence of lactase deficiency. A survey of milk intolerance and lactase deficiency in healthy adult males. JAMA 197:968–972.

Bayless, T. M., and N. S. Rosensweig. 1967. Topics in clinical medicine. Incidence and implications of lactase deficiency and milk intolerance in White and Negro populations. Johns Hopkins Med. J. 121:54–64.

Bayless, T. M., B. Rothfeld, C. Massa, L. Wise, D. M. Paige, and M. Bedine. 1975. Lactose and milk intolerance: Clinical implications. New Eng. J. Med. 292:1156–1159.

Bedine, M. S., and T. M. Bayless. 1973. Intolerance of small amounts of lactose by individuals with low lactase levels. Gastroenterology 65:735–743.

Berg, N. O., A. Dahlqvist, T. Lindberg, and A. Norden. 1970. Intestinal dipeptidases and disaccharidases in celiac disease in adults. Gastroenterology 59:575–582.

Bernier, J. J., J. C. Rambaud, and J. D. Sraer. 1967. Influence du lactose sur l'absorption intestinale du calcium. Arch. Mal. App. Digest. 56:195–205.

Birge, S. J., H. T. Keutmann, P. Cuatrecasas, and G. D. Whedon. 1967. Osteoporosis, intestinal lactase deficiency and low dietary calcium intake. New Eng. J. Med. 276:445–448.

Boellner, S. W., A. G. Beard, and T. C. Panos. 1965. Impairment of intestinal hydrolysis of lactose in newborn infants. Pediatrics 36:542–550.

Bolin, T. D., G. G. Crane, and A. E. Davis. 1968. Lactose intolerance in various ethnic groups in Southeast Asia. Aust. Ann. Med. 17:300–306.

Bolin, T. D., and A. E. Davis. 1969. Asian lactose intolerance and its relation to intake of lactose. Nature 222:382–383.

Bolin, T. D., and A. E. Davis. 1970a. Lactose intolerance in Australian-born Chinese. Australas. Ann. Med. 19:40–41.

Bolin, T. D., and A. E. Davis. 1970b. Primary lactase deficiency: Genetic or acquired? Am. J. Dig. Dis. 15:679–692.

Bolin, T. D., A. E. Davis, C. H. Seah, K. L. Chua, V. Yong, K. M. Kho, C. L. Siak, and E. Jacob. 1970a. Lactose intolerance in Singapore. Gastroenterology 59:76–84.

Bolin, T. D., A. McKern, and A. E. Davis. 1971. The effect of diet on lactase activity in the rat. Gastroenterology 60:432–437.

Bolin, T. D., R. M. Morrison, J. E. Steel, and A. E. Davis. 1970b. Lactose intolerance in Australia. Med. J. Aust. 4:1289–1292.

Bolin, T. D., R. C. Pirola, and A. E. Davis. 1969. Adaptation of intestinal lactase in the rat. Gastroenterology 57:406–409.

Bond, J. H., and M. D. Levitt. 1976. Quantitative measurement of lactose absorption. Gastroenterology 70:1058–1062.

Bose, D. P., and J. D. Welsh. 1973. Lactose malabsorption in Oklahoma Indians. Am. J. Clin. Nutr. 26:1320–1322.

Bradfield, R. B., D. B. Jeliffe, and A. Ifekwunigwe. 1975. Milk intolerance and malnutrition. Lancet 2:325.

Broitman, S., B. Thalenfeld, and N. Zamcheck. 1968. Alteration in gut lactase activity in young and adult rats fed lactose. Fed. Proc. 27:573.

Bryant, G. D., Y. K. Chu, and R. Lovitt. 1970. Incidence and aetiology of lactose intolerance. Med. J. Aust. 1:1285–1288.

Busk, H. E., B. Dahlerup,T. Lytzen, V. Binder, and E. Gudmand-Hoyer. 1975. The incidence of lactose malabsorption in ulcerative colitis. Scand. J. Gastroenterol. 10:263–265.

Cady, A. B., J. B. Rhodes, A. Littman, and R. K. Crane. 1967. Significance of lactase deficit in ulcerative colitis. J. Lab. Clin. Med. 70:279–286.

Cain, G. C., P. Moore, M. Patterson, and M. A. McElveen. 1969. The stimulation of lactase by feeding lactose. Scand. J. Gastroenterol. 4:545–550.

Calloway, D. H., and W. L. Chenoweth. 1973. Utilization of nutrients in milk- and wheat-based diets by men with adequate and reduced abilities to absorb lactose. I. Energy and nutrition. Am. J. Clin. Nutr. 26:939–951.

Calloway, D. H., E. L. Murphy, and D. Bauer. 1969. Determination of lactose intolerance by breath analysis. Am. J. Dig. Dis. 14:811–815.

Cavalli-Sforza, L. L. 1973. Analytic review: Some current problems of human population genetics. Am. J. Hum. Genet. 25:82–104.

Chua, K. L., and C. S. Seah. 1973. Lactose intolerance: Hereditary or acquired? Effect of prolonged milk feeding. Singapore Med. J. 14:29–33.

Chung, M. H., and D. B. McGill. 1968. Lactase deficiency in Orientals. Gastroenterology 54:225–226.

Condon, J. R., J. R. Nassim, F. J. C. Millard, A. Hilbe, and E. M. Stainthorpe. 1970. Calcium and phosphorus metabolism in relation to lactose tolerance. Lancet 1:1027–1029.

Cook, G. C. 1967. Lactase activity in newborn and infant Baganda. Brit. Med. J. 1:527–530.

Cook, G. C. 1973. Incidence and Clinical Features of Specific Hypolactasia in Man. In Intestinal Enzyme Deficiencies and Their Nutritional Implications, Borgstrom, M., A. Dahlqvist, and L. Hambraeus (Eds.), pp. 52–73. Stockholm, Almqvist and Wiksell.

Cook, G. C., and M. T. Al-Torki. 1975. High intestinal lactase concentrations in adult Arabs in Saudi Arabia. Brit. Med. J. 3:135–136.

Cook, G. C., N. G. Asp, and A. Dahlqvist. 1973. Activities of brush border lactase, acid β-galactosidase, and hetero-β-galactosidase in the jejunum of the Zambian African. Gastroenterology 64:405–410.

Cook, G. C., and A. Dahlqvist. 1968. Jejunal hetero-β-galactosidase activities in Ugandans with lactase deficiency. Gastroenterology 55:328–332.

Cook, G. C., and S. K. Kajubi. 1966. Tribal incidence of lactase deficiency in Uganda. Lancet 1:725–729.

Cook, G. C., A. Lakin, and R. G. Whitehead. 1967. Absorption of lactose and its digestion products in the normal and malnourished Ugandan. Gut 8:622–627.

Cox, J. A., and F. G. Elliott. 1974. Primary adult lactose intolerance in the Kivu Lake area: Rwanda and the Bushi. Amer. J. Dig. Dis. 19:714–724.

Cuatrecasas, P., D. H. Lockwood, and J. Caldwell. 1965. Lactase deficiency in the adult: A common occurrence. Lancet 1:14–18.

Dahlqvist, A. 1974. Enzyme Deficiency and Malabsorption of Carbohydrates. In Sugars in Nutrition, Sipple, H. L., and K. W. McNutt (Eds.), pp. 187–214. New York, Academic Press.

Dahlqvist, A., and B. Lindquist. 1971. Lactose intolerance and protein malnutrition. Acta Paediat. Scand. 60:488–494.

Davis, A. E. 1969. Milk intolerance in Southeast Asia. Natural History 78:54–55.

Davis, A. E., and T. Bolin. 1967. Lactose intolerance in Asians. Nature 216:1244–1245.

DeGroot, A. P., and P. Hoogendoorn. 1957. The dentrimental effect of lactose. II. Quantitative lactase determinations in various mammals. Neth. Milk Dairy J. 11:290–296.

DeRitis, F., G. G. Balestrieri, G. Ruggiero, E. Filosa, and S. Auricchio. 1970. High frequency of lactase activity deficiency in small bowel of adults in the Neapolitan area. Enzymol. Biol. Clin. 2:263–267.

Desai, H. G., A. V. Chitre, and K. N. Jeejeebhoy. 1967. Lactose loading. A simple test for detecting intestinal lactase deficiency. Evaluation of different methods. Gastroenterologia 108:177–188.

Desai, H. G., U. V. Gupte, A. G. Pradhan, K. D. Thakkar, and F. P. Antia. 1970. Incidence of lactase deficiency in control subjects from India. Indian J. Med. Sci. 24:729–736.

Dill, J. E., M. Levy, R. F. Wells, and E. Wezer. 1972. Lactase deficiency in Mexican-American males. Am. J. Clin. Nutr. 25:869–870.

Doell, R. G., and N. Kretchmer. 1962. Studies of small intestine during development. I. Distribution and activity of β-galactosidase. Biochim. Biophys. Acta 62:353–362.

Dubs, R., R. Gitzelmann, B. Steinmann, and J. Lindenmann. 1975. Catalytically inactive sucrase antigen of rabbit small intestine. Helv. Paediat. Acta 30:89–102.

Duncan, J. W., and E. M. Scott. 1972. Lactose intolerance in Alaskan Indians and Eskimos. Am. J. Clin. Nutr. 25:867–868.

Dunphy, J. V., A. Littman, J. B. Hammond, G. Forstner, A. Dahlqvist, and R. K. Crane. 1965. Intestinal lactase deficit in adults. Gastroenterology 49:12–21.

Dupuy, Y., P. Brun, and P. Fournier. 1962. Étude de l'activité du lactose, facteur exogéne de l'utilisation du calcium en fonction de la dose administrée. C. R. Acad. Sci. 254:2230–2232.

Editorial. 1975. Lactase deficiency. Lancet 2:910–911.

Eggermont, E., and H. G. Hers. 1969. The sedimentation properties of the intestinal α-glucosidases of normal human subjects and of patients with sucrose intolerance. Eur. J. Biochem. 9:488–496.

Ekström, K. E., N. J. Benevenga, and R. H. Grummer. 1975. Effects of diets containing dried whey on the lactase activity of the small intestinal mucosa and the contents of the small intestine and cecum of the pig. J. Nutr. 105:851–860.

Ekström, K. E., R. H. Grummer, and N. J. Benevenga. 1976. Effects of a diet containing 40% dried whey on the performance and lactase activities in the small intestine and cecum of Hampshire and Chester White pigs. J. Animal Sci. 42:106–113.

Elliott, F. G., J. Cox, and B. C. Nyomba. 1973. Intolérance au lactose chez l'adulte en Afrique centrale. Ann. Soc. Belg. Med. Trop. 55:113–132.

Elliot, R. B., and G. M. Maxwell. 1967. Lactose digestion in Australian Aboriginal children. Med. J. Aust. 1:46–49.

El-Schallah, M. O., H. W. Rotthauwe, and G. Flatz. 1973. Laktose-intoleranz in der arabischen Bevölkerung. Med. Welt 24:1376–1377.

Erkelens, D. W., and J. B. Bouman, and M. W. Jansen. 1972. Lactose-intolerantie en lactase-deficiente bij volwassen patienten op Curaçao. Ned. Tijdschr. Geneeskd. 116:1080–1085.

Ferguson, A., and J. Maxwell. 1967. Genetic aetiology of lactose intolerance. Lancet 2:188–190.

Figueroa, R. B., E. Melgar, N. Jo, Q. F. Garcia, and O. L. Garcia. 1971. Intestinal lactase deficiency in an apparently normal Peruvian population. Am. J. Dig. Dis. 16:881–889.

Fine, A., E. Willoughby, G. S. A. McDonald, D. G. Weir, and P. B. B. Gatenby. 1968. A family with intolerance to lactose and cold milk. Irish J. Med. Sci. 1:321–326.

Fischer, J. E. 1957. Effects of feeding a diet containing lactose upon β-D-galactosidase activity and organ development in the rat digestive tract. Am. J. Physiol. 188:49–53.

Fischer, W., and J. Zapf. 1965. Zur erworbenen Laktoseintoleranz. Klin. Wschr. 43:1243–1246.

Flatz, G., and H. W. Rotthauwe. 1971. Evidence against nutritional adaptation of tolerance to lactose. Humangenetik 13:118–125.

Flatz, G., and H. W. Rotthauwe. 1973. Lactose nutrition and natural selection. Lancet 2:76–77.

Flatz, G., and C. Saengudom. 1969. Lactose tolerance in Asians: A family study. Nature 224:915–916.

Flatz, G., C. Saengudom, and T. Sanguanbhokhai. 1969. Lactose intolerance in Thailand. Nature 221:758–759.

Fournier, P., Y. Dupuis, and A. Fournier. 1971. Effect of lactose on the absorption of alkaline earth metals and intestinal lactase activity. Isr. J. Med. Sci. 7:389–391.

Freiburghaus, A. U., J. Schmitz, M. Schindler, H. W. Rotthauwe, P. Kuitunen, K. Launiala, and B. Hadorn. 1976. Protein patterns of brush-border fragments in congenital lactose malabsorption and in specific hypolactasia of the adult. New Eng. J. Med. 294:1030–1032.

Garcia, G. J., J. M. R. Gomez, L. A. Quereda, S. M. A. Desfilis, and G. C. Gomez, 1974. Intolerancia a la lactosa en la poblacion espanola. Rev. Esp. Enferm. Apar. Dig. 42:367–382.

Garza, C., and N. S. Scrimshaw. 1976. Relationship of lactose intolerance to milk intolerance in young children. Am. J. Clin. Nutr. 29:192–196.

Gilat, T. 1971. Lactase – an adaptable enzyme? Gastroenterology 60:346–347.

Gilat, T., Y. Benaroya, E. Gelman-Malachi, and A. Adam. 1973. Genetics of primary adult lactase deficiency. Gastroenterology 64:562–568.

Gilat, T., R. Kuhn, E. Gelman, and O. Mizrahi. 1970. Lactase deficiency in Jewish communities in Israel. Am. J. Dig. Dis. 15:895–904.

Gilat, T., E. G. Malachi, and S. B. Schochet. 1971. Lactose tolerance in an Arab population. Am. J. Dig. Dis. 16:203–206.

Gilat, T., S. Russo, E. Gelman-Malachi, and T. A. M. Aldor. 1972. Lactase in man: A nonadaptable enzyme. Gastroenterology 62:1125–1127.

Girardet, P., R. Richterich, and I. Antener. 1964. Adaptation de la lactase intestinale à l'administration de lactose chez le rat adulte. Helv. Physiol. Acta 22:7–14.

Graham, G. G. 1975. Protein Advisory Group's recommendations deplored. Pediatrics 55:295–296.

Gray, G. M., and N. A. Santiago. 1966. Disaccharide absorption in normal and diseased human intestine. Gastroenterology 51:489–498.

Gray, G. M., and N. A. Santiago. 1969. Intestinal β-galactosidases. I. Separation and characterization of three enzymes in normal human intestine. J. Clin. Invest. 48:716–728.

Gray, G. M., N. A. Santiago, E. H. Colver, and M. Genel. 1969. Intestinal β-galactosidases. II. Biochemical alteration in human lactase deficiency. J. Clin. Invest. 48:729–735.

Gray, G. M., W. M. Walter, and E. H. Colver. 1968. Persistent deficiency of intestinal lactase in apparently cured tropical sprue. Gastroenterology 54:552–558.

Gudmand-Höyer E. 1971. Specific lactose malabsorption in adults. Thesis. Copenhagen, Fadl's Forlag.

Gudmand-Höyer, E., A. Dahlqvist, and S. Jarnum. 1969. Specific small-intestinal lactase deficiency in adults. Scand. J. Gastroenterol. 4:377–386.

Gudmand-Höyer, E., and S. Jarnum. 1969. Lactose malabsorption in Greenland Eskimos. Acta Med. Scand. 186:235–237.

Gudmand-Höyer, E., A. McNair, S. Jarnum, L. Broersma, and J. McNair. 1973. Laktosemalabsorption in Vestgrønland. Ugeskr. Laeger 135:169–172.

Gupta, P. S., R. C. Misra, K. A. Ramachandran, and H. K. Chuttami. 1970. Lactose intolerance in adults. J. Assoc. Physicans India 18:765–768.

Haemmerli, U. P., H. Kistler, R. Ammann, R. Marthaler, G. Semenza, S. Auricchio, and A. Prader. 1965. Acquired milk intolerance in the adult caused by lactose malabsorption due to a selective deficiency in intestinal lactase activity. Am. J. Med. 38:7–30.

Heilskov, N. S. C. 1951. Studies on animal lactase. II. Distribution in some of the glands of the gastrointestinal tract. Acta Physiol. Scand. 24:84–89.

Holzel, A. 1967. Sugar malabsorption due to deficiencies of disaccharidase activities and of monosaccharide transport. Arch. Dis. Child. 42:341–352.

Holzel, A., V. Schwarz, and A. W. Sutcliffe. 1959. Defective lactose absorption causing malnutrition in infancy. Lancet 1:1126–1128.

Hore, P., M. Landolt, and G. Semenza. 1972. Appendix to Schlegel-Haueter, G., P. Hore, K. R. Kerry, and G. Semenza. 1972. The preparation of lactase and glucoamylase of rat small intestine. Biochim. Biophys. Acta 258:506–519.

Huang, S. S., and T. M. Bayless. 1967. Lactose intolerance in healthy children. New Eng. J. Med. 276:1283–1387.

Huang, S. S., and T. M. Bayless. 1968. Milk and lactose intolerance in healthy Orientals. Science 160:83–84.

Huber, J. T., R. J. Rifkin, and J. M. Keith. 1964. Effect of level of lactose upon lactase concentrations in the small intestines of young calves. J. Dairy Sci. 7:789–792.

Jarrett, E. C., and G. H. Holman. 1966. Lactose absorption in the premature infant. Arch. Dis. Child. 41:525–527.

Jenkins, T., H. Lehmann, and G. T. Nurse. 1974. Public health and genetic constitution of the San ("Bushmen"): Carbohydrate metabolism and acetylator status of the Kung of Tsumkwe in the North-western Kalahari. Brit. Med. J. 2:23–26.

Jersky, J., and R. H. Kinsley. 1967. Lactase deficiency in the South African Bantu. S. Afr. Med. J. 41:1194–1196.

Johnson, J. D. 1973. Neutral hetero-β-galactosidase from rabbit small intestine. Biochim. Biophys. Acta 302:382–392.

Johnson, J. D., N. Kretchmer, and F. J. Simoons. 1974. Lactose malabsorption: Its biology and history. Adv. Pediat. 21:197–237.

Jones, D. P., F. R. Sosa, and E. Skromak. 1972. Effects of glucose, sucrose, and lactose on intestinal disaccharidases in the rat. J. Lab. Clin. Med. 79:19–30.

Jonxis, J. H. P. 1961. Some investigations on rickets. J. Pediat. 59:607–615.

Jussila, J. 1969a. Diagnosis of lactose malabsorption by the lactose tolerance test with peroral ethanol administration. Scand. J. Gastroenterol. 4:361–368.

Jussila, J. 1969b. Milk intolerance and lactose malabsorption in hospital patients and young servicemen in Finland. Ann. Clin. Res. 1:199–207.

Jussila, J., M. Isokoski, and K. Launiala. 1970. Prevalence of lactose malabsorption in a Finnish rural population. Scand. J. Gastroenterol. 5:49–56.

Kanaghinis, T., J. Hatzioannou, N. Deliavgyris, N. Danos, N. Zografos, A. Katsas, and C. Gardikas. 1974. Primary lactase deficiency in Greek adults. Am. J. Dig. Dis. 19:1021–1027.

Kern, F., and M. Heller. 1968. Blood galactose after lactose and ethanol: An accurate index of lactase deficiency. Gastroenterology 54:1250.

Keusch, G. T., F. S. Troncale, L. H. Miller, V. Promdath, and P. R. Anderson. 1969a. Acquired lactose malabsorption in Thai children. Pediatrics 43:540–545.

Keusch, G. T., F. J. Troncale, B. Thavaramara, P. Prinyanont, P. R. Anderson, and N. Bhamarapravathi. 1969b. Lactose deficiency in Thailand: Effect of prolonged lactose feeding. Am. J. Clin. Nutr. 22:638–641.

Kistler, H. 1966. Disaccharid-Malabsorption. Schweiz. Med. Wschr. 96:1349–1350.

Klaus, D., and H. Siebner. 1966. Laktose-Intoleranz beim Erwachsenen. Dtsch. Med. Wschr. 91:2174–2179.

Knudsen, K. B., M. D. Welsh, R. S. Kronenberg, J. E. Vanderveen, and N. D. Heidelbauch. 1968. Effect of a nonlactose diet on human intestinal disaccharidase activity. Am. J. Dig. Dis. 13:593–597.

Kocián, J., I. Skála, and K. Bakos. 1973. Calcium absorption from milk and lactose-free milk in healthy subjects and patients with lactose intolerance. Digestion 9:317–324.

Krasilnikoff, P. A., E. Gudmand-Hoyer, and H. H. Moltke. 1975. Diagnostic value of disaccharide tolerance tests in children. Acta Paediat. Scand. 64:693–698.

Kretchmer, N., and O. Ransome-Kuti. 1970. Lactose intolerance: An international problem. Proc. Inst. Med. Chic. 28:213–217.

Kretchmer, N., O. Ransome-Kuti, R. Hurwitz, C. Dungy, and W. Alakija. 1971. Intestinal absorption of lactose in Nigerian ethnic groups. Lancet 2:392–395.

Laws, J. W., and G. Neale. 1967. Radiology in the diagnosis of disaccharidase deficiency. Brit. J. Radiol. 40:594–603.

Lebenthal, E., I. Antonowicz, and H. Shwachmann. 1975. Correlation of lactase activity, lactose tolerance and milk consumption in different age groups. Amer. J. Clin. Nutr. 28:595–600.

Lebenthal, E., P. Sunshine, and N. Kretchmer. 1973. Effect of prolonged nursing on the activity of intestinal lactase. Gastroenterology 64:1136–1141.

Lebenthal, E., K. Tsuboi, and N. Kretchmer. 1974. Characterization of human intesti-

nal lactase and hetero-β-galactosidases of infants and adults. Gastroenterology 67:1107–1113.
Leese, H. J., and G. Semenza. 1973. On the identity between the small intestinal enzymes phlorizin hydrolase and glycosylceramidase. J. Biol. Chem. 248:8170–8173.
Leichter, J. 1971. Lactose tolerance in a Jewish population. Am. J. Dig. Dis. 16:1123–1126.
Leichter, J. 1972. Lactose tolerance in a Slavic population. Am. J. Dig. Dis. 17:73–76.
Leichter, J. 1973. Effect of dietary lactose on intestinal lactase activity in young rats. J. Nutr. 103:392–396.
Leichter, J., and M. Lee. 1971. Lactose intolerance in Canadian west coast Indians. Am. J. Dig. Dis. 16:809–813.
Leichter, J., and F. Tolensky. 1975. Effect of dietary lactose on the absorption of protein, fat and calcium in the postweaning rat. Am. J. Clin. Nutr. 28:238–241.
Lengemann, F. W., and C. L. Comar. 1961. Distribution of absorbed strontium-85 and calcium-45 as influenced by lactose. Am. J. Physiol. 200:1051–1054.
Lengemann, F. W., R. H. Wassermann, and C. L. Comar. 1959. Studies on the enhancement of radiocalcium and radiostrontium absorption by lactose in the rat. J. Nutr. 68:443–450.
Lifrak, I. L., R. Lev, and A. V. Loud. 1976. Substrate-induced acceleration of lactase synthesis in fetal rat intestine. Pediat. Res. 10:100–102.
Lifshitz, F., S. Diaz-Bensussen, V. Martinez-Garza, F. Abdo-Bassols, and E. Diaz del Castillo. 1971. Influence of disaccharides on the development of systemic acidosis in the premature infant. Pediat. Res. 5:213–225.
Lisker, R., B. Gonzalez, and M. Daltabuit. 1975. Recessive inheritance of the adult type of intestinal lactase deficiency. Am. J. Hum. Genet. 27:662–664.
Lisker, R., G. López-Habib, M. Daltabuit, I. Rostenberg, and P. Arroyo. 1974. Lactase deficiency in a rural area of Mexico. Am. J. Clin. Nutr. 27:756–759.
Littman, A., A. B. Cady, and J. Rhodes. 1968. Lactase and other disaccharidase deficiency in a hospital population. Isr. J. Med. Sci. 4:110–116.
Loiselet, J., and L. Jarjouhi. 1974. L'intolérance au lactose chez l'adulte libanais. J. Med. Liban. 27:339–350.
Loomis, W. F., 1967. Skin-pigment regulation of vitamin-D biosynthesis in man. Science 157:501–506.
Lorenz-Meyer, H., A. L. Blum, H. P. Haemmerli, and G. Semenza. 1972. A second enzyme defect in acquired lactase deficiency: Lack of small intestinal phlorizin hydrolase. Eur. J. Clin. Invest. 2:236–331.
Lufkin, E. G., F. B. Stifel, R. H. Herman, N. S. Rosensweig, and L. Hager. 1972. Effect of testosterone on jejunal pyruvate kinase activities in normal and hypogonadal males. J. Clin. Endocr. Metabol. 34:586–591.
Luyken, R., F. W. M. Luyken-Koning, and T. Immikhuizen. 1971. Lactose intolerance in Surinam. Trop. Geograph. Med. 23:54–58.
Madžarovová-Nohejlová, J. 1969. Activity of intestinal disaccharidases. Rev. Czech. Med. 15:212–234.
Malati, P., and K. R. Crane. 1969. Phlorizin hydrolase: A β-glucuronidase of hamster intestinal brush border membrane. Biochim. Biophys. Acta 173:245–256.
Marenco, G., D. Ghibaudi, and A. Meraviglia. 1970. Intolleranza al lattosio nell'adulto. Minerva Pediat. 22:505–513.
Masarei, J. R., P. Sharma, and A. A. Jansen. 1972. Lactose intolerance in Fijians and Indians. Fiji School Med. J. 7:166–171.
McCracken, R. D. 1970. Adult lactose tolerance. JAMA 213:2257–2260.
McCracken, R. D. 1971. Lactase deficiency: An example of dietary evolution. Current Anthropol. 12:479–500.
McGill, D. B., and A. D. Newcomer. 1967. Comparison of venous and capillary blood samples in lactose tolerance testing. Gastroenterology 53:371–374.
McGillivray, W. A. 1968. Lactose intolerance. Nature 219:615–616.
McMichael, H. B., J. Webb, and A. M. Dawson. 1966. Jejunal disaccharidases and observations on the cause of lactase deficiency. Brit. Med. J. 2:1037–1041.

Mendel, L. B., and P. H. Mitchell. 1907. Chemical studies on growth. I. The inverting enzymes of the alimentary tract, especially in the embryo. Am. J. Physiol. 20:81–89.

Mitchell, K. J., T. M. Bayless, D. M. Paige, R. W. Goodgame, and S. S. Huang. 1975. Intolerance of eight ounces of milk in healthy lactose-intolerant teen-agers. Pediatrics 56:718–721.

Morrison, W. J., N. L. Christopher, T. M. Bayless, and E. A. Dana. 1974. Low lactase levels: Evaluation of the radiological diagnosis. Radiology 111:513–518.

Murthy, M. S., and J. C. Haworth. 1970. Intestinal lactase deficiency among east Indians. An adaptive rather than a genetically inherited phenomenon? Am. J. Gastroenterol. 53:246–251.

Neale, G. 1968. The diagnosis, incidence and significance of disaccharidase deficiency in adults. Proc. Roy. Soc. Med. 61:1099–1102.

Neel, J. V., and W. J. Schull. 1954. Human Heredity. Chicago, University of Chicago Press.

Newcomer, A. D., and D. B. McGill. 1966. Distribution of disaccharidase activity in the small bowel of normal and lactase deficient subjects. Gastroenterology 51:481–488.

Newcomer, A. D., and D. B. McGill. 1967. Disaccharidase activity in the small intestine: Prevalence of lactase deficiency in 100 healthy subjects. Gastroenterology 53:881–889.

Newcomer, A. D., D. B. McGill, P. J. Thomas, and A. F. Hofmann. 1975. Prospective comparison of indirect methods for detecting lactase deficiency. New Eng. J. Med. 293:1232–1236.

Newcomer, A. D., P. J. Thomas, D. B. McGill, and A. F. Hofmann. 1977. Lactase deficiency: A common genetic trait of the American Indian. Gastroenterology 72:234–237.

Nordio, S., A. Berio, R. Gatti, and G. M. Lamedica. 1966. Relationships between lactase activity and calcium absorption. Ann. Paediat. 206:85–96.

Nordström, C., and A. Dahlqvist. 1973. Quantitative distribution of some enzymes along the villi and crypts of human small intestine. Scand. J. Gastroenterol. 8:407–416.

Olatunbosun, D. A., and B. K. Adadevoh. 1971. Lactase deficiency in Nigerians. Am. J. Dig. Dis. 16:909–914.

Paige, D. M., T. M. Bayless, and W. S. Dellinger. 1975a. Relationship of milk consumption to blood glucose rise in lactose intolerant individuals. Am. J. Clin. Nutr. 28:677–680.

Paige, D. M., T. M. Bayless, G. D. Ferry, and G. G. Graham. 1971. Lactose malabsorption and milk rejection in Negro children. Johns Hopkins Med. J. 129:163–169.

Paige, D. M., T. M. Bayless, and G. G. Graham. 1972a. Milk programs: Helpful or harmful to Negro children? Am. J. Publ. Health 62:1486–1488.

Paige, D. M., T. M. Bayless, S. S. Huang, and R. Wexler. 1975b. Lactose hydrolyzed milk. Am. J. Clin. Nutr. 28:818–822.

Paige, D. M., and G. G. Graham. 1971. Etiology of lactase deficiency: Another perspective. Gastroenterology 61:798–799.

Paige, D. M., E. Leonardo, B. Nakasima, B. T. Adrianzen, and G. G. Graham. 1972b. Response of lactose-intolerant children to different lactose levels. Am. J. Clin. Nutr. 25:467–469.

Pansu, D., and M. C. Chapuy. 1970. Calcium absorption enhanced by lactose and xylose. Calcif. Tissue Res. 4(suppl.):155–156.

Plimmer, R. J. A. 1906. On the presence of lactase in the intestines of animals and on the adaptation of the intestine to lactose. J. Physiol. 35:20–31.

Powell, G. K., M. Patterson, and M. McElveen. 1969. Induction of sucrase and maltase activity without increase in lactase with a high lactose diet. Gastroenterology 56:1190.

Protein Advisory Group of the United Nations. 1972. Low Lactase Activity and Milk Intake. New York, PAG Bulletin. Vol. 2, No. 2.

Rab, S. M., and A. Baseer. 1976. High intestinal lactase concentration in adult Pakistanis. Brit. Med. J. 1:436.

Rahimi, A. G., H. Delbrück, R. Haeckel, H. W. Goedde, and G. Flatz. 1976. Persistence of high intestinal lactase activity (lactose tolerance) in Afghanistan. Hum. Genet. 34:57–62.

Ransome-Kuti, O., N. Kretchmer, J. D. Johnson, and J. T. Gribble. 1972. Family studies of lactose intolerance in Nigerian ethnic groups. Pediat. Res. 6:359.

Ransome-Kuti, O., N. Kretchmer, J. D. Johnson, and J. T. Gribble. 1975. A genetic study of lactose digestion in Nigerian families. Gastroenterology 68:431–436.

Reche, O., and W. Lehmann. 1959. Die Genetik der Rassenbildung beim Menschen. In Die Evolution der Organismen, Heberer, G. (Ed.), pp. 1143–1191. Stuttgart, Fischer.

Reddy, B. S., J. R. Pleasants, and B. S. Wortman. 1968. Effect of dietary carbohydrates on intestinal disaccharidases in germ-free and conventional rats. J. Nutr. 95:413–419.

Reddy, V., and J. Pershad. 1972. Lactase deficiency in Indians. Am. J. Clin. Nutr. 25:114–119.

Rey, J., J. Schmitz, F. Rey, and J. Jos. 1971. Cellular differentiation and enzymatic deficits. Lancet 2:218.

Rosensweig, N. S. 1971. Adult lactase deficiency: Genetic control or adaptive response? Gastroenterology 60:464–467.

Rosensweig, N. S. 1974. Adaptive Effects of Dietary Sugars on Intestinal Disaccharidase Activity in Man. In Sugars in Nutrition, Sipple, H. L., and K. W. McNutt (Eds.), pp. 173–186. New York, Academic Press.

Rosensweig, N. S., and R. H. Herman. 1968. Control of jejunal sucrase and maltase activity by dietary sucrose or fructose in man: A model for the study of enzyme regulation in man. J. Clin. Invest. 47:2253–2262.

Rosensweig, N. S., and R. H. Herman. 1969a. Diet and disaccharidases. Am. J. Clin. Nutr. 22:99–102.

Rosensweig, N. S., and R. H. Herman. 1969b. Time response of jejunal sucrase and maltase activity to a high sucrose diet in normal man. Gastroenterology 56:500–505.

Rosensweig, N. S., and R. H. Herman. 1970. The dose response of jejunal sucrase and maltase activities to isocaloric high and low carbohydrate diets in man. Am. J. Clin. Nutr. 23:1273–1377.

Rosensweig, N. S., R. H. Herman, and F. B. Stifel. 1971. Dietary regulation of small intestinal enzyme activity in man. Am. J. Clin. Nutr. 24:65–69.

Rosensweig, N. S., R. H. Herman, F. B. Stifel, and Y. F. Herman. 1969. The regulation of human jejunal glycolytic enzymes by oral folic acid. J. Clin. Invest. 48:2038–2045.

Rosensweig, N. S., S. S. Huang, and T. M. Bayless. 1967. Transmission of lactose intolerance. Lancet 2:777.

Rotthauwe, H. W., M. O. El-Schallah, and G. Flatz, 1971a. Lactose intolerance in Arabs.

Rotthauwe, H. W., D. Emons, and G. Flatz, 1972a. Die Häufigkeit der Lactose-Intoleranz bei gesunden Erwachsenen in Deutschland. Dtsch. Med. Wschr. 97:376–380.

Rotthauwe, H. W., D. Emons, M. Kaeoplung, T. Tantachamroon, and G. Flatz. 1971b. Comparative study of intestinal disaccharidases in Thai and European subjects. Klin. Wschr. 49:503–504.

Rotthauwe, H. W., G. Flatz, D. Emons, and A. Heisig. 1972b. Trennung der intestinalen β-Galaktosidasen beim laktose-toleranten Erwachsenen durch Ultrazentrifugation im Dichtegradienten. Klin. Wschr. 50:258–259.

Rozen, P., and E. Shafrir. 1968. Behavior of serum free fatty acids and glucose during lactose tolerance tests. Isr. J. Med. Sci. 4:100–109.

Sahi, T. 1974a. Lactose malabsorption in Finnish-speaking and Swedish-speaking populations in Finland. Scand. J. Gastroenterol. 9:303–308.

Sahi, T. 1974b. The inheritance of selective adult-type lactose malabsorption. Scand. J. Gastroenterol. 9(Suppl. 30): 1–73.

Sahi, T., M. Isokoski, J. Jussila, and K. Launiala. 1972. Lactose malabsorption in Finnish children of school age. Acta Paediat. Scand. 61:11–16.

Sahi, T., M. Isokoski, J. Jussila, K. Launiala, and K. Pyörälä. 1973. Recessive inheritance of adult type lactose malabsorption. Lancet 2:823–826.

Sasaki, Y., M. Ilo, H. Kameda, H. Ueda, T. Aoyagi, N. L. Christopher, T. M. Bayless, and H. N. Wagner. 1970. Measurement of 14C-lactose absorption in the diagnosis of lactase deficiency. J. Lab. Clin. Med. 76:824–835.

Scheunert, A., and H. Sommer. 1956. Der Ernährungseffekt von Kohlenhydraten mit besonderer Berücksichtigung von Milchzucker und Galaktose. Biochem. Z. 327: 461–472.

Seetharam, B., and D. H. Alpers. 1976. Lactase deficiency maybe associated with an abnormal lactase protein? Gastroenterology 70:936.

Semenza, G., S. Auricchio, and A. Rubino. 1965. Multiplicity of human intestinal disaccharidases. I. Chromatographic separation of maltases and two lactases. Biochim. Biophys. Acta 96:487–497.

Semenza, G., H. J. Leese, V. Colombo, and H. Lorenz-Meyer. 1975. The Small Intestinal β-Glycosidase (Lactase-Glycosylceramidase) "Complex." In Modern Problems in Paediatrics, pp. 186–193. Basel, Karger.

Shatin, R. 1968. Evolution and lactase deficiency. Gastroenterology 54:992.

Sheehy, T. W., and P. R. Anderson. 1965. Disaccharidase activity in normal and diseased small bowel. Lancet 2:1–5.

Siddons, R. C. 1968. Carbohydrase activities in the bovine digestive tract. Biochem. J. 108:839–844.

Silverblatt, E. R., K. Conklin, and G. M. Gray. 1974. Sucrase precursor in human jejunal crypts. J. Clin. Invest. 53:76a.

Simoons, F. J. 1970. Primary adult lactose intolerance and the milking habit: A problem in biologic and cultural interrelations. II. A culture historical hypothesis. Am. J. Dig. Dis. 15:695–710.

Simoons, F. J. 1971. The antiquity of dairying in Asia and Africa. Geograph. Rev. 61: 431–439.

Simoons, F. J., 1973. New light on ethnic differences in adult lactose intolerance. Am. J. Dig. Dis. 18:595–611.

Sowers, M. F., and E. Winterfeldt. 1975. Lactose intolerance among Mexican Americans. Am. J. Clin. Nutr. 28:704–705.

Spanidou, E. L., and N. L. Petrakis. 1972. Lactose intolerance in Greeks. Lancet 2:872–873.

Sriratanaban, A., L. A. Symynkywicz, and W. R. Thayer, Jr. 1971. The effect of physiologic concentration of lactose on prevention of postweaning decline of intestinal lactase. Am. J. Dig. Dis. 16:839–844.

Stephenson, L. S. 1975. Lactose tolerance test as a predictor of milk intolerance. Am. J. Clin. Nutr. 28:86–88.

Stephenson, L. S., and M. C. Latham. 1974. Lactose intolerance and milk consumption: The relation of tolerance to symptoms. Am. J. Clin. Nutr. 27:296–303.

Stifel, F. B., R. H. Herman, and N. S. Rosensweig. 1969. Dietary regulation of glycolytic enzymes. IV. Differential hormonal effects in male and female rat jejunum. Biochim. Biophys. Acta 184:495–502.

Stifel, F. B., N. S. Rosensweig, D. Zakim, and R. H. Herman. 1968. Dietary regulation of glycolytic enzymes. I. Adaptive changes in rat jejunum. Biochim. Biophys. Acta 170:221–227.

Stoopler, M., W. Frayer, and M. H. Alderman, 1974. Prevalence and persistence of lactose malabsorption among young Jamaican children. Am. J. Clin. Nutr. 27:728.

Sunshine, P., and N. Kretchmer. 1964. Intestinal disaccharidases: Absence in two species of sea lions. Science 144:850–851.

Surjono, A., T. Sebodo, J. Sunarto, and P. Moemginah. 1973. Lactose intolerance among healthy adults. Paediat. Indones. 13:49–54.

Swaminathan, N., V. I. Mathian, S. J. Baker, and A. N. Radhakrishnan. 1970. Disaccharidase levels in jejunal biopsy specimens from American and South Indian control subjects and patients with tropical sprue. Clin. Chim. Acta 30:707–712.

Swaminathan, N., and A. N. Radhakrishnan. 1969. Studies on intestinal disaccharidases. III. Purification and properties of two lactase fractions from monkey small intestine. Indian J. Biochem. 6:101–105.

Troncale, F. J., G. T. Keusch, L. H. Miller, R. A. Olsson, and R. D. Buchanan. 1967. Normal absorption in Thai subjects with non-specific jejunal abnormalities. Brit. Med. J. 4:578–580.

Vaquez, C., H. Escobar, J. C. Vitoria, S. Carresco, and L. Suarez. 1976. Malabsorption of lactose in Spanish adults and children. Eur. Soc. Paediat. Gastroenterol. 9th Annual Meeting, Weimar (DDR).

Vazquez, G., J. J. Munoz-Conde, M. J. Guerrero, M. J. Garcia-Miguel, and L. Martin. 1976. Malabsorption of lactose in Spanish Gypsies. Eur. Soc. Paediat. Gastroenterol. 9th Annual Meeting, Weimar (DDR).

Welsh, J. D. 1970. Isolated lactase deficiency in humans: Report on 100 patients. Medicine 49:257–277.

Welsh, J. D., V. Rohrer, K. B. Knudsen, and F. F. Paustian. 1967. Isolated lactase deficiency. Correlation of laboratory studies and clinical data. Arch. Int. Med. 120: 261–269.

Welsh, J. D., O. M. Zschiesche, V. L. Willits, and L. Russel. 1968. Studies of lactose intolerance in families. Arch. Int. Med. 122:315–317.

Wen, C. P., I. Antonowicz, E. Tovar, R. B. McGandy, and S. N. Gershoff. 1973. Lactose feeding in lactose-intolerant monkeys. Am. J. Clin. Nutr. 26:1224–1228.

Yeh, K., and F. Moog. 1974. Intestinal lactase activity in the suckling rat: Influence of hypophysectomy and thyroidectomy. Science 183:77–79.

Zakim, D., R. H. Herman, N. S. Rosensweig, and F. B. Stifel. 1969. Clofibrate-induced changes in the activity of human intestinal enzymes. Gastroenterology 56:496–499.

Zografos, N., T. Kanaghinis, I. Hatzioannou, and C. Gardakis. 1973. Lactose intolerance in Greeks. Lancet 1:367.

6

Human Chromosome Heteromorphisms (Variants)

PATRICIA A. JACOBS

Department of Anatomy and Reproductive Biology,
University of Hawaii School of Medicine,
Honolulu, Hawaii

INTRODUCTION

Since the earliest days of the rebirth of human cytogenetics in the late 1950s, it has been recognized that morphologic differences exist between homologues of certain human chromosome pairs. These differences of morphology are without obvious clinical effect; they involve only heterochromatic chromosome regions; they are present in all cells of an individual; they are stable; and they are transmitted from parent to offspring in a Mendelian fashion. The advent of the various banding techniques in the 1970s has made possible a more precise definition of the variable or heteromorphic regions first noted on nonbanded preparations. In addition, many new heteromorphic regions not recognizable with conventional staining can now be resolved. Furthermore, the techniques of banding in conjunction with in situ hybridization are contributing to our understanding of the molecular architecture of the chromosome and the nature of the heteromorphic regions.

In the report of the Paris Conference (1971) on Standardization in Human Cytogenetics, it was recommended that the term "variant" be used in describing localized staining patterns which deviated from the norm of chromosome morphology. At that time eleven variable regions were recognized: ten on the autosomes and one on the Y chromosome. In the supplement to the Paris Conference (1975), the term "heteromorphic" was used to describe those chromosomes with variable bands and a system of nomenclature for describing heteromorphic bands was published. The descriptive terms "heteromorphic" and "heteromorphic chromosome" are used in this report; they seem preferable to the more commonly used terms "polymorphism" and "polymorphic chromosome," because they carry with them no implications with respect to frequency.

TYPES OF CHROMOSOME HETEROMORPHISMS

Heterochromatin, used in the most general sense, is associated with staining properties different from euchromatin. Constitutive heterochromatin is composed of moderately or highly repetitive DNA located in specific sites on the chromosome, and it is this type of heterochromatin that is associated with visible chromosome heteromorphisms.

Initially, using nonbanding techniques, it was observed that the chromatids of the proximal region of one arm of chromosome 1, 16, and one C group chromosome (subsequently shown to be number 9)

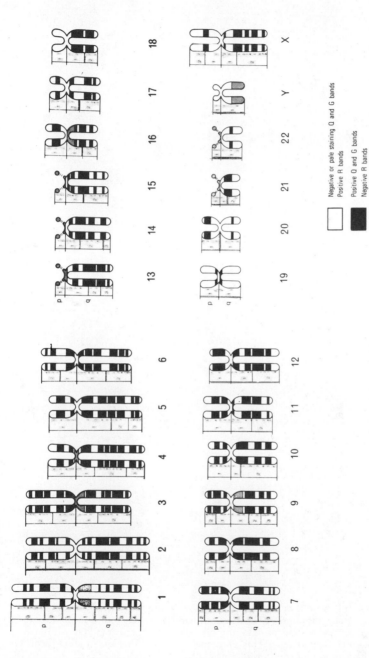

Figure 1. A diagram of the human chromosomes to show the position of the bands demonstrable by the Q, G, and R staining methods. The designation of each chromosome, chromosome arm, and band is by the internationally agreed "Paris Nomenclature." (Reproduced from Standardization in Human Cytogenetics. In Paris Conference Report, 1971, Bergsma D. (ed). White Plains, The National Foundation–March of Dimes, BD:OAS, VIII(7), 1972.)

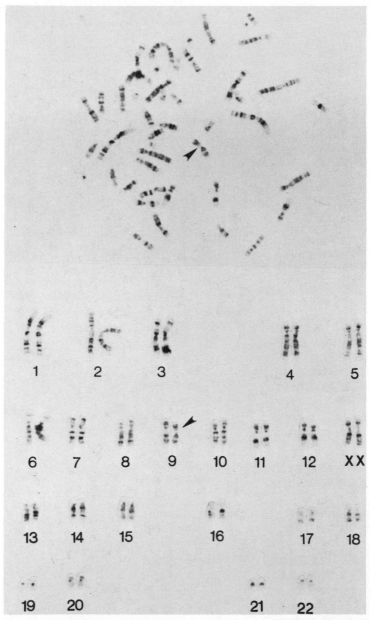

Figure 2. A cell from a female stained by the G-banding technique. There is a heteromorphism of chromosome 9. The variable band normally found in position q12 on the long arm is on the short arm, giving one chromosome 9 (marked with arrow) an almost metacentric appearance. This chromosome 9 was present in all cells of the individual and had been inherited from her father.

and the distal part of the Y chromosome frequently appeared thinner and were more palely stained than the rest of the chromosomes. Conventional staining techniques also demonstrated the presence of satellites on the ends of the short arms of many acrocentric chromosomes and showed that the short arms themselves, satellites, and satellite stalks were all heterochromatic. With the application of the various banding techniques it has been shown that every human chromosome contains one or more regions of constitutive heterochromatin usually associated with the centromeric region of the chromosome or the short arm of the acrocentric chromosomes (Fig. 1). The degree of variability in the extent and/or position of such heterochromatic areas forms the basis of the "normal" morphologic variation between homologous chromosomes (Fig. 2). In addition to varying in both size and position, heterochromatin from different locations can differ in appearance, depending on the type of cytologic technique employed. These dissimilarities presumably reflect differences in the composition of the underlying DNA and associated proteins (Evans, 1973). The major heteromorphic areas in the human chromosome complement, together with their staining properties and the type of DNA of which they are composed, are summarized in Table 1.

Numerous cytologic techniques can be used to demonstrate banding, each of which has its own particular advantages and disadvantages. The most common techniques used to demonstrate the basic banding patterns of the chromosomes are Q, G, and R banding. The first of these techniques employs the fluorochrome quinacrine mustard or quinacrine dihydrochloride as a stain, whereas the latter two involve pretreatment and subsequent Giemsa staining. All show the same basic pattern of bands (see Fig. 2), but the bands that stain brightly with Q-banding and darkly with G-banding appear pale with R-banding. The most commonly used techniques to demonstrate heteromorphisms are C-banding, in which the chromosomes undergo a very drastic pretreatment and are subsequently Giemsa stained, which stains most of the heterochromatin darkly (Fig. 3), and Q-banding, in which some heterochromatin fluoresces brilliantly, whereas some appears virtually unstained.

There are at least two major categories of constitutive heterochromatin — one composed of highly repetitive DNA, and one composed of moderately repetitive DNA. In man there are at least four main species of highly repetitive, simple sequence DNA, or satellite DNA, which have been isolated and characterized. Most evidence suggests that these DNAs are not transcribed, and in situ hybridization has shown that they are localized in the heterochromatin stained darkly by C-banding (Arrighi and Hsu, 1971), each satel-

Table 1. Some Properties of the Major Heteromorphic Bands of Human Chromosomes

Band No.	Staining Properties			Type of DNA
	C-Banding	Q-Banding	Lateral Asymmetry	
1q12	Dark	Negative	Simple or compound	Highly repetitive; major site of Sat II; also site of Sat I, III, and IV
3q12	Dark	Variable, brilliant→ med.	—	Highly repetitive
4cen	Dark	Variable, brilliant→ med.	—	Highly repetitive
9q12	Dark	Negative	Usually appears symmetrical; ?complex	Highly repetitive; major site of Sat I, II, III, and IV
13cen	Dark	Variable, brilliant→ med.	—	}Highly repetitive; site of Sat I, III, and IV
13p11	Variable	Variable, usually med.	—	
13p12	Variable, usually pale	Negative	—	Nucleolar organizing
13p13	Variable	Variable, brilliant→ pale	—	?Highly repetitive; nucleolar organizing
14p11	Variable	Variable, usually med.	—	Highly repetitive; site of Sat I, II, III, and IV
14p12	Variable, usually pale	Negative	—	Nucleolar organizing
14p13	Variable	Variable, brilliant→ pale	—	?Highly repetitive; nucleolar organizing
15p11	Variable	Variable, usually med	Simple	Highly repetitive; site of Sat I, II, III, and IV
15p12	Variable, usually pale	Negative	—	Nucleolar organizing
15p13	Variable	Variable, brilliant→ pale	—	?Highly repetitive; nucleolar organizing
16q11	Dark	Negative	Simple	Highly repetitive; site of Sat II
21p11	Variable	Variable, usually med.	—	Highly repetitive; site of Sat I, II, III, and IV
21p12	Variable, usually pale	Negative	—	Nucleolar organizing
21p13	Variable	Variable, brilliant→ pale	—	?Highly repetitive; nucleolar organizing
22p11	Variable	Variable, usually med.	—	Highly repetitive; site of Sat I, II, III, and IV
22p12	Variable, usually pale	Negative	—	Nucleolar organizing
22p13	Variable	Variable, brilliant→ pale	—	?Highly repetitive; nucleolar organizing
Yq12	Dark	Brilliant	Simple	High repetitive; major site of Sat I, II, III, and IV

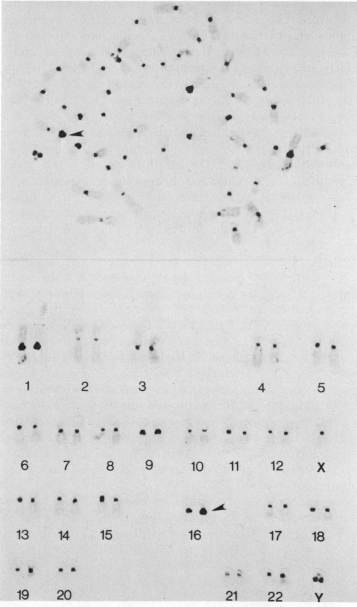

Figure 3. A cell from a male stained by the C-banding technique. The heterochromatin at the centromere of all 22 pairs of autosomes and the X and on the long arm of the Y appears darkly staining. The variability in the size of the centromeric heterochromatin from different chromosomes is clearly seen, that in chromosomes 1, 9, and 16 being particularly large. There is a pronounced heteromorphism in chromosome pair 16, one member of the pair having a very large heterochromatic band.

lite species having a characteristic distribution (Gosden et al., 1975). Darkly staining C-bands are demonstrable at the centromere of all the chromosomes except the Y, the Y having a dark band on the distal part of the long arm (Fig. 3). Chromosomes 1, 9, and 16 tend to have particularly large areas of chromatin at or very near the centromere, usually associated with the proximal region of the long arm. Occasionally such heterochromatic regions may be inverted and thus appear wholly or partly in the proximal part of the short arm. The short arms of the acrocentric chromosomes consist of three heterochromatic bands whose exact morphology is often rather hard to determine using C-banding. The satellite stalk is usually pale and is probably the site of the moderately repetitive nucleolar organizing DNA, whereas the short arms and satellites themselves may be medium or darkly stained, their appearance being constant in any one chromosome from a particular individual, but variable from person to person.

The heterochromatin stained darkly by the C-banding technique can be further resolved into at least two separate classes based on its appearance when the chromosomes are stained with the fluorochrome quinacrine mustard or quinacrine dihydrochloride (Caspersson et al., 1971). Using this dye, certain regions stained by C-banding may appear very brilliantly fluorescent, most notably the distal part of the Y chromosome, the centromeric regions of chromosomes 3, 4, and 13, and the short arms and satellites of at least some of the acrocentric chromsomes, whereas other regions, notably the large heterochromatic band on chromosomes 1, 9, and 16 and the satellite stalks, always appear nonfluorescent. The difference between the repetitive DNA which fluoresces brightly and that which does not fluoresce is not well understood, although it is thought to be a reflection of the number and distribution of the A-T base pairs in the DNA duplex (Weisblum, 1973).

Another technique, which differentiates between certain types of heterochromatin that stain darkly by C-banding, depends on the phenomenon of lateral asymmetry first described by Lin and his colleagues (1974). In this technique BrdU is substituted for thymine for a single DNA replication. Areas of the chromosome rich in BrdU can be visually differentiated after suitable treatment (Latt, 1973), and thus any marked asymmetry in the distribution of thymine, and therefore of substituted BrdU, between the single strands of the DNA duplex can be identified in chromatids at the first metaphase following BrdU substitution. Angell and Jacobs (1975) showed that the C-band heterochromatin of chromosomes 1, 15, 16, and the Y always showed lateral asymmetry, suggesting that it was composed of a class of repetitive DNA with marked sister strand asymmetry in distribution of thymine.

The second category of constitutive heterochromatin, that composed of moderately repetitive DNA, is present on the acrocentric chromosomes. The short arms of all five pairs of human acrocentric chromosomes have been shown to be the sites of genes coding for 18S and 28S ribosomal RNA (rRNA) (Henderson et al., 1972; Evans et al., 1974). Although there is still some uncertainty as to whether these genes are associated with satellite stalks and/or the satellites themselves, the weight of evidence suggests the satellite stalks as the major sites. It has been estimated that approximately 440 copies of the rRNA genes are distributed among the human acrocentric chromosomes (Bross and Krone, 1972). The exact relationship between the number of rRNA genes on a particular chromosome, the size of the heterochromatic region containing them, and the functional activity of the region remains to be defined. This class of constitutive heterochromatin differs from the heterochromatin composed of highly repetitive single sequence DNA in being actively transcribed.

CLASSIFICATION OF HETEROMORPHIC CHROMOSOMES

The differences between heteromorphic bands can be of size, position, staining intensity, or any combination of these variables. Unfortunately most of the variation is near the limits of resolution of the light microscope and therefore extremely difficult to quantify objectively. In the majority of studies of heteromorphisms the classification has been based on estimation rather than mensuration. More objective techniques are desirable; but on the few occasions when mensuration has been attempted, the methods have proved lengthy and have required the use of sophisticated image processing devices (Mason et al., 1975; Zimmerman and Johnston, 1976). Such methods are only in the developmental stage at present and cannot be used on a day-to-day basis in the laboratory.

The difficulty of measuring or estimating the size or staining ability of heteromorphic bands is compounded by the fact that their appearance is affected by the quality of the preparation and other technical variables, some of which are not easily controlled by the laboratory (Lubs et al., 1976). Furthermore, both to the human observer and to machines at their present level of sophistication, there usually appears to be a continuous gradation both in size and, for many Q-banded heteromorphisms, in staining intensity. Therefore any attempt at classification entails the adoption of some arbitrary scale. However, discrete bands can sometimes be observed within certain heteromorphic areas, especially those on chromosome 1 and the Y chromosome. Drets and Seuanez (1974) reported finding from one to five C-bands in the heteromorphic area of eight individuals with different-sized Y chromosomes, the number of bands being related to the size of the Y.

Although methods based on estimation rather than mensuration are of considerable utility if scored in a blind fashion and used for intralaboratory comparisons, they are of very limited use in comparisons between studies from different laboratories. The exceptions to this generalization are heteromorphisms involving alterations of position rather than alterations of size or staining characteristics. For example, there is a fairly common heteromorphism of chromosome 9 in which the entire darkly staining C-band appears on the short rather than the long arm. Provided that the same staining techniques are used for scoring this type of variation, there seems no reason why results from different laboratories and different populations should not be directly comparable.

FREQUENCIES OF HETEROMORPHISMS IN NORMAL POPULATIONS

In the majority of publications dealing with the frequency of heteromorphisms, the size or staining capacity of the variable bands has been estimated rather than measured. Therefore for the reasons given above, comparisons between different studies must be made with the greatest caution. The results of surveys of normal populations with respect to the frequencies of Q-banding intensity variations are shown in Table 2, and the frequency of variations in both size and position of C-bands is shown in Table 3.

As can be seen from Table 2, there are very wide variations among the various studies in the proportion of chromosomes having a brilliant or intensely fluorescent heteromorphism. This is seen most dramatically for chromosome 4, in which the proportion of chromosomes with a bright band at the centromere ranges from 2.7 to 48.3 percent, both figures being derived from largely Caucasian, Western European populations. It seems probable that the vast majority of the reported variation is due to differences of scoring technique rather than real differences between populations, although the latter possibility cannot be entirely discounted. If the different results of the various surveys were due largely to observers selecting

Table 2. Percentage of Brilliant or Intense Q-Band Heteromorphisms in Normal Individuals

Reference	Population	No. Studied	3q11	4cen	13 cen+p11	13 p13	14 p11	14 p13	15 p11	15 p13	21 p11	21 p13	22 p11	22 p13
Geraedts and Pearson (1974)	Normal individuals, Holland	221	48.4	2.7	50.0		14.3		21.5		24.4		21.9	
McKenzie and Lubs (1975)	Normal newborn babies, U.S.A.—Colorado	77	40.9	40.9	44.2	2.6	0	4.6	0	1.3	0	2.6	7.1	1.9
Mikelsaar et al. (1975)	Normal adults, U.S.S.R.—Estonia	208	65.0	27.8	84.4	4.1	0	9.8	0	6.2	0	8.0	35.9	8.0
Müller et al. (1975)	Newborn babies, U.S.A.—New York City	376	55.3	13.1	73.6	8.2	2.5	13.4	2.6	11.0	2.6	17.0	34.3	28.0
Buckton et al. (1976)	Newborn babies, U.K.—Edinburgh	482	64.9	48.3	38.0	8.8	0	10.3	0	12.5	0.7	9.6	3.0	15.0
Buckton et al. (1976)	14-year-old children, U.K.—Edinburgh	109	68.4	33.5	29.8	7.8	0	13.3	0	10.5	0.5	16.0	1.8	13.3
Lin et al. (1976)	Newborn babies, Canada—Ontario	930	55.0	14.0	31.0	1.9	0.8	0.2	0.1	0.9	0.1	1.1	0.3	0.3

Table 3. Percentage of Large, Small, and Inverted C-Band Heteromorphisms in Normal Individuals

Reference	Population	No. Studied	1q12				9q12				16q11			
			+	−	Partial Inv	Total Inv	+	−	Partial Inv	Total Inv	+	−	Partial Inv	Total Inv
Craig-Holmes et al. (1973)	Normal adults, U.S.A.	20	2.5	10.0	0	0	5.0	7.5	0	2.5	0	17.5	0	0
Tüür et al. (1974)	Normal adults, U.S.S.R. – Estonia	208	0.7	−	0	0.2	−	−	−	−	−	−	−	−
McKenzie and Lubs (1975)	Normal newborn babies, U.S.A. – Colorado	77	3.9	4.5	0	0	7.1	4.5		3.9	5.2	11.7	0	0
Müller et al. (1975)	Newborn babies, U.S.A. – New York City	376	8.1	0.6	1.6	0	8.0	0.4	10.7	0.6	6.5	23.6	1.4	0
Buckton et al. (1976)	Newborn babies, U.K. – Edinburgh	467	3	4.1	1.4	0	2.2	4.8	3.7	0.7	2.1	2.2	0	0
Buckton et al. (1976)	14-year-old children U.K. – Edinburgh	101	5.4	2.5	0.5	0	3.5	6.4	1.0	1.0	4.9	4.9	0	0
Ghosh and Singh (1976)	Normal individuals India	30	10.0	1.7	0	0	8.3	6.7	0	3.3	5.0	8.3	0	0

Heteromorphic Chromosome

different levels of fluorescent intensity to record as brilliant or intense, a more realistic comparison between studies would be obtained by comparing the relative rather than the absolute frequencies of different heteromorphisms. If chromosome number 4 is ignored, there is a reasonable measure of agreement among the surveys. All find chromosomes 3 and 13 to be the ones in which a bright heteromorphic band is most frequently seen, and all find the presence of brightly fluorescing material on the short arms of chromosomes 14, 15, and 21 to be a very rare occurrence.

The C-band heteromorphisms recorded in Table 3 show less variation among the surveys than the Q-band heteromorphisms. In each survey between 1 and 10 percent of chromosomes 1 and 9 are considered to have a large C-band and approximately the same proportion to have a small C-band. In chromosome 16 about 5 percent of the C-bands are considered to be large, whereas there is a greater range among the small C-bands on chromosome 16, from 2 percent in one survey to 24 percent in another. Again it is difficult to determine how much of this variation is real and how much due to technical factors.

With respect to the position variations, it appears that the total inversion of the C-band heteromorphism on chromosome 9 is a much more frequently occurring heteromorphism than the total inversion of the C-band on chromosomes 1 or 16. However, total inversions may be more difficult to detect on chromosomes 1 and 16 than on chromosome 9, because a transfer of chromosome material from the long to the short arm will not result in a dramatic change in chromosome morphology as seen by C-banding. Partial inversions can range in size from those having a very small amount of darkly staining material on the short arm, which may be confused with normal, to those having almost all the darkly staining material on the short arm, which may be confused with total inversions. Therefore unless the preparations are of comparable quality and the criteria for scoring partial inversions explicitly stated, it is difficult to compare results from different surveys.

It should be emphasized that the C-band heteromorphisms recorded in Table 3 are only the most frequently occurring and the most obvious ones. All C-bands appear to be heteromorphic. The variation in many of them is usually quite subtle, but can be striking as shown in Figure 4 and in the reports of a heteromorphic chromosome 19 by Crossen (1975) and of heteromorphic chromosomes 6 and 12 by Sofuni et al. (1974).

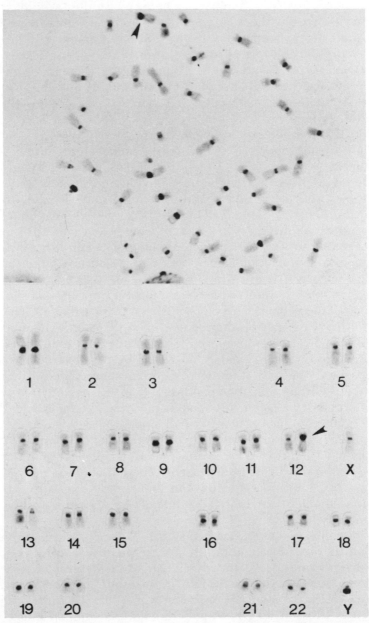

Figure 4. A cell from a male stained by the C-banding technique. One chromosome 12 has an unusually large heterochromatic band on the short arm. This chromosome was present in all cells of the individual and had been inherited from his father.

RACIAL VARIATION

Because of the difficulties of objectively assessing human heteromorphisms, comparisons between the results of different laboratories in which variations are attributed to the different ethnic backgrounds of the populations studied cannot be taken seriously at this time. However, differences in the frequency or types of chromosome heteromorphisms among ethnic groups, if demonstrated in an intra-laboratory study in which the scoring has been done blind, most probably reflect true differences among populations.

The first reported racial or ethnic differences in a chromosome heteromorphism was that of Cohen et al. (1966), who measured the Y chromosome of males from five ethnic groups and found the length of the Y of Japanese males to be significantly greater than that of males of the other four groups, whereas that of the non-Jewish Caucasians was significantly lower than that of the Japanese, Jews, and Negroes but not of the American Indians. In 1973 Angell reported finding the Y in Australian aborigines to be significantly smaller than that in Caucasians, and in 1975 Ghosh and Singh reported that the length of the Y chromosome from two Indian populations, the Rajputs and the Punjabis, differed—that of the Rajputs being significantly longer. Studies using quinacrine-stained chromosomes have shown that the variation in length of the Y chromosome is due entirely to differences in length of the brightly fluorescent heterochromatic distal segment, the remainder of the chromosome being the same length in all normal males (Bobrow et al., 1971).

Starkman and Shaw (1967) reported data which suggest that Negroes have a greater numer of acrocentric chromosomes with long short arms than a comparable group of Caucasians. Lubs and Ruddle (1971) reported findings on chromosome heteromorphisms detected by nonbanding techniques in 4366 consecutive neonates. They detected a metacentric C-group chromosome (probably a total inversion of the heterochromatic region of chromosome 9) in only two of 3176 Caucasians but in ten of 807 Negro babies. Furthermore, they found the frequency of long short arms and of large satellites in both the D and G group chromosomes and of a large chromosome 16 to be significantly greater in Negro than in White babies.

Lubs and his colleagues (1976) reported observations on heteromorphisms in a population of 200 White and 200 Black 7-year-old schoolchildren. They found significantly increased numbers of brightly fluorescing heteromorphisms among the Negroes for chromosome 3, for both the centromere and satellites of chromosome 13, and for the satellites of chromosome 22, whereas only in chromosome 4 were bright heteromorphisms more frequent in White than in Black children. Among the C-band heteromorphisms there were no significant differences between the races for extreme variations in size of chromosome 1, 9, or 16, although there was a significant increase of partial inversions of chromosome 1 in the Caucasians and of complete inversions of the C-band of chromosome 9 in the Negroes. This latter finding is in agreement with the earlier report (Lubs and Ruddle, 1971) of an increased frequency of a metacentric C group chromosome in Black newborn babies.

It seems clear, from the few reports in which individuals of different groups have been compared in a blind laboratory study, that there is considerable variation in chromosome heteromorphisms among different racial groups. Further investigation of this phenomenon would give valuable information on the origin, migration, and kinship of different ethnic groups.

CLINICAL SIGNIFICANCE

Numerous reports in the literature claim an association or a possible association between one or more particular heteromorphisms and clinical anomaly. However, the majority of these do not withstand critical examination, because the chromosomes of the patients were not examined in a blind fashion together with suitably matched normal controls. The majority of reports in which the methodology incorporated a blind controlled study show no convincing evidence of a phenotypic effect for any of the heteromorphisms examined. Thus Lubs and his colleagues (1976) studied both fluorescent and C-band heteromorphisms in a matched sample of children with IQ's above and below 85. They found no significant difference in frequency or type of any heteromorphism between the two groups. Schwinger and Wild (1974) and Benezech et al. (1976), in carefully controlled studies, were unable to confirm the finding of Nielsen and Friedrich (1972) that the Y chromosome was longer in criminal than noncriminal males.

However, in a few instances suggestive evidence for a possible phenotypic effect of a heteromorphism has been reported. Lubs and Ruddle (1970) found a four-fold increase in giant satellites in a G group chromosome in children who had a major congenital anomaly detected at birth by comparison with those who did not.

In a number of reports it is suggested that, although the presence of an extreme heteromorphism does not affect the phenotype of its carrier, it may predispose the carrier to produce children with chromosome abnormalities. Thus Nielsen and his colleagues (1974c) suggested that the frequency of the 9qh+ variant was significantly higher in the parents of children with major chromosome anomalies than in a random sample of newborn babies, whereas Bott and his colleagues (1975) claim to find an astonishingly high frequency of heteromorphisms in the parents of Down's syndrome patients by comparison with controls.

Finally, Jacobs and her colleagues (1975), in the analysis of reproductive fitness of individuals carrying an extreme variant chromosome detectable by nonbanding techniques, found both male and female carriers to have a lowered fertility by comparison with their first degree relatives who did not carry the variant.

The weight of evidence at this time suggests that there is no obvious phenotypic effect associated with any chromosome heteromorphism. However, some variants may have an effect on the reproductive capacity of their carriers, either by increasing their probability of having a chromosomally abnormal offspring or by lowering their fertility. The evidence for the latter suggestions is far from conclusive, and further carefully controlled studies will be necessary to test their validity.

GENETIC ANALYSIS

The classification of the majority of heteromorphisms is difficult, because it consists of more or less subjectively dividing an apparently continuous variation of size and/or brightness into categories. The difficulty of this is compounded by the fact that the variation is itself affected by a variety of technical factors (Lubs et al., 1976). Therefore at the present state of the art of classifying heteromorphisms, it seems premature to attempt to survey populations with respect to their heteromorphic chromosomes and then to test the results against Hardy-Weinberg expectations as if the factors being tested were discrete, recognizable entities. Some authors have attempted such an analysis (Müller et al., 1975), but it is difficult to take seriously the claims of different distributions of heteromorphisms between males and females (Mikelsaar et al., 1973) or failure of the data to fit Hardy-Weinberg equilibrium (Geraedts and Pearson, 1974).

However, the situation is quite different when we consider pedigree analysis, especially when the segregating heteromorphisms are at the extreme ends of the range. Such heteromorphisms are easy to see and are comparatively rare. Therefore they can be recognized by visual examination with great accuracy. In this situation formal segregation analysis and study of mutation rates are as valid as comparable studies of dominant genes with complete penetrance. In spite of this, little formal analysis of the segregation or mutation rate of heteromorphic chromosomes has been attempted. There are many reports of families in which an extreme heteromorphism is segregating, the majority being of single families studied to determine whether the unusual heteromorphism detected in the clinically abnormal proband is present in other family members and/or to test for linkage. In virtually all the reports, irrespective of the method of ascertainment, the heteromorphism has been found to be inherited, its segregation following simple Mendelian expectations with the trait being passed on to half the offspring of known carriers. A possible exception to simple Mendelian inheritance may be present in some kindreds in which a chromosome 9 with a very large C-band is segregating (Fitzgerald, 1973; Robinson et al., 1976). In these families there seems to be an excess of carriers, a nonsignificant excess if each family is considered separately but significant when data from all families are combined. However, the evidence that the 9qh+ chromosome may be preferentially segregating is based on small numbers of families and individuals, some of whom may have been selectively reported because of the unusual segregation. Hence, although the evidence is suggestive, it is obviously inconclusive.

The question of the origin or mutation rate for heteromorphisms is at present unanswered. In the vast majority of reports, the heteromorphism is familial and, when present, appears to be identical in all family members (de la Chapelle, 1974; Halbrecht and Shabtay, 1976). There are a few reports of individuals with a well-defined chromosome heteromorphism that was not present in the parents (Nielsen et al., 1974a, b). Unfortunately there is rarely any attempt to verify paternity in these apparent mutants, and, although some may well be a result of de novo mutation, there is no way of estimating the mutation rate from this type of anecdotal reporting.

However, in a small number of reports the segregation and mutation rates of chromosome heteromorphisms have been studied in a systematic way. Craig-Holmes and her colleagues (1975) published a study of familial patterns of C-band heteromorphisms in five pedigrees comprising ten segregating sibships. They found 99 variants in the ten sibships, of which 85 appeared to be transmitted unchanged from parent to child and 14 were not. They suggested that the alterations found in transmission were due to mutational events involving unequal crossing over at meiosis. Furthermore, they thought that mosaicism for C-band heteromorphisms was present in the population and believed it to result from somatic crossing over between homologues. If these results are confirmed, it would suggest an astonishingly high mutation rate for C-band heteromorphisms.

Jacobs and her colleagues (1975) reported on the reproductive fitness of individuals having a structural chromosome abnormality or pronounced heteromorphism detected using nonbanding techniques. They studied 31 kindreds in the latter category having a total of 275 sibships. Their data on these families showed the segregation frequency of the heteromorphic chromosome to be 0.447 ± 0.039, a figure not statistically different from the expected frequency of 0.5, and they found not a single individual who was a mutant for the heteromorphism being studied.

Robinson and her coworkers (1976) published an investigation of the segregation of chromosome heteromorphisms detected by Q- and C-banding in 32 families. They found that the segregation of inversions for C-band heteromorphisms followed a simple Mendelian pattern, in agreement with the previous report of Madan and Bobrow (1974). They also found the great majority of C-band size variants to follow a Mendelian distribution and considered the majority of the exceptions to be more likely the result of technical artifacts than of abnormal segregation, although they thought that chromosome 9qh+ might show preferential segregation. There appears to be an excess of brilliant variants among the fluorescent heteromorphisms, but this was significant only at the 5 percent level and only if the results from all chromosomes were summed. The authors are inclined to the view that the results are artifacts caused by a combination of a small amount of data and scoring error. In no family was a fluorescent or C-band heteromorphism found which was not present in one or the other of the parents.

At present it is clear that there are many unanswered questions concerning the segregation and mutation rate of chromosome heteromorphisms in man. It appears that the vast majority of heteromorphisms, with the possible exception of a large C-band on chromosome 9, segregate in a simple Mendelian fashion. There are virtually no adequate data on mutation rates. Craig-Holmes and her colleagues (1975) reported an extremely high mutation rate, while two studies from Edinburgh (Jacobs et al., 1975; Robinson et al., 1976) fail to find a single mutant individual in a relatively large number of sibships. If the population is at equilibrium with respect to chromosome heteromorphisms, this latter finding is at variance with the report of the reduced reproductive fitness among carriers of at least certain types of heteromorphisms. Jacobs et al. (1975), in an attempt to reconcile these two apparently conflicting observations, suggested that "new heteromorphisms" may only rarely arise as a single step event in a "normal" gamete, but probably arise most frequently as a series of very small changes, each one below our current level of resolution. More data, collected in as unbiased a way as is practicable, are needed on the inheritance patterns of chromosome heteromorphisms. In time such data should help elucidate the mechanism of origin and the clinical and evolutionary significance of chromosome heteromorphisms in our species.

USES OF CHROMOSOME HETEROMORPHISMS

Chromosome heteromorphisms, especially the more unusual and extreme variations, are very useful characters for identifying chromosomes, cells, and individuals. Their use as a marker depends on the fact that they are inherited, are stable, and are presumed to have a low mutation rate. Cytogenetic heteromorphisms have been used extensively in the past few years in linkage studies. Indeed, the first assignment of a gene to an autosome in man, that of the Duffy blood group to chromosome 1, was made by showing that the Duffy blood group gene and a large heteromorphic region on chromosome 1 were linked (Donahue et al., 1968). Subsequently a number of genes and linkage groups have been assigned to specific chromosomes by the study of families in which obvious heteromorphisms were segregating (Magenis et al., 1970).

Since the great majority of chromosome heteromorphisms are situated at or near the centromere, they are minimally affected by crossing over and therefore are extremely good markers for tracing the origin of chromosome aberrations involving the heteromorphic chromosomes. There are numerous reports in which heteromorphisms have been used to trace the origin of the extra chromosome in Down's syndrome (Robinson, 1973; Mikkelsen et al., 1976), to trace the origin of a mutational event giving rise to chromosome structural rearrangement (Jacobs et al., 1974), and to trace the origin of the extra set of chromosomes in triploid fetuses (Lauritsen, 1976). However, care must be exercised in attempting this type of analysis, because information is more readily obtained for certain mechanisms of origin than for others. This may give rise to a serious bias unless the information from all analyzed matings is reported. Methodology for analyzing the origin of additional chromosomes by the use of heteromorphisms has recently been discussed by Langenbeck et al. (1976) and Jacobs and Morton (1977).

The distribution of heteromorphisms is an excellent discriminator between the cells of one individual and those of another. In this way heteromorphisms have been used to establish paternity (de la Chapelle et al., 1967) and to distinguish maternal from fetal cells in cultures of amniotic fluid (Hauge et al., 1975).

SUMMARY

The study of heteromorphisms in the chromosomes of man has been given an enormous impetus by the development of banding techniques. However, heteromorphisms are difficult to quantify objectively, and their appearance is affected by a large number of technical variables. Therefore great caution must be exercised before claiming a phenotypic effect for a heteromorphism and in comparing results from different laboratories, or from the same laboratory if the scoring was not done in a blind fashion.

There is clear evidence that the distribution of at least some heteromorphisms is different in different racial groups, but there is no convincing evidence at present that chromosome heteromorphisms have any obvious phenotypic effect. However, there is some suggestion that the extreme variants may lower the reproductive fitness of their carriers.

The segregation of human heteromorphisms, with the possible exception of a large heteromorphism on chromosome 9, follows a simple Mendelian distribution. The mechanism of origin of heteromorphisms is not understood, and the data on mutation rates are few and conflicting, although the weight of evidence suggests a very low occurrence of de novo heteromorphisms.

In spite of the difficulties of objectively classifying heteromorphisms, they are invaluable as chromosome markers. They have been used in linkage studies, in determining the origin of chromosome abnormalities, in establishing paternity, and in determining the origin of cells in tissue culture. When objective methods of mensuration are available, heteromorphisms will take their place alongside conventional blood group and enzyme polymorphisms as tools in formal and population cytogenetics.

References

Angell, R. 1973. The Chromosomes of Australian Aborigines. In The Human Biology of Aborigines in Cape York, Kirk, R. L. (Ed.). Canberra, Australian Institute of Aboriginal Studies.

Angell, R. R., and P. A. Jacobs. 1975. Lateral asymmetry in human constitutive heterochromatin. Chromosoma 51:301–310.

Arrighi, F. E., and T. C. Hsu. 1971. Localization of heterochromatin in human chromosomes. Cytogenetics 10:81–86.

Benezech, M., B. Nöel, E. Travers, and J. Mottet. 1976. Antisocial behaviour and variations in length of Y chromosome. Hum. Genet. 32:77–80.

Bobrow, M., P. L. Pearson, M. C. Pike, and O. S. El-Alfi. 1971. Length variation in the quinacrine-binding segment of human Y chromosomes of different sizes. Cytogenetics 10:190–198.

Bott, C. E., G. S. Sekhon, and H. A. Lubs. 1975. Unexpectedly high frequency of paternal origin of trisomy 21. Am. J. Hum. Genet. 27: Abs. Am. Soc. Hum. Genet. #20A.

Bross, K., and W. Krone. 1972. On the number of ribosomal RNA genes in man. Humangenetik 14:137–141.

Buckton, K. E., M. L. O'Riordan, P. A. Jacobs, J. A. Robinson, R. Hill, and H. J. Evans. 1976. C- and Q-band polymorphisms in the chromosomes of three human populations. Ann. Hum. Genet. 40:99–112.

Caspersson, T., G. Lomakka, and L. Zech. 1971. The 24 fluorescence patterns of the human metaphase chromosomes – distinguishing characters and variability. Hereditas 67:89–102.

Cohen, M. M., M. W. Shaw, and J. W. MacCluer. 1966. Racial differences in the length of the human Y chromosome. Cytogenetics 5:34–52.

Craig-Holmes, A. P., F. B. Moore, and M. W. Shaw. 1973. Polymorphism of human C-band heterochromatin. I. Frequency of variants. Am. J. Hum. Genet. 25:181–192.

Craig-Holmes, A. P., F. B. Moore, and M. W. Shaw. 1975. Polymorphism of human C-band heterochromatin. II. Family studies with suggestive evidence of somatic crossing over. Am. J. Hum. Genet. 27:178–189.

Crossen, P. E. 1975. Variation in the centromeric banding of chromosome 19. Clin. Genet. 8:218–222.

de la Chapelle, A., J. Fellman, and V. Unnerus. 1967. Determination of human paternity from the length of the Y chromosome. Ann. Genet. 10:60–64.

de la Chapelle, A., J. Schroder, K. Stenstrand, J. Fellman, R. Herva, M. Saarni, I. Anttolainen, I. Tallila, L. Tervila, L. Husa, G. Tallqvist, E. B. Robson, P. J. L. Cook, and R. Sanger. 1974. Pericentric inversions of human chromosomes 9 and 10. Am. J. Hum. Genet. 26:746–766.

Donahue, R. P., W. B. Bias, J. H. Renwick, and V. A. McKusick. 1968. Probable assignment of the Duffy blood group locus to chromosome 1 in man. Proc. Nat. Acad. Sci. 61:949–955.

Drets, M. E., and H. Seuanez. 1974. Quantitation of Human Heterochromatin. In Physiology and Genetics of Reproduction, Coutinho, E. M., and F. Fuchs (Eds.), Part A, pp. 29–52. New York, Plenum Press.

Evans, H. J. 1973. Molecular architecture of human chromosomes. Brit. Med. Bull. 29:196–202.

Evans, H. J., R. A. Buckland, and M. L. Pardue. 1974. Location of the genes coding for 18S and 28S ribosomal RNA in the human genome. Chromosoma 48:405–426.

Fitzgerald, P. H. 1973. The nature and inheritance of an elongated secondary constriction on chromosome 9 of man. Cytogenet. Cell Genet. 12:404–413.

Geraedts, J. P. M., and P. L. Pearson. 1974. Fluorescent chromosome polymorphisms: Frequencies and segregations in a Dutch population. Clin. Genet. 6:247–257.

Ghosh, P. K., and I. P. Singh. 1975. Morphological variability of the human chromosomes in two Indian populations – Rajputs and Punjabis. Humangenetik 29:67–78.

Ghosh, P. K., and I. P. Singh. 1976. Morphologic variability of human chromosomes: Polymorphism of constitutive heterochromatin. Hum. Genet. 32:149–154.

Gosden, J. R., A. R. Mitchell, R. A. Buckland, R. P. Clayton, and H. J. Evans. 1975. The location of four human satellite DNAs on human chromosomes. Exp. Cell Res. 92:148–158.

Halbrecht, I., and F. Shabtay. 1976. Human chromosome polymorphism and congenital malformations. Clin. Genet. 10:113–122.

Hauge, M., H. Poulsen, A. Halberg, and M. Mikkelsen. 1975. The value of fluorescence markers in the distribution between maternal and fetal chromosomes. Humangenetik 26:187–191.

Henderson, A. S., D. Warburton, and K. C. Atwood. 1972. Location of ribosomal DNA in the human chromosome complement. Proc. Nat. Acad. Sci. 69:3394–3398.

Jacobs, P. A., K. E. Buckton, S. Christie, M. Newton, and D Matthe. 1974. A family with two translocations and a polymorphism involving chromosome 14. J. Med. Genet. 11:65–68.

Jacobs, P. A., A. Frackiewicz, P. Law, C. J. Hilditch, and N. E. Morton. 1975. The effect of structural aberrations of the chromosomes on reproductive fitness in man. II. Results. Clin. Genet. 8:169–178.

Jacobs, P. A., and N. E. Morton. 1977. Origin of human trisomics and polyploids. Hum. Hered. In press.

Langenbeck, U., I. Hansmann, B. Hinney, and V. Hönig. 1976. On the origin of the supernumerary chromosome in autosomal trisomics — with special reference to Down's syndrome. Hum. Genet. 33:89–102.

Latt, S. A. 1973. Microfluorometric detection in deoxyribonucleic acid replication in human metaphase chromosomes. Proc. Nat. Acad. Sci. 70:3395–3399.

Lauritsen, J. G. 1976. Aetiology of spontaneous abortion. A cytogenetic and epidemiological study of 288 abortuses and their parents. Acta Obstet. Gynecol. Scand. Supplement 52:1–29.

Lin, C. C., M. M. Gedeon, P. Griffith, W. K. Smink, D. R. Newton, L. Wilkie, and L. M. Sewell. 1976. Chromosome analysis on 930 consecutive newborn children using quinacrine fluorescent banding technique. Hum. Genet. 31:315–328.

Lin, M. S., S. A. Latt, and R. L. Davidson. 1974. Microfluorometric detection of asymmetry in the centromeric region of mouse chromosomes. Exp. Cell Res. 86:392–394.

Lubs, H. A., and F. H. Ruddle. 1970. Applications of Quantitative Karyotyping to Chromosome Variations in 4,400 Consecutive Newborns. In Human Population Cytogenetics, Jacobs, P. A., W. H. Price, and P. Law (Eds.): pp. 119–142. Pfizer Medical Monographs No. 5. Edinburgh, University of Edinburgh Press.

Lubs, H. A., and F. H. Ruddle. 1971. Chromosome polymorphism in American Negro and White populations. Nature 233:134–136.

Lubs, H. A., S. R. Patil, W. J. Kimberling, J. Brown, M. Cohen, P. Gerald, F. Hecht, N. Myrianthopoulos, and R. L. Summitt. 1976. Q and C Banding Polymorphisms in 7 and 8 Year Old Children. Racial Differences and Clinical Significance. In Population Cytogenetics, Hook, E. B., and I. H. Porter (Eds.). New York, Academic Press.

Madan, K., and M. Bobrow. 1974. Structural variation in chromosome no. 9. Ann. Genet. 17:81–86.

Magenis, R. E., F. Hecht, and E. W. Lovrien. 1970. Heritable fragile site on chromosome 16: Probable localization of haptoglobin locus in man. Science 170:85–87.

Mason, D., I. Lauder, D. Rutovitz, and G. Spowart. 1975. Measurement of C-bands in human chromosomes. Comput. Biol. Med. 5:179–201.

McKenzie, W. H., and H. A. Lubs. 1975. Human Q and C chromosomal variations: Distribution and incidence. Cytogenet. Cell Genet. 14:97–115.

Mikelsaar, A.-V. N., M. E. Käosaar, S. J. Tüür, M. H. Viikmaa, T. A. Talvik, and J. Lääts. 1975. Human karyotype polymorphism: III. Routine and fluorescence microscopic investigation of chromosomes in normal adults and mentally retarded children. Humangenetik 26:1–24.

Mikelsaar, A.-V. N., S. J. Tüür, and M. E. Käosaar. 1973. Human karyotype polymorphism: I. Routine and fluorescence microscopic investigation of chromosomes in a normal adult population. Humangenetik 20:89–101.

Mikkelsen, M., A. Hallberg, and H. Poulsen. 1976. Maternal and paternal origin of extra chromosome in trisomy 21. Hum. Genet. 32:17–21.

Müller, H. J., H. P. Klinger, and M. Glasser. 1975. Chromosome polymorphism in a human newborn population. II. Potentials of polymorphic chromosome variants for characterizing the idiogram of an individual. Cytogenet. Cell Genet. 15:239–256.

Nielsen, J., and U. Friedrich. 1972. Length of the Y chromosome in criminal males. Clin. Genet. 3:281–285.

Nielsen, J., U. Friedrich, and A. B. Hreidarsson. 1974a. Frequency and genetic effect of 1qh+. Humangenetik 21:193–196.

Nielsen, J., U. Friedrich, A. B. Hreidarsson, and E. Zeuthen. 1974b. Frequency and segregation of 16qht+. Clin. Genet. 5:316–321.

Nielsen, J., U. Friedrich, A. B. Hreidarsson, and E. Zeuthen. 1974c. Frequency of 9qh+ and risk of chromosome aberrations in the progeny of individuals with 9qh+. Humangenetik 21:211–216.

Paris Conference, 1971. Standardization in Human Cytogenetics. Birth Defects: Original Articles Series, VIII:7, 1972. New York, The National Foundation.

Paris Conference, 1971. Supplement (1975). Standardization in Human Cytogenetics. Birth Defects: Original Articles Series, XI:9, 1975. New York, The National Foundation.

Robinson, J. A. 1973. Origin of extra chromosome in trisomy 21. Lancet 1:131–133.

Robinson, J. A., K. E. Buckton, G. Spowart, M. Newton, P. A. Jacobs, H. J. Evans, and R. Hill. 1976. The segregation of human chromosome polymorphisms. Ann. Hum. Genet. 40:113–121.

Schwinger, E., and P. Wild. 1974. Length of the Y chromosome and antisocial behavior? Humangenetik 22:67–69.

Sofuni, T., K. Tanabe, K. Ohtaki, H. Shimba, and A. A. Awa. 1974. Two new types of C-band variants in human chromosome (6ph+ and 12ph+). Jap. J. Hum. Genet. 19:251–256.

Starkman, M. N., and M. W. Shaw. 1967. Atypical acrocentric chromosomes in Negro and Caucasian mongols. Am. J. Hum. Genet. 19:162–173.

Tüür, S., M. Käosaar, and A.-V. N. Mikelsaar. 1974. 1q+ variants in a normal adult population (one with a pericentric inversion). Humangenetik 24:217–220.

Weisblum, B. 1973. Why centric regions of quinacrine-treated mouse chromosomes show diminished fluorescence. Nature 246:150–151.

Zimmerman, S. O., and D. A. Johnston. 1976. Automated Cytogenetics at the M. D. Anderson Hospital. In Automated Cytogenetics, Menelsohn, M. L. (Ed.), pp. 85–89. Springfield, Virginia, National Technical Information Service.

AUTHOR
INDEX

275

SUBJECT INDEX

Note: Page numbers in *italics* indicate illustrations; folios followed by "t" refer to tabular material.